T0327520

VIRAL DISEASES OF CATTLE

SECOND EDITION

VIRAL
DISEASES
OF CATTLE

SECOND EDITION

Robert F. Kahrs

Iowa State University Press / Ames

Robert F. Kahrs received the DVM and PhD degrees from Cornell University. He has served on the faculties of veterinary medicine at Cornell University, the University of Florida, and the University of Missouri, where he served as dean for ten years. He spent seven years developing animal health policies and negotiating international trade agreements for the U.S Department of Agriculture. He has written more than one hundred articles and lectured widely on viral diseases of cattle, investigation of animal disease outbreaks, and international trade in animals and animal products. He currently resides in Saint Augustine, Florida.

Iowa State University Press
2121 South State Avenue, Ames, Iowa 50014

Orders: 1-800-862-6657
Office: 1-515-292-0140
Fax: 1-515-292-3348
Web site: www.isupress.com

First edition, 1981
Second edition, 2001

Library of Congress Cataloging-in-Publication Data

Kahrs, Robert F.,
    Viral diseases of cattle / Robert F. Kahrs.—2nd ed.
       p. cm.
    Includes bibliographical references and index (p.).
    ISBN 0-8138-2591-1
    1. Cattle—Virus diseases. I. Title.

SF961 .K26 2001
636.2'089625—dc21   00-053961

The last digit is the print number: 9 8 7 6 5 4 3 2 1

CONTENTS

PREFACE

Dynamic technological and societal changes have occurred since *Viral Diseases of Cattle* was initially published in 1981. These transformations involve new knowledge about viruses, major modifications in cattle rearing and marketing methods, and changing attitudes of people about the livestock industry and foods of animal origin.

Most information in the first edition was acquired by animal inoculations and use of emerging cell culture technology. These methods expanded capabilities for isolating and identifying viruses, detecting antibodies, and developing vaccines.

The last 20 years have provided improved sensitivity and automation of serologic tests that reveal the presence of cross-reacting serotypes, strains, and subtypes of many bovine viruses. The 1980s and 1990s saw the introduction of genetic technology and computer-automated nucleic acid sequencing. The technology has attained levels of specificity that divided and subdivided bovine viruses into new categories, requiring changes in nomenclature and taxonomy.

Immunologic and genetic research conducted during the 1990s created new levels of understanding that answered some questions posed in the first edition. Unfolding knowledge raised the possibility that conclusions of some early experiments may have been flawed by inability to recognize viral strains or subtypes, or by use of coinfected cultures. More recent findings have corrected some erroneous details and elucidated the genealogy and genetic diversity of viral lineages but altered few fundamental principles.

While viral technology was advancing, the significance of bovine viral diseases was affected by complex changes in animal science and society. These included advances in animal husbandry, nutrition, and genetics (including widespread application of embryo transfer). Also important were increased public concern about food safety and transmission of animal diseases to humans, awareness of newly discovered or emerging diseases, and emphasis on wildlife reservoirs of livestock diseases. In addition governing and controlling regulatory styles have been replaced with government-stakeholder partnering; there has as well been a movement to highly competitive globally oriented free-market economies that require maximum production efficiency.

These changes have been accompanied by intensification of cattle-raising practices and changes to production, processing, and distribution methods. There have been major shifts in international trade in animals and animal products that make health requirements (sanitary measures) a major force in the global trade. Meeting these requirements is essential for future expansion of the collective bovine industries.

Increasing international trade in animals and animal products dictates that disease control efforts must now respond to concerns of foreign markets that set prices and international health standards that determine product acceptability.

The accelerating movement of bovine practice from individual animal therapy to herd health consultation sometimes forces individual disease diagnosis to take second place to overall management. Nonetheless, veterinarians successful in managerial roles must be experienced diagnosticians, knowledgeable about the clinical, immunologic, and epidemiological characteristics of viral diseases.

There are a number of viruses, such as caliciviruses and Cache Valley virus, that infect cattle without producing significant disease or for which minimal amounts of disease data are available. In future decades these and others may emerge as major pathogens but their current status does not justify a full chapter. They are mentioned in the appropriate virus families in the section on virus classification in Chapter 1 and throughout the text.

Four new chapters—"Bovine Spongiform Encephalopathy," "Bovine Lentivirus (Bovine Immunodeficiency-like Virus)," "Disinfectants and Disinfection," and "The Impact of Viral Diseases on International Trade"—have been added.

This edition, like the first edition, is intended as a readily understandable reference and study guide for anyone requiring quick access to species-oriented disease-specific information.

I have tried to combine day-to-day applications with scientific principles into a readable treatise on bovine viral diseases and a primer in virology to serve as a review and update for practitioners, students, teachers, diagnosticians, animal scientists, regulatory officials, trade negotiators, and scientists of all ages.

I am grateful to colleagues at Cornell University, the University of Florida, the University of Missouri, the United States Department of Agriculture, and practitioners and academicians throughout the country whose thoughts, comments, constructive criticisms, and questions have shaped the directions of this work.

The book is dedicated to my wife, Evelyn, whose inspiration, support, understanding, and love have made my career and this book possible.

VIRAL DISEASES OF CATTLE

SECOND EDITION

1

VIRUSES AND VIROLOGY

INTRODUCTION

Viruses, formerly called filterable viruses because they pass filters that retain bacteria, are among the smallest disease-producing agents known. Most are smaller than 300 nanometers (nm) in diameter.

Historically, viruses were recognized by the signs or lesions resulting from infection of animals, cell cultures, or embryonating eggs, and by immunologic procedures. More recently, genetic analyses and viral nucleic acid detection methods have been applied to recognize viruses and distinguish among them.

Individual viral particles cannot be seen with ordinary light microscopes, but viruses and their complex structural details can be visualized by electron microscopy.

The properties, characteristics, and taxonomy of viruses have been reviewed by Murphy et al. (1999) and by Butel et al. (1999).

VIRUS STRUCTURE

Viruses consist of a nucleic acid genome (genetic component) surrounded by a symmetric shell of protein (the capsid) composed of morphologic units (capsomeres) in geometric arrays.

The genome contains either deoxyribonucleic acid (DNA) or ribonucleic acid (RNA) but usually not both. The genome and surrounding capsid are collectively called the nucleocapsid. In some cases (nonenveloped viruses), the nucleocapsid is the complete infective particle.

A virion is a complete infective particle comprising the nucleocapsid plus any outer covering essential for infectivity.

The poxviruses have complex outer coats. Many other viruses possess less complex but nonetheless essential lipid-containing outer layers called envelopes. The presence of an envelope can be detected by testing for ether sensitivity.

Capsids assume a variety of sizes and shapes, all of which are variations on two basic symmetrical forms: icosahedral (twelve-cornered) symmetry and helical (spiral) symmetry.

VIRUS REPLICATION AND SURVIVAL

Virus synthesis in host cells is called replication. The materials, biosynthetic pathways, and required energy are all provided by host cells, which synthesize viral proteins and nucleic acids and assemble them using genetic instructions provided by the infecting virus.

Viruses require living cells close to body temperatures for replication but can survive without replicating when appropriate virus–cell equilibrium is achieved, as occurs in persistently infected animals or cell cultures. In addition they can survive for long periods without replicating in nonliving environments if frozen in appropriate media, as in preservation of laboratory cultures; when they are lyophilized and vacuum packed, as in vaccine production; or when surrounded with stabilizing substances such as serum or scabs. Ordinarily, outside of living cells, infectivity is lost rapidly through exposure to heat, drying, dilution, or alterations of pH. The resistance of viruses to environmental influences varies greatly.

VIRUS CLASSIFICATION

Viruses are arranged in families and genera based on nucleic acid type (DNA or RNA) present in the genome, the nature of the genome, and the mode of replication in host cells (Murphy et al. 1999). These criteria are more exacting but less clinically significant than those of earlier classification schemes.

Less consistent attributes like size, shape, and structural detail; immunological relationships; physiochemical properties; and modes of transmission are used to further describe viruses and set them aside one from another, but they are not usually used in viral taxonomy.

Viruses in the same family or genus sometimes have similarities in clinical features (signs or lesions); epidemiological characteristics, (mechanisms of transmission and survival); diagnostic attributes (such as inclusion bodies); and susceptibilities to disinfectants or antiviral drugs. The many exceptions to such generalizations, however, make these features unreliable as taxonomic criteria.

Virus classification has been detailed by Butel et al. (1999), Murphy et al. (1999), and the Western Hemisphere Committee on Animal Virus Characterization (Murphy et al. 1995). The following characterization of bovine viral families and genera introduces the nomenclature applicable to viruses of all species. As new data appear, changes may occur in classification schemes themselves as well as in placement of viruses within them.

A TAXONOMY OF BOVINE VIRUSES

In most viral classifications the first major dichotomy is based on nucleic acid type, and the two major virus groups are DNA-containing and RNA-containing viruses.

Families of DNA Viruses

The DNA-containing bovine viruses are in the families Adenoviridae, Herpesviridae, Papovaviridae, Parvoviridae, Poxviridae, and Retroviridae.

The Family Adenoviridae

The family Adenoviridae, initially isolated from human adenoids, are 80 to 100 nm, cubically symmetrical, nonenveloped, ether-resistant viruses. They produce intranuclear inclusion bodies, and are distinguished immunologically and by species of origin.

The family has two genera: *Aviadenovirus,* which infects avian species, and *Mastadenovirus,* which infects mammals and includes, among others, infectious canine hepatitis and the bovine adenoviruses discussed in Chapter 9.

Adenovirus-associated viruses, which depend on adenoviruses for replication are mentioned briefly in Chapter 9. They are actually members of the family Parvoviridae.

The Family Herpesviridae

The family Herpesviridae contains enveloped, cubically symmetrical, medium-sized viruses and has two subfamilies with bovine members.

The subfamily Alphaherpesvirinae contains bovine herpes virus-1, the cause of infectious bovine rhinotracheitis and infectious pustular vulvovaginitis (Chapter 18), bovine herpes virus-2, the cause of bovine herpes mamillitis (Chapter 17), and bovine herpesvirus-5, which causes encephalitis (mentioned in Chapter 18).

The subfamily Betaherpesvirinae contains bovine herpesvirus-3, the herpes virus of malignant catarrhal fever (Chapter 19), bovine herpesvirus-4 (Chapter 18), a bovine origin virus of uncertain pathogenicity, and porcine herpesvirus-1, which causes pseudorabies (Chapter 24), a disease that can be fatal to cattle.

Almost every animal species has one or more herpesviruses. Most are characterized by development of latent persistent infections that are intermittently reactivated with shedding of virus. Herpes simplex, the human cold-sore virus, is the most studied herpesvirus and is the type to which others are compared.

The Family Papovaviridae

The Papovaviridae are small (45-55 nm), cubically symmetrical, etherresistant, nonenveloped viruses that are relatively thermostable and acid resistant and usually cannot be propagated in cell cultures. There are two genera:

Polyomavirus and *Papillomavirus*. The genus *Papillomavirus* contains bovine papillomavirus, which has at least six types based on nucleotide sequence homology, and causes bovine fibropapillomatosis (warts) (Chapter 16).

The Family Parvoviridae

The Parvoviridae are small (25 nm), icosahedrally symmetrical, non-enveloped, ether-resistant viruses that induce production of intranuclear inclusion bodies and vary in their resistance to temperature changes. Bovine parvoviruses (Chapter 22) are classified in the genus *Parvovirus*.

The family Parvoviridae also includes the adeno-associated viruses (mentioned in Chapter 9), the porcine parvoviruses, canine parvovirus, and the virus of feline panleukopenia.

The Family Poxviridae

The family Poxviridae contains large, brick-shaped or ovoid viruses that are covered by a complex outer layer. They usually replicate in the cytoplasm and frequently cause intracytoplasmic inclusion bodies.

The three genera with bovine representatives are the genus *Orthopoxvirus*, which includes vaccinia and cowpox viruses (Chapter 23); the genus *Capripoxvirus*, which includes lumpy skin disease (Chapter 33); and the genus *Parapoxvirus*, which includes paravaccinia or pseudocowpox virus (Chapter 23) and papular stomatitis virus (Chapter 20).

The Family Retroviridae

The family Retroviridae is so named because its members require RNA-dependent reverse DNA polymerase for replication. Members of the family Retroviridae are unique, enveloped, medium-sized, icosahedrally symmetrical viruses associated with leukemias and immunodeficiency diseases in many species.

The understanding and differentiation of members of the family Retroviridae is based largely on mechanisms of replication and genetic distinctions. These phenomena have been explored extensively in search of solutions to the global problem of human immunodeficiency virus-1, the cause of acquired immunodeficiency syndrome (AIDS).

Bovine members of the family Retroviridae are the bovine leukemia virus (BLV) (Chapter 12), the type species of the genus *Deltaretrovirus*, and bovine lentivirus (bovine immunodeficiency-like virus) (Chapter 11), a member of the genus *Lentivirus*, which also contains the *Jembrana* virus (discussed briefly in Chapter 11).

Other animal retroviruses, immunologically distinct from BLV and bovine lentivirus are the viruses that cause equine infectious anemia and caprine arthritis-encephalitis.

Families of RNA-containing Viruses

The RNA-containing virus families with members infective for cattle are the family Astroviridae, the family Bornaviridae, the family Bunyaviridae, the family Caliciviridae, the family Coronaviridae, the family Paramyxoviridae, the family Picornaviridac, the family Reoviridae, the family Rhabdoviridae, and the family Togaviridae.

The Family Astroviridae

Viruses of the family Astroviridae, so named for their star-like appearance, are small (25–30 nm) and icosahedrally symmetrical. They are found in the feces of most mammals, including cattle, and may occasionally cause diarrhea. Their significance (if any) remains to be elaborated (Woode 1990a).

The Family Bornaviridae

Borna disease virus, currently the only member of the genus *Bornavirus* of the family Bornaviridae causes a neurologic disease of horses that is usually fatal or leaves permanent neurologic residua.

The virus has been reported to cause fatal encephalomyelitis in cattle in Europe (Bode et al. 1994). It is characterized by anorexia, circling, paresis, paralysis, and death.

As information on Borna disease in cattle emerges, Borna disease will assume a role in the differential diagnosis of bovine neurological disease.

The Family Bunyaviridae

The family Bunyaviridae contains more viruses than any other viral family. They are spherical, heat-labile, ether-sensitive, helically symmetrical, enveloped viruses ranging from 80 to 100 nm in diameter. Most family members are arthropod-borne and are highly selective regarding mammalian reservoirs, insect host preferences, and ecosystems habitations.

The genus *Bunyavirus* contains the Akabane (Chapter 30), Aino, Peaton, Douglas, and Timaroo viruses that cause congenital defects similar to those of Akabane. It also contains the Cache Valley virus, a mosquito-borne agent, which produces inapparent infections, congenital anomalies, and possibly abortion in cattle and is endemic in North America (Edwards 1994).

The genus *Phlebovirus* contains the Rift Valley fever virus (Chapter 34).

The Family Caliciviridae

Viruses of the family Caliciviridae cause hemorrhagic disease of rabbits, feline calicivirus infection (a respiratory disease), and San Miguel sea lion disease, which is probably related to vesicular exanthema of swine. Caliciviruses are being associated with gastroenteritis in some species including swine and cattle (Woode 1990c).

The Family Coronaviridae

The family Coronaviridae contains medium-sized (80–220 nm), helically symmetrical, ether-sensitive viruses that have a lipid-containing envelope and a characteristic morphology featuring surface projections that form a crown-like halo surrounding a central core.

The genus *Coronavirus* contains the bovine coronavirus (Chapter 14), which is associated with neonatal calf diarrhea, winter dysentery, and respiratory signs.

The genus *Torovirus* of the family Coronaviridae contains the Breda virus, named for the Iowa town in which it was found in a calf with diarrhea (Woode 1990b). The Breda virus is immunologically distinct from bovine coronavirus and can cause diarrhea in experimental calves. It may eventually emerge as another factor in neonatal calf diarrhea.

The Family Flaviviridae

The family Flaviviridae are spherical enveloped, probably icosahedrally symmetrical, small (50 nm) enveloped viruses that are sensitive to heat and many disinfectants.

The bovine viral diarrhea (BVD) virus (Chapter 13) is the type species of the genus *Pestivirus,* which also contains the viruses of hog cholera and border disease of sheep. Border disease follows infection of pregnant ewes with a BVD-like virus and induces birth of lambs with a congenital syndrome characterized by tremors, fleece abnormalities, unthriftiness, and early mortality.

The genus *Flavivirus* contains Wesselsbron virus, which causes an important disease of sheep and subclinical bovine infections and resembles Rift Valley fever (Chapter 34), even though the viruses are unrelated.

The genus *Flavivirus* also contains the virus of louping ill, which causes a neuroparalytic infection of sheep and occasionally infects humans and cattle (Kreuger and Reid 1994). It also contains the West Nile virus, introduced into the United States in 1999 where it killed crows, humans, and horses, and caused inapparent infections in cattle.

The Family Paramyxoviridae

The family Paramyxoviridae contains medium-to-large-sized (150–300 nm), pleomorphic, enveloped, and ether-sensitive viruses that are related genetically but immunologically distinct. The genus *Respirovirus* contains bovine parainfluenza-3 virus (Chapter 21), the genus *Morbillivirus* includes rinderpest virus (Chapter 35), and the genus *Pneumovirus* contains respiratory syncytial virus (Chapter 26).

The Family Picornaviridae

The family Picornaviridae are small (approximately 30 nm), cubically symmetrical, nonenveloped viruses with varying sensitivities to pH and disinfectants; they are usually associated with mammalian respiratory or alimentary tracts. The type species of the genus *Aphthovirus* is foot-and-mouth disease virus (Chapter 32). The genus *Enterovirus* is discussed in Chapter 15, and members of the genus *Rhinovirus* are covered in Chapter 27.

The Family Reoviridae

The Reoviridae are medium-sized (60–80 nm), icosahedrally symmetrical viruses that are ether resistant and that lack an essential envelope.

Bluetongue virus (Chapter 10) is the type species of the genus *Orbivirus*, which also contains Ibaraki and Polyam viruses, and the virus of epizootic hemorrhagic disease of deer (all mentioned in Chapter 10).

The genus *Rotavirus* contains the bovine rotavirus associated with calf diarrhea (Chapter 28).

The Family Rhabdoviridae

The family Rhabdoviridae are helically symmetrical, bullet-shaped, lipid-containing, enveloped viruses, measuring 70 by 180 nm, that frequently infect arthropods.

Vesicular stomatitis virus (Chapter 29) is the type species of the genus *Vesiculovirus* and rabies virus (Chapter 25) is the type species of the genus *Lyssavirus*.

Bovine ephemeral fever virus (Chapter 31) is the type species of the genus *Ephemerovirus*. Signs similar to those of ephemeral fever are sometimes attributed to two less-studied rhabdoviruses, namely Kotonkan virus found in parts of Africa and Puchong virus in Malaysia. Other antigenically related, but less common and apparently nonpathogenic Rhabdoviridae include Kimberly virus, Berrimah virus, and Adelaide River virus.

The Family Togaviridae

The family Togaviridae includes many arthropod-borne viruses. They are ether-sensitive, enveloped viruses approximately 70 nm in diameter. The genus *Alphavirus* includes eastern equine encephalitis virus, which occasionally causes subclinical infections in cattle.

Prions

Prions are subviral disease-producing agents that seem to lack nucleic acids and that do not strictly fulfill current taxonomic criteria for viruses. Bovine spongiform encephalopathy and other prion-induced diseases are discussed in Chapter 36.

THE STUDY OF VIROLOGY

The study of virology has progressed markedly because of advances in immunology, development of tissue-culture technology, and the application of viral genetics. In addition to seeking disease information, virology has expanded into molecular biology, cellular and subcellular biochemistry, and molecular genetics.

Today, virologists are involved in a broad spectrum of activities from studies of the biochemical basis of life to the diagnosis, treatment, and prevention of disease. Thus for scientists and practitioners it is a rapidly advancing field requiring constant study.

REFERENCES

Bode L, Durrwald R, Ludwig H, 1994. Borna virus infections in cattle associated with fatal neurological disease. *Vet. Rec.* 135:283–284.

Butel JS, Melnic JL, Zee YC, 1999. General Properties of Viruses. In *Veterinary Virology,* edited by DC Hirsch, YC Zee. Malden, MA: Blackwell Science Publishers, pp. 311–327.

Edwards JF, 1994. Cache Valley virus. *Vet. Clin. North. Am.* 10(3): 515–524.

Kreuger N, Reid HW, 1994. Detection of louping ill virus in formalin-fixed paraffin-wax-imbedded tissues of mice, sheep and a pig by the avidin-biotin-complex immunoperoxidase technique. *Vet. Rec.* 135:224–225.

Murphy, FA, Faquet CM, Bishop DHL, Ghabrial SA, Jarvis AW, Martelli GP, Mayo MA, Summers MD, 1995. *Virus taxonomy: The classification and nomenclature of viruses. The sixth report of Western Hemisphere Committee on Animal Virus Characterization.* Vienna: Springer Verlag.

Murphy FA, Gibbs EPJ, Horzinek MC, Studdert MJ, 1999. *Veterinary virology,* 3rd ed. San Diego: Academic Press.

Woode GN, 1990a. Astroviruses. In *Infectious diseases of ruminants,* edited by Z Dinter, B Morein. Amsterdam: Elsevier Scientific Publishers, pp. 543–546.

Woode GN, 1990b. Breda virus. In *Infectious diseases of ruminants,* edited by Z Dinter, B Morein. Amsterdam: Elsevier Scientific Publishers, pp. 311–316.

Woode GN, 1990c. Calicivirus-like agents. In *Infectious diseases of ruminants,* edited by Z Dinter, B Morein. Amsterdam: Elsevier Scientific Publishers, pp. 519–522.

2

CONCEPTS FOR STUDYING VIRAL INFECTIONS

INTRODUCTION

Action appropriate for diagnosis, prevention, and treatment of viral diseases requires knowledge of facts and understanding of concepts. Facts and concepts are not mutually exclusive and cannot always be separated. In the search for facts, however, concepts are frequently overlooked. Thus, a brief look at concepts can profitably precede the study of bovine viral diseases.

CLINICAL LOOK-ALIKES

The signs and syndromes caused by many bovine viral infections are similar to one another and to those caused by some bacteria or toxins. It is difficult to obtain an etiologic diagnosis solely on clinical observations or physical examinations of sick cattle because few signs or lesions of bovine viral infections are pathognomonic. The more complete the diagnostic efforts, the higher the probability of accuracy. The hierarchy of diagnostic specificity consists of the clinical diagnosis based on history and clinical signs, the pathologic diagnosis based on examination of lesions, and the etiologic diagnosis based on establishing that a specific virus infection caused the disease. The credibility of diagnoses is determined by the level attained in this hierarchy.

A clinical diagnosis is adequate for immediate therapeutic action and corrective management recommendations. Vaccination discussions, diagnosis of exotic diseases, publication of case reports, and legal testimony require a specific etiologic diagnosis based on laboratory tests. Thus, it is best to acknowledge a certain degree of ignorance at the clinical level. If animals are necropsied, it is fitting to describe lesions and render a pathologic diagnosis.

When laboratory identification of a viral infection is obtained, the hierarchy has been completely ascended. Arguments over cause-and-effect relationships, however, frequently leave an element of doubt, as do the etiologic roles of environment and secondary or simultaneous infections.

ENDEMIC AND EXOTIC INFECTIONS

In addition to taxonomic considerations and anatomic systems affected, viruses can be discussed in epidemiologic categories. These categories are based on the degree of equilibrium attained with cattle populations in a geographic area. In this work, viral infections are categorized as endemic or exotic in North America. Exotic viruses are not present in regions because they have never been introduced, the area lacks a supportive ecosystem, or they have been eradicated and measures are in place to prevent their reintroduction and establishment.

Endemic Viral Infections

Infections indigenous to North America, such as infectious bovine rhinotracheitis (IBR), bovine viral diarrhea (BVD), bovine parainfluenza-3 (PI-3), and bovine leukemia virus are firmly established and continually perpetuated in cattle populations. At any time a portion of the cattle population is partially immune; a smaller portion is experiencing primary acute infection; and with some viruses another portion is persistently infected. Clinical disease is sporadic and occasionally occurs in herd outbreaks, but involvement of multiple herds and major geographic areas is unusual. Infections with endemic viruses are frequently mild or inapparent, and clinical signs are frequently nondescript and lack uniqueness required for easy clinical diagnosis. Most viruses endemic in North America are also globally endemic.

Exotic or Epidemic Viral Infections

On a worldwide basis, striking losses from bovine viral infections occur from epidemics of foot-and-mouth disease, rinderpest, ephemeral fever, Rift Valley fever, and Akabane. They occur in epidemic waves, spread rapidly in susceptible populations, and produce clinical disease in a high percentage of infected cattle or their fetuses. Relatively speaking, epidemic and exotic viral infections are less likely to be inapparent than the endemic infections, although clinical manifestations are partially contingent on characteristics of the infected cattle. Most infections exotic to North America behave as epidemics when initially introduced but can evolve to endemicity if left unchecked after establishment.

The Office International Des Epizooties (OIE) categorizes animal diseases with respect to their potential for global spread and economic loss and their public health significance. List A comprises diseases considered most serious by these criteria and contains 15 diseases. List A diseases of cattle are foot-and-mouth disease, rinderpest, vesicular stomatitis, bluetongue, Rift Valley fever, and lumpy skin disease.

INAPPARENT INFECTIONS

Simple singular infection of susceptible cattle with some viruses, particularly OIE List A diseases, can result in serious clinical disease. In the case of most endemic viruses, however, simple singular infection is frequently mild. Most mild infections go unobserved because they are associated with little inflammation, degeneration, or cell necrosis and are called inapparent or nonclinical infections.

Cattle respond immunologically to inapparent and clinical infections by developing local or humoral antibody. The endemic viruses causing inapparent infections have high antibody prevalences but low clinical attack rates. The goal of modified live virus (MLV) vaccines is to produce inapparent infection accompanied by partial immunity.

Inapparent infection of pregnant cattle frequently causes abortion or defects in fetal development because, until midgestation, fetal immune mechanisms are inadequate to resist viral infections. The interval between exposure of the dam and abortion or birth of malformed calves can be several months and the cause often remains obscure.

Frequently, infections that would be inapparent in some cattle are associated with severe disease in others, perhaps because of altered immunologic capability, concomitant infections, or detrimental environmental influences such as stress or use of immunosuppressive drugs. Thus, clinical disease associated with endemic viruses frequently has a complex multifactorial etiology.

EMERGING DISEASES

About the time humankind thinks it knows all the infectious agents on the planet, a new one, like human immunodeficiency virus or bovine spongiform encephalopathy (BSE), appears or is discovered. Many bovine viruses first recognized in the 1900s were undoubtedly previously present as subclinical or unrecognized infections and became apparent under intensive cattle rearing practices or as pathogenic strains emerged through mutations, genetic recombinations, or transmission and adaptation to new host species.

TRANS-SPECIES TRANSMISSION PAST AND POTENTIAL

Most bovine viruses can successfully infect other species, with or without clinical signs. Genetic analyses indicate close ancestral relationships between viruses that are in the same family or genus.

The question of which species was the original host often remains unresolved. Undoubtedly advancing technology will reveal new relationships between bovine infections and diseases of other species, including humans.

COMPLICATIONS FROM ADVANCING TECHNOLOGY

Things were simple when all information about bovine viruses was acquired from clinical or pathological observations and supported by inoculation of animals with blood or tissues of sick cattle. Before the mid-1900s, many questions were eventually addressed through cell culture technology, immunofluorescent methods using monoclonal antibodies, and by electron microscopy. The advent of molecular biology and genetic technology employing polymerase chain reactions answered many questions, cast doubt on some earlier conclusions, provided new methods for addressing old questions, and introduced terminology comprehensible only to new-generation scientists. Subsequent cycles of technology will continue to raise new questions and challenge the status quo.

MULTIFACTORIAL ETIOLOGY

Following infection by an endemic virus, some cattle experience inapparent infection, others develop mild disease and survive, and still others develop severe disease and succumb. The many factors involved in susceptibility and resistance to endemic viral infections lead to the generalization that many clinical syndromes require multiple causes for their expression. This multifactorial etiology can be described as a complex agent-host-environment interaction. Specific data on these interactions are scarce, however, and many attempts to explain them are speculative.

Some syndromes appear only if two or more organisms are present simultaneously (concomitant infections). Others may require that one infection precede the other (secondary infection).

Most veterinarians are familiar with the so-called shipping fever equation, which suggests that pulmonic pasteurellosis results from a combination of viral infection, stress, and bacteria. Various viral infections (frequently PI-3, IBR, bovine respiratory syncytial virus, respiratory coronaviruses, adenoviruses), stresses (usually movement of cattle), and bacteria (usually *Pasteurella*) can be fitted logically into the equation. The implications are disquieting because acceptance of this hypothesis indicates that this syndrome is not controllable by simply eliminating a single viral or bacterial infection or a single stress factor.

Epidemiology and research support the concept of multifactorial etiology and the role of endogenous and exogenous influences on the ability of cattle to contain infections by viruses that are usually relatively nonpathogenic.

Of the syndromes associated with viral infections, bovine respiratory disease (BRD) most readily fits the multifactorial etiology model because intimate contact of respiratory mucosa with the environment makes concomitant and secondary infections easy to acquire. The alimentary tract is similarly exposed and discussions of the role of viruses as enteric pathogens (particularly in the neonate) usually emphasize the role of secondary or concomitant infections, dietary disturbances, and immunologic deficits in disease pathogenesis.

The concept of multifactorial etiology is particularly appealing with the less pathogenic viruses because it is difficult to consistently induce clinical disease by experimental inoculation of large doses of viruses into cattle deemed susceptible by immunologic methods. It has been difficult to evaluate vaccines because of inconsistent pathogenicity of viral strains used for challenging vaccinated and unvaccinated cattle.

In many instances, simple singular infection of pregnant cattle with abortogenic viruses is adequate to cause fetal death or anomalies. The role of multifactorial etiology of abortion must also be considered, however, because multiple fetal infections can be detected by virus isolations or identification of multiple viral antibodies in fetal serum.

The practical significance of multifactorial etiology is the difficulty it causes in establishing the etiologic role of viruses or other agents isolated from diseased cattle or aborted fetuses. Unless they are associated with distinctive lesions, a classic clinical syndrome, or serologic evidence of an acute primary infection, the possibility that a virus isolated may be the result of a long-standing asymptomatic persistent infection or previously administered MLV vaccines must always be considered.

Recognition of contributions of multifactorial etiology to the economic impact of endemic bovine viruses indicates that simple singular control procedures are usually inadequate to prevent many syndromes and that many viruses produce identical clinical signs.

CLINICAL DIAGNOSIS

People who work with cattle rapidly learn that many bovine viral diseases are indistinguishable clinically, and that often laboratory tests are necessary to make a definitive diagnosis.

Clinicians called to examine sick cattle are confronted with problems such as reduced feed consumption or productivity, respiratory disease, diarrhea, skin lesions, eye problems, or lameness. A thorough physical examination can identify distinguishing signs and propose an anatomic-pathologic diagnosis such as pneumonia or enteritis. Therapy and control procedures must be initiated with this information before the specific cause (etiologic diagnosis) is known.

Clinical diagnosis of vesicular diseases, and of other diseases affecting the bovine mucosa (DABM), respiratory disease, and abortion is particularly challenging. Clinical signs associated with these syndromes are similar. The cautious diagnostician is aware that few signs or gross lesions are pathognomonic and makes a diagnosis of "undifferentiated" respiratory or enteric disease, DABM of unknown etiology, or "idiopathic abortion."

Given a principal complaint and anatomic-pathologic diagnosis, the veterinarian must consider all possible etiologies (including exotic infections) that could produce the observed syndrome. The clinical diagnosis thus obtained usually suffices as a basis for therapeutic measures, particularly where individual cattle are involved. When additional cases appear or evidence emerges to suggest need for a specific etiologic diagnosis, laboratory tests are employed. Such tests are often done, however, after the ideal time for efficient utilization of laboratories has passed.

The clinical diagnosis devoid of laboratory substantiation is frequently the most efficient method of delivery of veterinary medical service to cattle raisers. Such diagnoses are tenuous, though, and rarely survive the scrutiny of litigation or professional publication.

IMMUNITY AND PARTIAL PROTECTION

Resistance to viral infection and clinical disease is subject to individual variation. Cattle exposed to some viruses develop long-lived immunity capable of preventing subsequent infection. More generally, however, natural infection or vaccination with MLV vaccines induces immunologic responses that afford partial protection and that may reduce the likelihood of reinfection and the seriousness of resulting disease. Cattle with partial protection from previous exposure or vaccination with some viruses can experience superficial infections of mucosal surfaces, but in general they are less likely to experience severe systemic disease or abortion than susceptible cattle undergoing primary infection.

The understanding of bovine viral diseases is tied to immunologic advances that indicate a multiplicity of immunoglobulins and immunocompetent cells, and complex local and humoral immune responses. Thus, in discussions of bovine viral diseases, the word "immunity" should be replaced by "partial protection" to express realistically the immunologic implications of vaccination or natural exposure and clarify their impact on disease control.

PRIMARY, ACUTE, PERSISTENT, LATENT, AND CHRONIC INFECTIONS

The term "primary infection" describes infection of susceptible cattle that have had no previous exposure to the virus in question. It can occur in utero or anytime in life. Primary infections are considered "acute" when they are of recent origin, rapidly developing, or produce a sudden onset of clinical signs.

The term "chronic infection" suggests a long-lasting situation and in virologic terms usually implies the presence of virus in an animal. The terms chronic and persistent are used interchangeably and sometimes in combination to indicate long-lasting infection.

Following primary viral infection, host defenses may clear the virus from the animal's body. Frequently, however, viral replication continues, resulting in chronic persistent infections that last for prolonged periods, often a lifetime, with continuous or intermittent virus shedding detectable by laboratory tests. In active persistent infections, virus can be shed by normal cattle or by unthrifty, chronically affected cattle. Active persistent infections occur with bovine viral diarrhea virus, bovine parainfluenza-3 virus, bovine leukemia virus, bovine lentivirus, and enteroviruses.

Latent persistent infections differ from active persistent infections. For example, after primary IBR infection, serum antibody usually appears, virus replication and excretion cease, intact virus can not be isolated from the animal, but the virus is not permanently eliminated. Instead, viral DNA or viral genome remains in a latent state that is capable of subsequent reactivation, sometimes many years after primary infection. Generally, reactivations are associated with stress but they can be induced by steroid injections. The clinical signs (if any) associated with reactivations are generally milder than those occurring with primary infections, but cattle experiencing these "recrudescenses" constitute a reservoir of virus and a potential source of infection for herdmates.

The presence of persistent infections (both latent and active) complicates the control and diagnosis of viral diseases by providing a source of virus many months after primary infection.

The mechanisms of persistent infections are complex. Active persistent infections are sometimes associated with immunologic deficits but may result from an equilibrium between virus and host or from viral sequestration in places inaccessible to effective immunologic activity.

Persistent infections also occur in experimental animals and cell cultures where they complicate experiments and diagnostic procedures, and can contaminate vaccines.

VIRUS VACCINES FOR CATTLE

Many MLV and inactivated vaccine combinations exist for administration to cattle by various routes. Each product has advantages and disadvantages and unique indications and contraindications.

Vaccination along with management-based disease control measures needs to be placed in perspective and not be regarded as a panacea. Partial protection stimulated by vaccination reduces the likelihood of catastrophic losses but will not prevent all infections or all disease. Intelligent and effective use of vaccines requires application of the concepts elaborated in Chapter 5.

The "facts" associated with bovine vaccines are tainted by marketing efforts and altered by frequent emergence of new information and improved products. Thus, there are legitimate disagreements regarding the safety, efficacy, and conditions under which individual and combination vaccines should be administered.

Vaccination programs must be tailored to specific areas and production-management systems, and vaccine users should adhere to manufacturers' recommendations and local regulations.

In international trade matters, use of vaccine in a country or region is usually considered evidence of the presence of the disease and tends to negate claims of disease-free status.

CRITERIA FOR ERADICATION OR CONTROL

Eradication implies elimination of a virus and all possible sources of infection including nonbovine reservoirs. Eradication efforts can be conducted on a herd, area, country, or regional basis. Local eradication implies continued efforts to prevent reintroduction into clean areas. National or regional eradication requires government programs, and enforcement of regulations requiring monitoring, surveillance and reporting systems; border security; diagnostic activity; and emergency preparedness programs. National or regional eradication programs should be undertaken only after careful study.

Control, on the other hand, implies reduction of losses to an economically acceptable level. Any effort to reduce the occurrence of disease or infection constitutes control. Control measures can be directed at many phases of the virus-host-environment interaction and can be undertaken haphazardly and unilaterally in individual herds at the whim of the owner, and with only fragmentary information about the biology of the virus. Most bovine viral diseases are amenable to a wide variety of control procedures.

On the other hand, economic and political realities make eradication of many bovine viruses an ideal that has low probability of fulfillment in most parts of the world.

Consideration of eradication programs must be predicated on thorough knowledge of the virus and its reservoir hosts, its mode of transmission, and its mechanisms for perpetuation in nature. There must be a simple, inexpensive, sensitive, and specific test for detecting infection on an individual and population basis. In addition, unless the infection causes serious human disease, or disease-free animals or germ plasm command exceptional prices, the cost of eradication must be far less than the cost of the disease. Additionally, the eradication procedure must have strong support of cattle owners.

3

THE EPIDEMIOLOGY OF BOVINE VIRAL INFECTIONS

INTRODUCTION

Epidemiology is the branch of medical science that records distributions of diseases (or infections) in populations, explains the observed patterns, and applies the conclusions in control strategies.

Epidemiological procedures evaluate disease, infections, or related indicators such as death, illness, abortions, seropositivity, or production data in terms of time (temporal distribution), place (spatial or geographic distribution), and individual characteristics of affected and unaffected individuals or populations. Epidemiologic analysis involves comparing affected and unaffected groups one with another and with exposure to potential risk factors.

Applications of epidemiology to bovine health include field investigations of herd problems or suspected emerging or exotic diseases, statistically designed surveys, and long-term population studies. In all cases, they must be conducted systematically, logically, and without predetermined conclusions.

Outbreak investigations (detailed in Chapter 4), use the knowledge, skill, and wisdom of experienced clinicians and laboratory workers to determine the cause, source, and extent of disease outbreaks or production shortfalls.

Long-term epidemiological methods such as serological surveys, risk analyses, vaccine field trials, cohort studies, case-control studies, and longitudinal population studies are usually conducted in academic or regulatory environments. They evaluate preventive strategies or seek etiologic associations between disease prevalence, economic losses, and potential risk factors. Such studies are used to prioritize disease-control expenditures, determine the most efficient production practices, or evaluate claims of freedom from disease or endemicity. They require elaborate preplanning to ensure efficient use of resources and appropriate sample sizes and sampling procedures. Statisticians must be involved initially and throughout these studies to clarify hypotheses, determine appropriate statistical methods, and analyze data.

Statistical epidemiological methods are sometimes more applicable to human medicine than to bovine virology, because in cattle they can be bypassed by virus inoculations of animals and sequential necropsies. This option is not available in human studies.

Nonetheless, both descriptive (qualitative) and analytic (quantitative) epidemiological methods are applicable to bovine viral diseases and useful in practice, regulatory medicine, diagnostic services, academic research, and trade activities.

In private bovine practice, population considerations frequently overshadow diagnosis and treatment of individual animals as practitioners increasingly focus on preventive medicine and use epidemiologic questioning techniques in customizing health maintenance through management strategies.

Epidemiological methods are used constantly in regulatory programs that focus on maintaining healthy domestic populations, excluding exotic diseases, investigating potential animal health emergencies, and conducting monitoring, surveillance, and reporting (MS&R) activities. These data are needed to prioritize use of resources and to fulfill the expectations of domestic stakeholders and the international community (Kahrs 1999).

The veterinary diagnostic community supports epidemiologic activities of practitioners and regulators. The diagnostic community can be most helpful and conduct the most appropriate tests when an epidemiologic history accompanies each specimen.

In academic research, epidemiologic data provide focused questions for experimental study.

MS&R data collection and risk analysis are expanding uses of epidemiologic techniques. They are crucial to international trade in dairy and beef products because most trade barriers imposed on those commodities are based on health (sanitary) concerns.

Epidemiologic thought modes essential for dealing with bovine viral diseases include the disease iceberg concept and appreciation of the complex agent-host-environmental interactions involved in viral infections. This background is needed because viral infections must be addressed on a population basis, and pre-exposure strategies are essential because individual treatments are usually ineffective. The epidemiology of viral diseases has been reviewed by Murphy et al. (1999).

THE DISEASE ICEBERG

The disease iceberg principle is basic to bovine viral epidemiology. It indicates that a complex series of unobserved virus-host-environment interactions occurs below the clinical threshold that is represented by the waterline in the iceberg analogy. Clinical disease is just the tip of the iceberg.

The more pathogenic viruses (the so-called epidemic viruses) exceed the clinical threshold more frequently than do less pathogenic and endemic viruses.

Effective diagnosis and control of viral infections requires understanding not only of clinical diseases but also of the precipitating activities below the clinical threshold. These activities include infections of individuals and herds with ubiquitous viruses and the agent-host-environmental interactions.

Viral Infection of Individuals

Following exposure, some individual cattle are infected while others are not. These outcomes are determined by the immune status of individuals, the virulence and dose of virus, routes of inoculation, and other factors.

Following infection, virus replication occurs, and immunocompetent cells, which initiate immunologic responses, acquire viral antigen.

The clinical consequences of exposure are determined by complex virus-host-environment interactions. Ideally, immune mechanisms result in clearing of viruses from the animal's system. If clearing occurs promptly, the infection is aborted, no disease occurs, and the result is an inapparent infection. If the cow or calf is susceptible and the sufficient viral replication occurs, cell damage and clinical disease may result. The proportion of exposures causing disease or inapparent infection varies from virus to virus.

In either case, the aftermath for survivors is partial protection, the magnitude and duration of which is determined by viral characteristics and host capabilities. If all infected cattle were immunized, or more correctly partly protected, and subsequently refractive to reinfection, they would rarely infect other cattle once they had recovered from primary infection. Persistent infections, however, upset this scheme.

Herd Infections

Susceptible herds are infected through introduction of cattle with active primary, active persistent, or recurrent latent persistent infections or through introduction of virus on animate or inanimate objects. Infected cattle excrete virus. If contact is close enough, all cattle are exposed and infected and whether or not clinical disease is recognized, the population of susceptibles is replaced by a population of partially protected individuals. When this event occurs, new infections cease and, unless persistent infections develop, the virus is cleared from the herd.

A solidly immune herd rarely exists because individual immunity is only partial. Furthermore, herd immunity is transient because partially protected individuals are replaced continually by susceptibles. This replacement occurs through diminution of partial protection in individuals and cattle entering the herd by birth or purchase.

The percentage of partially protected individuals is further reduced by culling cattle present during the original exposure. The time required for a partially protected herd to revert to susceptibility is related to the duration of partial protection in individual animals, the rate of culling of partially protected cattle, and the rate of introduction of susceptibles. In a dairy where 25% of the total population is culled annually, time required for reversion to almost complete herd susceptibility is about 4 years unless rapid waning of partial protection in individual cattle makes the time shorter or reinfection or vaccination prolongs it.

Perpetuation of Viral Infections in Populations

Viruses survive in populations through cow-to-cow transmission of new infections (clinical and inapparent), by presence of persistently infected cattle, and by intermittent reactivation of latent persistent infections. All these increase the probability of exposure to viruses and add to the unpredictability of outbreaks.

Ubiquitousness of Endemic Viruses

Serologic and virologic evidence indicates widespread, probably global, distribution of bovine viral diarrhea virus, infectious bovine rhinotracheitis virus, adenoviruses, coronavirus, enteroviruses, rhinoviruses, respiratory syncytial virus, and parainfluenza-3 virus. This constant exposure leaves widely distributed, partially protected bovine populations. Unlike the viruses of foot-and-mouth disease and rinderpest, these endemic viruses rarely cause devastating epizootics because they are less virulent and cause inapparent infections, leaving large populations of partially protected animals.

The probability of exposure of individual herds to ubiquitous endemic viruses is influenced by the amount of immigration and the movement of people and equipment that have recently been in contact with cattle.

AGENT-HOST-ENVIRONMENT INTERACTIONS

Clinical disease attributable to viruses (the tip of the iceberg) is best explained as a dynamic interaction among three major components: the agent, the host, and the environment. In the case of habitat-adopted, insect-borne viral infections, vectors and their environmental requirements add additional components.

The three components of these interactions will be described separately. They cannot, however, be fragmented into mutually exclusive elements because of their complex interrelationships.

Agent Factors

The agent characteristics that influence the epidemiology and economic impact of viral diseases are pathogenicity and virulence, transmissibility or infectiveness, and the ability to establish persistent infections.

Pathogenicity is the ability to produce detectable disease. The term *virulence,* (the degree of pathogenicity of an agent) is frequently used to compare the pathogenicity of different viruses or strains of the same virus. Pathogenicity and virulence interact with host characteristics to mutually determine the outcome of exposure to viruses.

Transmissibility (the capacity to spread from one animal to another) is sometimes expressed as the fraction of susceptibles estimated to be infected by each animal shedding virus. Transmissibility, along with virulence, can be modified by host and environmental influences.

The likelihood of transmission is related to the likelihood of exposure: it is greater with viruses causing chronic persistent infections with continual viral excretion, or latent persistent infections capable of reactivation. Persistent or latent persistent infections in nonbovine reservoir hosts can also be sources of exposure.

Transmission of vector-borne diseases requires adequate populations of susceptible cattle and threshold levels of competent vectors; the latter sometimes occurs when excess rain causes insect population explosions. More specific discussions of the epidemiology of insect-transmitted infections are found in the chapters on bluetongue, ephemeral fever, lumpy skin disease, Rift Valley fever, and vesicular stomatitis.

The variable resistance of viruses to environmental conditions like exposure to drying, alterations in pH, and disinfectant applications (see Chapter 7) helps determine their survival in nature and their transmissibility.

Host Factors

Individual host characteristics cannot be separated from those of host populations that are merely aggregates of individual cattle. Host factors bearing on bovine viral infections are age, breed, sex, and immune status.

Aside from immune status, age is probably the most important host factor bearing on the outcome of viral infections, particularly if one assumes life begins at conception. In the protected uterine environment, the fetus is vulnerable to infection because the bovine placenta permits virus transmission from dam to unborn calf but holds back protective immunoglobulins. If nursing occurs within 12 hours of birth, the immunoglobulins thus acquired endow the newborn calf with a moderate degree of protection against postnatal exposure to viruses with which its dam has had previous contact. In some environments, like veal calf operations that assemble calves from multiple sources, failure of colostrum acquisition or absorption means the calf will probably die.

Certain virus infections, like foot-and-mouth disease, are more pathogenic for neonatal calves than for adult cattle. Age, however, cannot be discussed as an isolated variable, because it is related to immunocompetence, colostrum acquisition, and probability of exposure.

Few data are available on the effect of breed per se as a determinant of the outcome of bovine viral infections. The environment imposed on individuals of certain breeds such as aggregation in feedlots is a factor, however.

Except for specific reproductive and gynecological conditions, there is little evidence indicating that sex per se has bearing on the outcome of viral infections. However, the environments imposed on individuals by virtue of sex (dairy cows, feedlot steers, or bulls in insemination units) are important determinants of the economic impact of viral infections.

Use of age, sex, and breed distribution in epidemiologic investigation of outbreaks on specific farms to compare the characteristics of sick and unaffected animals can provide clues to the source of infection or toxicosis. They can also help determine the mode of transmission, and practical immediate and future control strategies. Although frequently irrelevant to specific situations, these characteristics sometimes dictate modes of housing and lead to identification of spatial differences in disease distribution. When combined with environmental factors, they provide a template for systematic outbreak investigation (Kahrs 1978) and for developing regulatory strategies.

Immunity and susceptibility to viral infections are important determinants of the outcome of exposure or infection. There is interaction between age and susceptibility, which involves the partial protection imparted by active and passive immunity and nonimmunologic resistance factors. With most viruses, animals regarded as "immune" by serologic tests have been previously exposed or vaccinated. Frequently, such cattle can be infected, although subsequent infections are usually less severe than primary infections. Resistance to clinical disease is a complex matter subject to many individual variations.

Population immunity, expressed as the percentage of individuals possessing some degree of partial protection from previous exposure or vaccination, can be measured by serologic surveys and has dimensions beyond the exposure status of individuals. As immunity waxes and wanes in populations, the probability of successful reintroduction and establishment of infections rises and falls, as does the likelihood of infection's causing clinical signs. Population immunity is influenced by the stresses of aggregation and the rate of new entries into a herd.

Environmental Factors

Environmental factors are significant determinants of the outcome of infection in both individuals and populations.

The epidemic viruses are of such virulence for susceptible populations that they frequently can cause clinical disease regardless of the environment.

In the case of endemic viruses, however, the environment is probably the most significant determinant of the outcome of infection in both individuals and populations. The environment influences both the agent and the host. It alters the opportunity for exposure and the probability that exposure will produce infection, clinical disease, or death. If left to feed and breed naturally, with adequate space, feed, and water, cattle would probably establish an ecological balance with the endemic viruses. The environmental influences to be discussed individually actually act collectively.

Population density and size and associated stresses are important determinants of the outcome of viral infections. Extreme crowding (as exists in veal units, feedyards and some large dairies) plays a role in determining infection and mortality rates associated with endemic viral infections.

Density is an important factor in neonatal mortality. Mortality in the first 14 weeks of age is frequently attributed to bacterial infections that are secondary to viral infections but must be regarded in conjunction with colostrum deprivation, diet, ventilation, and ambient temperature.

Calves nursing dams on the range experience less mortality than those concentrated in veal units or feedlots. The endemic viral infections contribute significantly to losses in feedyards, where many fatalities are attributable to pulmonic pasteurellosis, which is triggered by viral infections.

Availability of feed and water and nutritional status directly affect the outcome of exposure or infection of cattle with viruses. This factor, however, is a hard one to measure. Central feeding and watering areas expedite cow-to-cow transmission, and anxiety and apprehension associated with competition for limited water and feed contribute to the epidemiology of viral infections.

Introduction of new animals into populations (regardless of size or density) inevitably results in introduction of viral infections from actively or persistently infected cattle.

An important effect of immigration is stress associated with socialization and peck order realignment. In stocker operations, which assemble newly weaned, recently transported calves, some calves never adjust to new environments and die from exhaustion and starvation after continual wailing, bawling, and fence walking. Less dramatic effects of intermingling are hard to assess but certainly enhance the pathogenic effects of endemic infections that could be nonclinical in healthy, well-nourished, unstressed cattle in established social systems.

Housing also affects outcomes of viral infections. In nature, cattle graze open spaces and seek protection by turning from the wind and huddling in groups. Manufactured housing can introduce confinement, crowding, inadequate ventilation, and fluctuations of temperature and humidity, which expedite transmission of viral infections and secondary bacterial invaders.

Management practices influence economic losses associated with endemic viral infections. In turn, the spread and virulence of these infections are to a large extent determined by stresses and environmental influences imposed by the production-management systems under which the cattle are reared.

RISK ANALYSIS

Risk analysis gained prominence as an emerging epidemiologic technique in the 1990s. International trade agreements decreed that sanitary (health) measures imposed on imports of animals or animal products must be in accord with international standards or based on scientifically sound risk analyses (see Chapter 8). Risk analysis is sometimes defined as comprising risk assessment, risk management, and risk communication.

Risk assessment, the key component of risk analysis, is an epidemiological approach to import decision making and development of animal health regulations. It can be a very simple or very complex procedure depending on the method selected and political sensitivity of the issue involved.

Import risk assessments are documents used to justify import measures that are more stringent than international standards. Similar techniques are suitable to underlie new animal health regulations.

At a minimum, import risk assessments should define acceptable levels of risk, identify the risks (diseases) potentially associated with commodities proposed for importation, estimate the likelihood that the disease agent can enter and become established in the recipient country, and enumerate risk-mitigating measures such as processing, testing, or quarantines that can permit the import to occur safely.

Zero risk is unattainable. Thus past strategies of attempting to eliminate all risk are being replaced by determinations of acceptable levels of disease-specific risks.

Acceptable level of risk is a term sometimes used synonymously with acceptable level of protection. Even though countries have sovereign rights to unilaterally establish acceptable levels of risk, the international community can't agree on its definition.

When quantitative risk assessments are conducted, acceptable levels of risk can be expressed numerically for each disease. For example, a 1:1,000,000 likelihood of introduction or establishment of one disease agent may be acceptable to an importing country, while a 1:100,000,000 risk may be deemed acceptable for a second disease.

Acceptable levels of risk may also be expressed nonnumerically. For example, a country may accept an import if it is determined in a qualitative risk assessment that the risk is negligible. For qualitative risk determinations, it is appropriate to define a continuum of risk levels such as maximum risk, high risk, moderate risk, low risk, slight risk, or negligible risk. The criteria for each category should be defined in terms of origin factors such as disease prevalence, monitoring and surveillance systems, diagnostic capacity, border security, and animal health. Infrastructure of the exporting country and destination factors such as potential pathogenicity, transmissibility, economic impact, and eradicability of the disease from the recipient country are also relevant.

SUMMARY

The complexity of the virus-host-environment interactions influencing bovine viral diseases complicates their diagnosis, control, and prevention and makes it apparent that they must be addressed on a population basis. The handling of outbreaks and development of control strategies are best approached systematically using tested epidemiologic approaches.

REFERENCES

Kahrs RF, 1978. Techniques for investigating outbreaks of livestock disease. *J. Am. Vet. Med. Assoc.* 173:101–103.

Kahrs RF, 1999. The international animal health community's expectations of the U.S. national animal health reporting system (NAHRS). *Proc. U.S. Anim. Health. Assoc.* 103:100–109.

Murphy FA, Gibbs EPJ, Horzinek MC, Studdert MJ, 1999. Epidemiology of virus diseases. In *Veterinary Virology,* 3rd ed. San Diego: Academic Press, pp. 245–258.

4

DIAGNOSTIC AND INVESTIGATIVE TECHNIQUES

INTRODUCTION

The diagnosis of bovine disease utilizes physical exams, necropsies, epidemic investigations, and laboratory tests.

Physical exams achieve a clinical diagnosis; necropsies produce a pathologic diagnosis; laboratory tests achieve an etiologic diagnosis; and epidemic investigations determine the source and extent of outbreaks. All help in resolving existing problems and preventing recurrences.

Diagnosis of viral diseases has been reviewed by Castro and Heuschele (1992) and Murphy et al. (1999).

PHYSICAL EXAMINATION

Proficiency in physical examination and clinical diagnosis requires concentration, skill, experience, and constant verification by necropsy and laboratory tests.

Proficient diagnosticians minimize oversights by following a systematic procedure involving observation from a distance and hands-on examination each time they examine individual cattle, regardless of how irrelevant some steps may seem or how obvious the diagnosis may seem.

Examination at a Distance

Before they are handled, undisturbed cattle should be observed in their usual surroundings to determine spatial relationships with each other and the environment.

Selected individuals are then observed from a distance to determine the anatomic system involved. This determination is made by examination of their posture, attitude, body and skin condition, stance, and gait. From a distance, the examiner can discern if normal patterns of respiration are present or if there are locomotive abnormalities or abnormal oral, nasal, ocular, vaginal, or preputial discharges. Distant examination can also be used to detect gross external lesions or swellings and determine if defecation and urination are occurring normally. All this evaluation is best accomplished before the cattle are handled or restrained.

Hands-on Examination

A thorough physical examination includes recording the temperature and pulse rate. The vaginal mucosa must be examined for lesions, pallor or discharges. The udder should be palpated and all four quarters milked onto a strip plate. The area between legs and udder (scrotum in males) and area lymph nodes should be palpated.

Auscultation with the stethoscope will determine the nature, frequency, and magnitude of rumen contractions and other visceral activity. The entire rib cage on both sides should be auscultated to determine the presence, nature, and location of any abnormal cardiac or pulmonary sounds. The entire trachea should be auscultated for the presence of stenosis and to correlate tracheal sounds to thoracic sounds. The skin and superficial lymph nodes should be palpated. The muzzle and visible portions of the nasal mucosa should be examined for lesions and discharges. The oral mucosa, including tongue, hard and soft palates, cheeks, and gums, are examined using a flashlight. The feet and interdigital spaces must also be examined.

POSTMORTEM EXAMINATIONS

Necropsies can be conducted in the field but are best carried out in diagnostic laboratories where facilities and expertise permit harvesting appropriate tissues for histopathology, electron microscopy, and microbiological tests and where approved methods are available for carcass disposal.

The postmortem lesions of viral infections are described in the chapters on each disease.

DIFFERENTIAL DIAGNOSIS

The differential diagnosis developed by the procedures described above includes diseases, syndromes, or etiologic designations that may ultimately constitute the final diagnosis. Misdiagnoses more frequently result from incomplete examinations than from misinterpretation of observations. The investigator must be cautious about developing tentative differential diagnoses before visiting the premises, because predeterminations bias observations.

EPIDEMIOLOGICAL INVESTIGATION OF HERD OUTBREAKS

Detailed systematic epidemiological investigations provide information that might otherwise be overlooked. They are undertaken when outbreaks are severe or unusual, resemble exotic infections, or appear to have legal or regulatory implications.

The objectives of epidemiologic investigations are to determine the cause (etiologic diagnosis), source (method of exposure), and extent of the problem, take immediate corrective action, and make recommendations to prevent recurrences.

These objectives are best achieved by systematically delineating the characteristics of affected and unaffected cattle and observing, recording, and analyzing the distribution of the disease with respect to time, place, and a variety of exposure factors and environmental influences. This information must be correlated with physical examinations, necropsy findings, and laboratory tests.

Outbreak investigations are often initiated after standard diagnostic or therapeutic efforts have failed to provide solutions. A unique systematic process should be employed even if it repeats some procedures conducted previously.

An epidemiologic investigation begins with an interview of owners or managers and involved veterinarians. Then follows an inspection of the premises and examination of healthy and affected animals. The investigation is completed when data are assembled and analyzed and conclusions and recommendations are presented.

Procedures for outbreak investigation are detailed by Kahrs (1978) and Ribble et al. (1998).

Interview and Questionnaire

The interview identifies the ownership and location of the farm, clarifies the principal complaint, and evaluates its impact. At the outset, the investigator should determine the attributes to be tabulated. These are traits attributable to disease, that is, disease-dependent variables such as clinical signs, lesions, events (such as abortion or death), carefully defined syndromes, or test results. The attributes selected must be easily identified, because the tabulations require that each animal on the premises be distinguishable as possessing or lacking each attribute.

When the size or inaccessibility of the population prohibits direct observation and tabulation for each animal, more accessible (but indirect) indicators may be used. Thus, distribution of disease in large herds can be estimated by tabulating attributes by pen, pasture, or age groups or from records of weight gain, milk production, reproductive performance, or drug and biologics use.

Interviews are best conducted with standard questionnaires containing basic questions and with space for comments.

During the interview, the investigator orients the episode in time and space by establishing the location and identification of the first case (index case), the day when it was first recognized (index date), and the time and place of subsequent onsets.

Possible exposure factors and their temporal relationship to the onset of disease are recorded. These include the source of replacement cattle, vaccination and feeding programs; methods of crop or pasture fertilization, irrigation, and insecticide applications; and changes in employees. The interviewer should inquire about illness among employees or their families and similar diseases in the area.

The interview, which lasts several hours, yields a list of all cattle on the farm. This line listing should include age, sex, breed, use, origin, feeding, and breeding status of each animal or group of animals.

Examination of the Farm or Ranch

Examination of the premises follows the interview. It is crucial that the premises be examined before animal inspections are made and diagnostic efforts are undertaken to prevent biased searching for substantiating factors.

Premises examination includes inspection of water sources, feed supplies, pastures, and storage areas for equipment, lubricants, chemicals and fertilizers, and trash-disposal methods. It should include an evaluation of local geography (including potential insect habitats), flow direction of streams, and location of wells and ponds. Tactful questioning should reveal the managerial practices and what changes, if any, have been instituted. This information may be sensitive. Leading questions or potentially incriminating lines of interrogation should be avoided to minimize bias.

Examination of Healthy Cattle

Even if previous clinical examinations have occurred, complete epidemiologic investigations require documentation of clinical signs and lesions. Physical examination of healthy cattle should precede examination of sick cattle to avoid spreading infections and to minimize bias. Sometimes reportedly healthy animals are found to be involved. If not, it is essential to determine why they were spared. It is also desirable to collect blood for serology and hematology from a few unaffected cattle.

Examination of Sick Cattle

Examination of representative sick cattle should be conducted carefully and thoroughly (see Physical Examination). Tentative diagnoses are usually offered by herdsmen or veterinarians, but investigators should also examine some affected cattle. When herd size permits, 10% to 20% of sick animals (at least five or six patients) should be identified and subjected to a complete physical examination. Clinical descriptions and a list of possible diagnoses should be recorded. Blood for serology, hematology, and other tests should be collected.

Assembling and Analyzing Data

Line listing permits evaluation of the distribution of the disease with respect to various population characteristics such as age, sex, breed, and use. In addition, by means of line listing, the temporal and spatial relationships of affected and unaffected animals are compared with each potential exposure factor.

Temporal relationships are best visualized using histograms (epidemic curves) that express the onset of new cases to time. Convention requires inclusion of each sick animal only on the date first observed ill. The shape of epidemic curves suggests the nature of exposure and modes of transmission. When numbers of cases are adequate, a propagated outbreak with cow-to-cow transmission usually produces a bell-shaped curve.

A point outbreak (all cases appearing at one point in time and space) presents an abrupt-onset pattern, which occurs following simultaneous exposure to a common source via a common vehicle. Point outbreaks of enteritis or gastroenteritis are almost always food or water borne. Nondescript configurations may reflect poor observation, erratic exposure patterns, variable exposure-onset intervals, multiple causative factors, or inadequate case numbers.

The relationship of sick and healthy cattle to various exposure factors is determined on the farm, using the line listing of individual cattle or population exposure charts that deal with groups of cattle housed together. In this format, target or high-likelihood exposure factors are readily identified when there is complete correspondence between the disease and a risk factor (i.e., all sick subpopulations were exposed and all unexposed subpopulations were spared). When multiple target exposure factors are identified, the search can be narrowed by examination of the temporal relationship of the target risks to the onset of disease.

Frequently, several exposure factors, such as purchase of cattle or change of feed, occur immediately preceding the onset of clinical disease. In such events, the investigator must search for further evidence to identify the source of infection.

Quantitative Description of Outbreaks

The extent of outbreaks is determined by defining the base population and calculating clinical attack rates (percentages of populations affected), death rates (percentages of populations that died), and specific attack rates by age, sex, breed, and other relevant distributions. It should be stated whether disease distributions by age, breed, sex, and use differ from that of the study population.

Reporting Results of Outbreak Investigations

Data can occasionally be assembled on the premises, and immediate tentative conclusions provided. Usually, however, data organization and analysis takes time, and presentation of a comprehensive report must await laboratory reports. The final report should include the cause, source, and extent of the problem and the basis for the conclusions. Statistical analysis of numerical data occasionally adds useful dimensions but should only support biologically feasible conclusions.

Utility of Outbreak Investigations

Outbreak investigations provide solutions to many bovine health problems. Some produce more questions than answers and problems may be unresolved despite tedious and expensive efforts.

LABORATORY TESTS

An array of laboratory tests is evolving for bovine viruses and their antigens, nucleic acids, and antibodies. These tests vary in sophistication, availability, cost, and in their applicability to diagnosis, regulatory programs, disease reporting, research, and trade.

Serologic Testing and Serum Antibodies

Serologic testing is used for diagnosis of illness or abortion, for determining the geographic distribution of viruses, and for estimating efficacy of vaccines. Serology is a valuable diagnostic tool but has serious limitations and must be correlated with clinical observations, physical examinations, histories, and necropsy findings.

The key to appreciating virus serology lies in understanding it is largely a retrospective educational tool. Serologic diagnosis usually requires two specimens from the same animal plus a wait for reports that require skillful interpretation.

In response to viral infection cattle produce a variety of specific immune globulins that appear in blood and milk and bathe mucous membranes where they react with stimulating viruses.

Antibodies are a heterogeneous group of macromolecules with different characteristics that are manifested by variable reactions to different tests, varying effects on infectious agents, and varying sites of activity.

The principal immunoglobulins are immunoglobulin M (IgM), a large molecule that is the major component of primary immune responses and appears in serum immediately after infection; several types of classic immunoglobulins (IgG), which appear later in infection and comprise the majority of serum, milk, and colostral antibodies; and immunoglobulin A (IgA), which usually is produced locally in tissues and mucous membranes and comprises a smaller proportion of humoral immunoglobulins.

The stage of infection determines the type of globulins most prominent in serum. Most primary exposures induce an early IgM response followed by production of IgG and IgA.

Antigen–antibody reactions can be detected by neutralization tests, complement fixation tests, hemagglutination-inhibition tests, agar gel immunodiffusion (AGID) tests, enzyme-linked immunoabsorbent assay (ELISA), western blot, and other tests.

Serum antibody usually implies some degree of protection against subsequent infections. It may be actively produced in response to exposure or vaccination or passively acquired by transfer of antibody synthesized by one animal (donor) to a second (recipient) animal.

Passive antibody acquisition can result from blood transfusions, and inoculations of antiserums or globulin concentrates. In cattle, however, it most commonly occurs when newborn calves ingest colostrum.

Colostrally Acquired Antibodies

Unlike human infants, who acquire their mother's immune status transplacentally, calves are born without serum antibodies unless they are prenatally infected in utero. Immunoglobulins are concentrated in colostrum, and calves nursing immediately after birth ingest antibodies that reach the bloodstream by absorption through gastrointestinal mucosa. They then have a temporary immune status similar to that of their dams and react to serologic tests even if never infected or vaccinated.

The concentration of antibodies in the cow's milk declines following parturition. Calves lose their immunoglobulin-absorbing ability shortly after birth and must acquire their passive immunity on the first day of life. Calves that fail to nurse and are not fed colostrum immediately after birth are vulnerable to infections. Colostrally acquired immunoglobulins are metabolically dissipated at fairly uniform rates so the interval between ingestion of colostrum and the loss of passive immunity is determined largely by the amount of immunoglobulin a calf absorbs on the first day of life. Calves with high initial titers will be seropositive longer than calves with lower titers.

Some people erroneously believe calves are immune as long they are nursing. Some calves are weaned about the time their colostrally acquired maternal antibody diminishes but such timing is coincidental. Diseases associated with weaning are related to dietary change, stress, aggregation, and shipment.

Test kits for screening calf blood for IgG, the principal immunoglobulin in colostrum, are used to identify colostrum-deprived day-old calves that are at high risk of infections so they can be fed stored colostrum and observed carefully.

Effect of Age on Serology

Evidence of antibodies in calves indicates previous exposure, vaccination, or colostrally acquired immunity; these means are indistinguishable by most tests. Most colostrally acquired viral antibody disappears within 8 months but there are exceptions. Single serum samples have minimal diagnostic value in calves so virus isolation, antigen identification, or paired serums are needed.

Importance of Paired Serums

Serologic diagnosis of clinical disease usually requires paired samples. When history, clinical signs, and lesions suggest a specific disease, a positive serologic diagnosis can be based on two specimens from the same animal. The first (acute sample) is collected at the first sign of infection. The second (convalescent sample) is collected 1–4 weeks after the first. A negative acute sample followed by a positive convalescent sample, sometimes called seroconversion, is considered diagnostic.

Negative paired samples eliminate the virus in question. Positive paired samples are diagnostically meaningless unless, having been titrated simultaneously, the second specimen has a titer at least four times higher than that of the first, constituting a fourfold titer increment or a "significant rise in titer." Efforts to demonstrate significant rises in titer are frequently frustrating, and diagnoses obtained this way are less convincing than diagnoses based on seroconversion, because fourfold titer increments can result from laboratory variations, cross-reactions, secondary immune responses, or stress-induced reactivation of latent infections. When coupled with virus isolation, seroconversion presents strong evidence of an acute primary infection.

Some laboratories test for virus-specific IgM in acute-phase serums. Because IgM is indicative of early infection, its presence is regarded as diagnostic of acute infection. Such findings must be interpreted cautiously, because IgM is also detectable in some persistently infected animals.

Diagnostic Utility of Single Serums

Often it is not possible to collect paired serum samples. Single samples are of value only as a part of the diagnostic process of elimination, and interpretation is difficult because the relationship between infection and the time of collection is usually unknown.

A negative serum collected 3 or more weeks after a suspected infection indicates that the animal was still susceptible when the sample was drawn, and the disease was probably not related to the virus in question. If the single negative serum was collected less than 3 weeks following the event, it is possible that the animal was infected but had not yet produced detectable antibodies. In this case, a later sample would be positive.

Without information about time relationships between the clinical disease and collection of serum specimens, a single positive test has limited diagnostic value because serum antibodies can result from clinical disease, inapparent infection, vaccination, or passive immunity. Unless a marker vaccine is used, most serologic tests cannot distinguish between vaccination titers and infection titers.

Single serums are useful in some retrospective studies, diagnosis of exotic infections, and serological surveys.

Serological Surveys

Single specimens from cattle populations provide data about the extent and geographic distribution of infections and for estimating the degree to which a virus produces inapparent infections. The results of single sample surveys produce point estimates of antibody prevalence (the percentage of populations with antibody at a given time). Unless there is a distinctive age distribution of positive cattle, antibody prevalence estimates give no information of the time of infection. For export purposes, statistically designed serosurveys can serve as evidence of regional freedom from infection.

Interpretation of Herd Tests

The expense of testing entire herds can be prohibitive, and some laboratories limit sample sizes to conserve resources. Herd antibody prevalence is a useful parameter in epidemiologic studies, and a small sample often provides an indication of a herd's immune status. Tests adaptable to bulk milk samples can provide preliminary indications of the presence of antibody or virus presence in herds.

Diagnosing Abortion or Congenital Defects with Dam's Serum

Serologic tests on aborting cows must be interpreted cautiously because antibodies against abortifacient viruses are common, abortions or birth of calves with virus induced congenital anomalies can occur months after infection and, usually when fetal damage is recognized the dam's titer has stabilized excluding seroconversion or rising titers.

Single positive serums collected on the day of abortion have limited diagnostic value particularly for viruses with high antibody prevalence.

If a day-of-abortion serum is negative, it usually eliminates the suspected virus but a second negative specimen, taken 3 weeks later, makes this interpretation more convincing. If the second specimen contains specific antibodies, indicating seroconversion, infection occurred in the test interval. This finding suggests, but does not prove, the virus is involved.

Diagnosis Using Serums from Fetuses and Neonates

Unlike the dam's serum, fetal and neonatal serums have excellent diagnostic potential if properly interpreted. The bovine fetus can respond immunologically by mid-gestation and fetal antibody usually indicates transplacental intrauterine infection from a dam undergoing primary infection during pregnancy. Possible mistakes in this conclusion are test error, unobserved colostrum acquisition, and occasional antibody leakage across a damaged placenta.

Fetal serology is underutilized because fetal serum is difficult to obtain, usually hemolyzed, contaminated, or mixed with substances toxic to test systems. Fluids collected from fetal body cavities are equally toxic.

Failure to detect suspect antibody in an aborted fetus is not always grounds for eliminating a virus from etiologic consideration because infection can occur before fetal immunocompetence and some acute fetal infections, such as infectious bovine rhinotracheitis, can cause fetal death before antibody production occurs.

Presence of antibody in fetuses or presuckle serum from neonates indicates fetal infection but not necessarily a cause-and-effect relationship with any specific virus because fetuses (like adult cattle) experience numerous inapparent infections and can have antibodies against multiple viruses.

Bovine neonates lack maternally bestowed antibodies prior to nursing. In serologic diagnosis of prenatal infection in calves born alive, it is critical to determine that the specimen was collected before nursing. This is possible if someone is present at birth or if the fetus is aborted or stillborn. If calves are standing when first seen, the cow's teats can be examined for evidence of nursing. Ascertainment of colostrum deprivation can be determined at necropsy if a calf has no milk in its stomach.

Collection of Blood Samples for Virus Serology

Serums tested for viral antibodies should be clear and free from hemolysis and contaminants that can render them unsuitable for testing. The blood should be collected in sterile, sealed vials, allowed to clot and held at 65–75° F until the clot contracts exuding the serum. When clot retraction is completed, the specimen should be refrigerated. Cattle serums can be submitted with the clot because they do not hemolyze rapidly, and the risk of contamination involved in decanting the serum or removing the clot may outweigh the hazard of slight hemolysis.

The logistics of paired serum testing should be worked out with individual laboratories.

Serologic Test Procedures

Laboratory techniques for bovine serology vary with the virus. Standardization is common in accredited laboratories and where regulatory programs are involved. The techniques for detecting antibodies against specific viruses are outlined in the *Manual of Diagnostic Tests and Vaccines,* published by the Office International Des Epizooties (OIE 2000).

Serologic tests permit visualization of reactions occurring when known viruses or antigens combine with specific antibodies. The relative concentration of antibodies (titer) is determined by testing serial serum dilutions to find the point (dilution) at which the visible reaction ceases. Serologic tests for bovine viruses were reviewed by Castro and Heuschele (1992).

Virus Neutralization Test

When combined with specific serum antibody, viruses are neutralized and rendered unable to infect cell cultures and other assay systems. The virus neutralization test, sometimes called the serum neutralization test, is the traditional serologic test for bovine viruses and the one to which other tests are compared. It employs known viruses to detect antibodies or specific antiserums to identify viruses. It involves inoculating cultures or test animals with virus–serum mixtures and comparing the observed effects with those of appropriate controls.

Complement Fixation Test

Complement is a series of serum proteins that mediates many antigen–antibody reactions in which it is fixed (used up) in forming immune complexes.

The presence of complement (usually provided by addition of guinea pig serum) is detectable by its ability to lyse sensitized red blood cells.

The complement fixation (CF) test is an indirect test for specific serum antibodies. It measures utilization of added complement by reaction of serum antibodies with known viruses. It is gradually being replaced by newer techniques.

Hemagglutination Inhibition Test

Some viruses agglutinate certain red blood cells. This reaction, known as hemagglutination (HA) can be quantitated and adapted for indicating presence of specific antibodies in serum mixed with a known virus and then added to red cell suspensions. Hemagglutination inhibition (HI), in adequately controlled systems, indicates the presence of specific antibody.

Agar Gel Immunodiffusion Test

Many antigen–antibody reactions cause precipitation, when antigen–antibody complexes form after diffusion through agar.

The AGID test uses this phenomenon to assay viral antibodies. It is conducted using punched-out wells in agar filled with known virus suspensions that diffuse toward wells filled with test serums.

Fluorescent Antibody Tests

The term "fluorescent antibody (FA) test" denotes a variety of tests that use fluorescent-tagged specific immune serums. When the labeled antibody reacts with tissues or cultures containing virus, the binding capacity withstands washing leaving only combined (positive) reactants for visualization by fluorescent microscopy. Direct FA tests detect antigen in tissues, discharges, or cultures and a positive FA test means virus is present.

The indirect FA (IFA) test detects serum antibody when it binds with known test virus making it unavailable to combine with fluorescein-labeled antibodies. The IFA test requires careful standardization of reagents, multiple control reactions, and special equipment.

Enzyme Immunoassays

Conjugation of enzymes to specific antiserums produces reagents that can be visualized by color changes when enzymes react with suitable substrates. This principle is used to detect antigen by direct methods and specific antibody by indirect methods. The most commonly used enzyme immunoassay, the ELISA is performed in plastic microtiter plates and, for some viruses, is available in test kits.

Diagnostic Value of Serology

Excessive reliance on serology is unwarranted and frustrating. Serologic tests are useful if their significance and limitations are appreciated and when correlated with clinical observations, history, necropsy, and virus isolation.

Virus Isolation and Identification

Direct laboratory diagnosis of viral infections utilizes isolation of viruses, identification of viruses or viral antigens, or detection of viral nucleic acids. These procedures use several approaches each with multiple variations, adaptations, combinations, and limitations.

If virus isolation or identification is to be attempted, advanced instructions for collecting, packaging, and transporting specimens should be obtained from the laboratory.

Virus Isolation

Virus isolation, the best way of identifying new viruses, is the time-tested procedure for diagnosing infection with known viruses, and the standard to which other techniques are compared. It involves producing recognizable infections in assay systems (such as cell cultures, laboratory animals, or embryonating eggs) that support replication of viruses if they are present in infective doses in the specimen.

Specimens for virus isolation can be tissues from live or dead cattle; blood; vesicular fluids; feces; or swabs of nasal, ocular, oral, or reproductive tract mucosa. Infectivity is preserved by placing specimens in viral transport media or freezing. Freezing tissues reduces their value for histopathology, so a second specimen is placed in fixative for histologic study.

A serum sample is taken at the time specimens are collected for virus isolation and again 2 to 3 weeks later to permit testing for seroconversion to any virus isolated.

Specimens are ground, diluted with antibiotic and antifungal agents, centrifuged to remove extraneous material, and again to concentrate virus, and filtered to remove contaminating organisms.

The presence of virus in specimens is evident by appearance of characteristic disease, or development of gross or histologic lesions. In cell cultures, these lesions are called cytopathogenic changes or cytopathic effects (CPE).

Failure to isolate virus can result from miscalculation anywhere in the procedure. Thus, negative virus isolation attempts are not evidence that viruses were not present in animals.

Virus isolation procedures are complete when the virus is identified immunologically or genetically. The complexity of virus identification leads to specialization, because few laboratories have reagents and expertise for all viruses.

Immunologic Identification of Viruses

Identification of viruses isolated from diagnostic specimens can be accomplished by employing monospecific antiserums or monoclonal antibodies. Monoclonal antibodies are secreted by immunoglobulin-producing hybridomas that are produced by hybridizing antibody-producing cells (usually plasma cells) with tumor cells. When maintained in cultures or implanted in laboratory mice, hybridomas produce large quantities of highly specific immunoglobulins that combine with homologous viruses in a variety of identifiable reactions, including neutralization, AGID, ELISA, direct FA, immunohistochemistry, latex agglutination, and other detection systems.

Virus Identification by Electron Microscopy

Virus identification can sometimes be achieved quickly by electron microscopy (EM) on fluids, tissue extracts, or cell cultures containing high virus concentrations. In skilled hands, EM identification is fairly accurate for poxviruses, rotaviruses, coronaviruses, rabies virus, and vesicular stomatitis virus.

Immunoelectron microscopy employs specific antiserum or convalescent serum from animals providing specimens to aggregate virus particles, that may be widely dispersed in specimens, to expedite their detection by electron microscopy.

Genetic and Molecular Technology in Viral Diagnosis

A variety of molecular and genetic techniques that identify viral nucleic acid sequences instead of antigenic markers are used in viral classification and identification. This technology uses labeled molecular probes to identify viruses by detecting virus-specific nucleic acid sequences in clinical samples, fixed tissue specimens, or cell cultures.

Molecular probes, sometimes called DNA probes, nucleic acid probes, or genetic probes are labeled virus-specific nucleic acid sequences that combine (hybridize) with complementary sequences in test preparations and remain to be detected by a variety of procedures after rinsing that washes away unbound materials. The nucleic acid sequences used in probes are extracted from purified cultures of known viruses; once their base sequences are known, it is possible to synthesize them.

The polymerase chain reaction (PCR) is a method of amplifying nucleic acid sequences in test materials to achieve quantities detectable by a variety of procedures. It is useful for viruses that are difficult to cultivate; for specimens with levels of virus that are undetectable by other methods or because they have been inactivated by time, temperature, or other influences; for diseases in which viral nucleic acids persist after infective virus has been cleared; and for detection of latent persistent infections.

The PCR procedure involves automated enzymatic amplification of nucleic acid strands through stepwise heating and cooling.

The term PCR suggests a specific test procedure, but actually PCR technology is a key preliminary step in a variety of identification and quantification methods involving hybridization; detection by diffusion or electrophoresis in membrane or agar substrates; and readings by enzymatic, colorimetric, or radiographic indicators. PCR-based tests, which can be automated, are rapid and sensitive, and test positivity can persist after replicating virus is no longer present in animals or tissues.

Because molecular probes can be specific to family, genus, virus, and even subtype, one key to probe technology is searching for the right viruses particularly if animals have clinical signs common to multiple viral infections. Some laboratories develop batteries of probes for use in testing materials from cattle with multiple cause syndromes like respiratory or enteric disease. Many PCR-based tests are incorporated into diagnostic test kits.

Nucleotide fingerprinting procedures, commonly called DNA fingerprinting but also modifiable for RNA viruses, are sensitive methods of detecting minute genetic shifts or comparing virus subtypes for determination of the origin of outbreaks.

"Fingerprinting" involves side-by-side gel electrophoresis of enzymatically separated nucleic acid fragments from test samples and known viruses and comparison of their diffusion patterns (fingerprints) for similarity.

CONCLUSION

Determination of the cause, source, and extent of viral diseases and initiation of the most appropriate control measures requires integration of a variety of clinical, epidemiologic, and laboratory findings. Their interpretation is complex and requires appreciation of the limitations of each approach as well as understanding of the pathogenesis of individual infections.

REFERENCES

Castro AE, Heuschele WP (eds.), 1992. Diagnostic techniques—bovine. In *Veterinary Diagnostic Virology: A Practitioners Guide*. St. Louis: Mosby Yearbook, pp. 1–132.

Kahrs RF, 1978. Techniques for investigating outbreaks of livestock disease. *J. Am. Vet. Med. Assoc.* 173(1):101–103.

Murphy FA, Gibbs EPJ, Horzinek MC, Studdert MJ (eds.) 1999. Diagnosis of viral diseases. In *Veterinary Virology,* 3rd ed. San Diego: Academic Press, pp. 193–225.

OIE 2000. Office International Des Epizooties (OIE). *Manual of Diagnostic Tests and Vaccines,* 6th ed., with annual updates. Paris: OIE: pp. 1–389.

Ribble CS, Janzen ED, Campbell J, 1998. Disease outbreak investigation in the beef herd: defining the problem. *Bovine Practitioner* (31):121–127.

5

VACCINES AND VACCINATION

INTRODUCTION

Vaccination against viral diseases is a generally effective control measure that is made complex by the multiplicity of bovine viruses, the many available vaccines, the numerous production systems in which they can be used, the variable responses of cattle to vaccination, and constantly changing information. These aspects of bovine vaccination were reviewed by Schultz (1998) and the principles of veterinary vaccinology are detailed by Pastoret et al. (1999)

Excessive reliance on vaccines should be avoided because they are not substitutes for sound management.

The three major classes of bovine viral vaccines are modified live virus (MLV) vaccines, inactivated virus vaccines, and genetically engineered vaccines. Each has unique production methods, applications, advantages, disadvantages, and hazards.

MODIFIED LIVE VIRUS VACCINES

MLV vaccines induce mild immunizing infections and provide efficacy at the expense of safety and stability. Because replication of MLV vaccine virus occurs in vaccinated cattle, one successful vaccination provides immunologic stimulation comparable to multiple doses of inactivated vaccines.

Attenuation

Attenuation is modification to reduce virulence (relative disease-producing capacity). It can be achieved by gene deletions or by serial passage in alien hosts. Attenuation is relative and virus strains attenuated for one host may be virulent in another.

Gene-deletion attenuation, which is gradually being adopted, removes genes associated with virulence and produces stable avirulent vaccine virus strains that are incapable of reversion to virulence.

Traditionally, most bovine vaccines have been attenuated by serial passage in cell cultures. Attenuation is accomplished by growing viruses to peak titer, harvesting, and inoculating new cell cultures repeatedly. The inoculations continue until tests reveal the virus strain no longer produces disease but is still antigenic.

Serial passage causes other changes so the resulting virus strains are actually modified rather than simply attenuated and the resulting vaccines are called MLV vaccines.

While exceptions occur, usually serial passage also causes loss of antigenicity. Thus vaccine developers walk a tightrope between maximum attenuation with minimal antigenicity and maximum antigenicity with minimal attenuation. When a satisfactory balance is achieved, the virus is tested in animals for safety and efficacy and in the laboratory for purity and potency. When these requirements are met to the satisfaction of manufacturers and regulatory agencies, large "seed stocks" are grown and stored at ultra-low temperatures. Production batches can be started from seed stocks without further animal testing.

Components of MLV Vaccines

In addition to the antigenic component, MLV vaccines often contain portions of the cell cultures and nutrient fluids in which vaccine virus was propagated, including an array of carbohydrates, amino acids, vitamins, minerals, and antibiotics. Sometimes, serum or polysaccharide stabilizers are added to protect the infectivity of MLV vaccines.

The conditions for production of MLV vaccine viruses are suitable for maintenance and replication of unwanted extraneous viruses, which can enter as contaminants carried in cell cultures or serum. Extraneous viruses in MLV vaccines can be hard to detect and can cause problems.

Potential Shortcomings of MLV Vaccines

There are numerous potential shortcomings of MLV vaccines that require caution in their use. Under certain conditions, some vaccine strains or vaccine contaminants can cause abortion or clinical disease, be shed and spread to contact animals, or establish latent or persistent vaccine virus infections that can spread or be mistaken for natural infections by some laboratory tests. In addition, seropositivity engendered by vaccination can be a trade impediment.

Postvaccination Disease

Normally, after vaccination with MLV vaccines, immune responses result, partial protection develops, and vaccine virus is cleared by the animal. Sometimes MLV vaccine strains persist in vaccinated cattle and shedding of vaccine virus results. A small percentage of cattle, frequently individuals with immunologic deficits, develop clinical disease from infection with MLV vaccines. Some postvaccination disease is actually the result of natural infection present at the time of vaccination.

Shed and Spread of MLV Vaccines

Vaccine virus can be spread by product spillage or brief leakage from vaccination sites.

"Vaccine shed" implies exteriorization of vaccine after replication in cattle vaccinated with MLV vaccines. Shed can also occur from intermittent reactivation of latent persistent infectious bovine rhinotracheitis (IBR) vaccine virus infections; from chronic persistent vaccine virus infection developing after vaccination of cattle unable to clear attenuated vaccine virus; or from a brief post-vaccination shed of replicating marginally attenuated vaccine virus before normal cattle respond immunologically and clear the virus.

When vaccine viruses attenuated by serial passage are shed by vaccinated individuals and infect other animals, they can sometimes revert to virulence after repeated field transmission, but this situation rarely occurs. Reversion to virulence should not be a problem with vaccines with virulence genes deleted.

Resistance Induced by MLV Vaccines

Vaccine-induced resistance, best described as partial protection, results from nonclinical infection with vaccine virus. Successful vaccination prior to exposure should protect against abortion and severe systemic manifestations. Successful vaccination will not necessarily prevent infection of mucosal surfaces or establishment of latent persistent infections with vaccine and field viruses. Previous successful vaccination, though, should engender enough resistance (through local resistance factors, humoral antibody, or anamnestic immune response) that animals survive uncomplicated exposures.

In the case of PI-3 and the rotavirus and coronavirus associated with neonatal diarrhea and other ubiquitous viruses of uncertain pathogenicity, both the solidarity and duration of partial protection are limited.

INACTIVATED VACCINES

Inactivated vaccines stimulate antibody responses more slowly than MLV vaccines and require two initial inoculations and semiannual or annual boosters. The safety and relative stability of inactivated vaccines compensates for their immunologic inferiority.

Inactivation processes usually eliminate contaminants and extraneous agents. Preservatives in killed vaccines retard growth of bacteria introduced after the vial has been opened.

Inactivated vaccines can be used on pregnant cattle without fear of vaccine-induced abortion and can be used in situations where use of live virus vaccines may be ill-advised because cattle are stressed, exposed to infectious diseases, or pregnant. In short, inactivated vaccines provide maximum safety at the expense of efficacy.

Inactivated (killed) vaccines do not replicate in vaccinated cattle, and the entire antigenic mass must be provided in the vaccine. This fact partly explains why inactivated virus vaccines are harder to produce in adequate dosage forms and why repeated vaccination is required for them to be effective.

Components of Inactivated Vaccines

Various immunostimulators and adjuvants are added to inactivated vaccines to slow their dissemination after injection or expedite their uptake by immunocompetent cells. Antibiotics or preservatives may be added to minimize bacterial growth.

The inactivators used in preparing killed vaccines are usually adequate to inactivate extraneous viruses. For this reason, killed vaccines have considerable safety advantages over MLV vaccines.

The multiple components of inactivated vaccines occasionally stimulate tissue reactions detected as blemishes at slaughter, so inoculated cattle should not be slaughtered until withdrawal times indicated on labels have passed.

GENETICALLY MANIPULATED VACCINES

Molecular technology provides subunit, gene-deleted, and vectored vaccines. These are sometimes called genetically engineered vaccines. Although not without challenging technologic intricacies, these products appear to be the key to the future of veterinary vaccinology (Pastoret et al. 1999).

Subunit vaccines consist of purified antigenic virion proteins that are mass-produced by several cloning mechanisms. They use protein-specific genes to direct self-replicating DNA molecules (plasmids) in bacteria, yeasts, or mammalian cells to generate the antigenic protein. Subunit vaccines have been developed for infectious bovine rhinotracheitis (IBR) and foot-and-mouth disease.

Gene-deleted vaccines are created by utilizing enzymatic reactions to remove specific genes from vaccine viruses. Deletions of genes controlling antigenic properties produce marker vaccines that allow serologic tests to distinguish vaccinated animals from naturally infected cattle. Marker vaccines for IBR and bovine viral diarrhea (BVD) are used in Europe by countries attempting to eradicate these diseases.

Deletion of virulence genes offers a controlled method of attenuating vaccine viruses. This process usually ensures that they will not revert to virulence during serial cow-to-cow passage in the field.

Vectored vaccines require insertion of genes from one virus (the vaccine) into a carrier (vector) agent, a process that infects animals without causing disease. Inserted genes instruct host animals to generate immune responses to the vaccine virus. This process requires the vector to infect vaccinated animals so if they are immune to the vector virus, the process may be aborted. Vaccinia virus–vectored oral rabies vaccine incorporated in baits has been used to vaccinate wildlife in Europe and the United States.

BASIC PRINCIPLES OF BOVINE VACCINATION

Vaccination is an area where it is difficult to separate fact from philosophy. Vaccination philosophies must recognize that vaccines are useful in long-term health maintenance on a population basis but will not prevent all viral infections. Properly used, they help avoid viral abortion storms and herd outbreaks.

Vaccine axioms include the distinction between vaccination (inoculation) and immunization (the immunologic response), the reality that no vaccine is 100% safe or effective, and the fact that vaccination will not replace sound management. The analogy of vaccination to insurance fails because vaccine benefits are not guaranteed and there is no compensation for losses.

Objectives of Vaccination

The objective of vaccination is to generate herd resistance so that death, sickness, abortion, and neonatal mortality are minimized. This objective is accomplished by vaccinating healthy cattle for long-range benefits.

Objectives vary with geographic area, management practices, and production goals. Specific programs must be designed for each herd to maximize protection, minimize risks, and adhere to label recommendations.

Elements of Viral Vaccination Programs

Sound use of vaccine requires common sense and appreciation of disease risks in specific production-management systems. It also requires understanding of the pathogenesis of bovine viral infections and knowledge of the indications and hazards of available vaccines.

Using this information, specific vaccination programs can be devised that define the vaccines used and the best time and age of the animal for vaccination and the frequency of vaccination.

Potential Hazards of Vaccination

Potential hazards such as vaccine-induced disease or abortion must be considered in vaccination planning.

More subtle hazards of vaccination are inefficient utilization of funds for nonefficacious or unneeded vaccines and neglect of sound management practices due to the illusion of security vaccination provides. Other hazards are forfeiture of laboratory diagnoses because vaccine-induced antibodies often cannot be distinguished from those induced by natural infection, injection site lesions or abscesses, the risk of transmitting infections with vaccinating instruments, and the impact of stress from assembly and restraint for vaccination. Although it occurs rarely, fatal anaphylaxis can follow vaccination.

Livestock owners tend to blame vaccines for any problems that develop after vaccination. Even when unfounded, such accusations blemish the reputations of products.

Failure to observe withdrawal times rarely causes problems with MLV vaccines but can complicate use of inactivated vaccines.

Regulation of Vaccines

Many national governments license vaccine production and require vaccines to be pure, potent, safe, and effective.

Purity (freedom from bacterial or viral contamination) is usually determined by bacteriological culture and viral detection techniques.

Vaccine potency implies a vaccine dose adequate to engender an immunologic response and is determined by titration or detection of antibody production in vaccinated cattle.

Purity is usually determined by culture and potency by titration in the laboratory.

Safety means the vaccine is free of hazard to vaccinated animals or herdmates and its demonstration requires controlled vaccination of cattle.

Efficacy implies the vaccine protects against the disease. Efficacy is usually evaluated by inoculation of vaccinated cattle with a standardized challenge-strain virus capable of producing defined clinical signs in unvaccinated susceptible control cattle.

Some subnational jurisdictions license and regulate animal biologics but usually national governments retain the right to exclude entry, sale, or use of vaccines and diagnostic reagents. In the United States, the Center for Veterinary Biologics, Animal and Plant Health Inspection Service of the US Department of Agriculture (USDA), is responsible for biologics (Espeseth and Myers, 1999).

International standards for veterinary vaccines are outlined by the Office International Des Epizooties (OIE) in the *Manual of Diagnostic Tests and Vaccines* (OIE 2000).

Antigenicity of Vaccines

Vaccines contain active components and other materials to support and preserve them.

Antigen (virus or virus fraction) must be delivered to the lymphoreticular system of vaccinated cattle for an immunologic response to occur. The expression "required antigenic mass" has evolved to represent quantities of virus or antigenic particles required for immunologic stimulation.

BASIC PRINCIPLES OF VACCINE USE

Safe, effective, cost-efficient use of vaccines requires conscientious efforts, planning, and understanding of the objectives and limitations of vaccination. Directions for storage, refrigeration, reconstitution, routes of injection, and indications and contraindications on labels and package inserts must be studied and meticulously followed.

Because of possible incompatibilities, only recommended diluents should be used. Vaccines should not be mixed or given with the same syringe unless they are designed and labeled as combined vaccines. Extreme caution must be used with disinfectants to avoid inactivation of MLV vaccines. Dilution beyond the manufacturer's recommendations is intolerable. The entire contents of a vial should be used at one time.

To avoid transmitting infections by vaccination, healthy, unexposed cattle should be vaccinated with sterile equipment. Individual needles are essential to minimize spread of anaplasmosis, bovine leukemia virus, and bovine immuno-deficiency virus.

Vaccination Concepts

Design and implementation of vaccination programs require understanding of the concepts detailed in Chapters 2 and 3. These concepts deal with the inter-actions between viruses, cattle, and the environment; emphasize multifactorial etiology and complex diagnosis of viral infections; indicate that viral infections are virtually ubiquitous, frequently inapparent, and possessed of mechanisms for perpetuation in individuals and populations. Also important is the concept that exposure or vaccination confers only partial protection. These concepts underlie the following principles of vaccination.

Vaccine Selection

The availability and use of vaccines varies throughout the world. In the United States, bovine vaccines are available for IBR, BVD, parainfluenza-3 (PI-3), bovine respiratory syncytial virus (BRSV), and the rotaviruses and coronaviruses associated with neonatal calf diarrhea. Vaccination planning requires consideration of objectives and potential health hazards of a specific production-management system rather than a simple check-off of available vaccines.

Vaccine Safety and Efficacy

Successful vaccination requires use of high-quality products manufactured and maintained under stringent conditions and delivered appropriately to healthy cattle capable of maximum immune responsiveness. No vaccine is totally safe or effective.

Usually, there is no way to predict vaccination failures, but stressed, recently assembled, moved, and sick animals are prime candidates for a "wreck." The likelihood of satisfactory vaccine performance declines if expiration dates pass; if vaccine has been improperly handled, stored, or damaged; or if vacuum is lost from vacuum-packed products. If vials lack vacuum when punctured, assume air, moisture, and contamination have entered and inactivation has occurred. Such vials should not be used.

Vaccination of Infected, Exposed, or Stressed Cattle

Vaccines are intended for use on healthy, unexposed, uninfected animals prior to exposure. Vaccination after onset of disease promulgates the erroneous philosophy that vaccines are curative and control procedures can be postponed until disease appears. The difficulty in clinical diagnosis of bovine viral dis-eases provides uncertainty about which vaccine to choose if considering vacci-nation of sick animals or their herdmates.

The restraint required for vaccination can induce stress, a recognized component of bovine respiratory disease, and the value of adding further stress to outbreak situations is questionable.

Natural disease occurring after administration of vaccines to incubating cases can be attributed erroneously to vaccine. This apparent lack of vaccine safety serves as a deterrent to use on healthy animals and hampers disease-control efforts. Abortion following vaccination of pregnant animals in the face of outbreaks may be blamed on the vaccine.

When conducted in the urgency of disease outbreaks, vaccination is frequently a belated one-time procedure. Following vaccination under these circumstances, disease control is subsequently forgotten. Good judgment suggests conservative approaches to vaccine use during outbreaks.

Vaccination for Exotic Diseases

Vaccination for exotic diseases is usually contraindicated because vaccine titers confuse surveillance programs. If an exotic disease enters a region, ring, or zone vaccination may be part of control strategies but is usually discontinued as eradication approaches.

Countries claiming disease-free status for trade purposes rarely vaccinate and if they do, they must explain why vaccination is needed if the disease is not present.

VACCINATION GUIDELINES AND RECOMMENDATIONS

General vaccination guidelines for various production management systems can be based on the above considerations. These must be modified for local situations and adjusted as new information appears.

General Vaccination Guidelines

Vaccinations are intended to minimize major disease outbreaks, protect pregnant cattle from virus-induced abortions and fetal wastage, and increase the specific immunoglobulin content of colostrum for protection of newborn calves. They are also intended to immunize calves against disease after decline of maternally bestowed antibodies and prepare calves for the rigors of transport to stocker and feeder operations, as well as protect feedlot cattle from the ravages of viral infections. Package inserts define product limitations and deviations render users vulnerable and culpable.

Self-Contained Dairy Herds Raising Replacements

In self-contained dairy herds, disease outbreaks and virus-induced fetal wastage can be minimized by vaccinating all calves for IBR, BVD, PI-3, and BRSV sometime after 6 months of age, when most interfering colostral antibody has dissipated, and revaccination at 10-12 months of age or well before breeding. Under this schedule, adequate herd immunity should persist, but some people advocate annual revaccination particularly if inactivated vaccines are part of the mixture.

To help control neonatal diarrhea, oral vaccination with rotavirus-coronavirus on the day of birth is applicable. If it is desired to boost immunoglobulin levels in colostrum, vaccination a month prior to anticipated parturition dates with inactivated or nonabortifacient vaccines can be conducted.

Dairy Herds that Purchase Replacements

Dairy herds that purchase replacements present a challenge because disease-control programs are compromised by continual introduction of new viral infections and the stress of immigration and constantly changing peck orders. Addition of replacements from mixed sources not only introduces new viruses and potential diseases but also provides some inconsistent herd immunity. It cannot, however, be counted on to constitute a vaccination program.

Veterinarians should inform owners that this type of management involves tremendous hazard from a disease standpoint. They should discuss the alternative of raising replacements or establishing controlled replacement sources where calfhood vaccination is guaranteed.

If owners insist on vaccinating pregnant cattle, inactivated or nonabortifacient vaccines should be used. Herds with purchased replacements usually have high BVD antibody prevalence, and some persistently infected carrier cattle.

Cow–Calf Operations

Vaccination programs can establish and maintain herd immunity in breeding animals by vaccination of heifers kept for breeding for IBR, BVD, and PI-3 after 6 months of age and again prior to breeding.

If market premiums can be arranged, a preconditioning program consisting of dehorning and castration several months before weaning and vaccination at least 3 weeks before weaning can be instituted (Cortese 1999). It should also include postweaning acclimation to dry feed before distribution to backgrounding operations or feedlots. The possible premium price for calves so treated must exceed the cost of vaccination.

Heifers to be kept as brood cows should be vaccinated prior to the first breeding and revaccinated periodically.

Veal Growers and Operations Assembling Neonatal Calves

Veal operations assemble 3- to 7-day-old calves. The lack of colostrum, the stress of assembly, and unnatural dietary and housing conditions combine with buildup of microbiologic flora to produce disastrous situations that are rarely amenable to control by vaccination.

In the first 14 weeks, assembled calves suffer considerable mortality from stress-induced syndromes associated with colibacillosis, salmonellosis, and pasteurellosis.

Any vaccination procedure must be carefully thought out, and under most circumstances, MLV vaccines are probably contraindicated.

Because they should be administered at birth, vaccines against rotavirus and coronavirus should not be expected to markedly alter mortality patterns in these operations.

A wide variety of bacterins and vaccines have been used in neonatal calf assembly operations with varied success.

Calves that survive until 6 months of age should then be vaccinated as described above, depending on their ultimate destination.

Feedlots

A substantial part of vaccination rationale involves preventing fetal wastage—not a consideration in feedlots, where respiratory infections are major concerns. If possible, IBR, BVD, BRSV, and PI-3 vaccination should be completed well prior to movement to assembly points, backgrounding areas, or feedlots. For economic reasons, this schedule is usually not followed, and cattle of unknown vaccination and exposure status arrive in feedlots.

Most operators initiate various vaccinations upon entry concomitant with the stress of movement, reassembly, and dietary adjustment. Data can be found to support almost any suggested program, but despite continued progress, a satisfactory solution to feedlot respiratory diseases has not evolved. Feedlot vaccination practices are often based on clinical impressions and are controversial. Administration of intranasal vaccine for IBR and PI-3 immediately upon arrival is sometimes recommended, and avoidance of BVD MLV vaccines in feedlot situations is a standard recommendation.

Until beef production becomes integrated, like the pork and poultry industries, and calves are controlled from birth to slaughter through suitable preconditioning regimes, respiratory and enteric disease will diminish efficiency and competitiveness of feedlot produced beef in global markets.

Exhibited Cattle

Cattle moving to shows and fairs must meet specific state and local health and vaccination requirements. Veterinarians must consider the health of the valuable purebred exhibited cattle, the health of other cattle at the show, and the hazard of herd exposure upon return. Owners showing cattle should consider giving combination IBR, PI-3, and BVD vaccine to nonpregnant show cattle at least 90 days prior to departure. Because of the legal implications, the difficulty in enforcement, and possible effects on subsequent value for export, particularly for bulls, vaccination for livestock shows should be a recommendation, not a requirement. Its feasibility should be examined on an individual basis.

Show-quality cattle are potential donors of semen and embryos and stand to suffer from vaccine-induced seropositivity. For this reason, owners should consider keeping them home from shows and isolating them from returning cattle.

Artificial Insemination Units

Vaccination programs for artificial insemination units present unique problems. The concern for the health of the bulls is important, but this consideration is sometimes overwhelmed by export requirements for seronegative semen donors.

Designing vaccination programs should involve antibody prevalence studies for IBR and BVD and careful evaluation of potential risks of attempting to maintain IBR- and BVD-free studs to preserve markets in countries that are attempting to eradicate these diseases.

Donor Cattle for Embryo Transfer

Donor cattle for embryo transfer should be treated like semen donors.

CONCLUSION

Carefully planned appropriate use of vaccines against endemic viral infections is a useful adjunct to bovine herd-health programs in a variety of production-management systems. Vaccination requires considerable attention to basic principles and concepts of vaccine usage and to manufacturers' instructions.

Healthy, well-nourished calves vaccinated prior to breeding for IBR, BVD, BRSV, and PI-3 will have reduced probability of aborting or suffering severe diseases from endemic viruses.

Vaccination in the presence of exposure and disease or during adjustment to changes in feed or environment is risky and should be approached conservatively.

REFERENCES

Cortese VS, 1999. Vaccination programs: Fundamentals. *Proc. Cornell Conf. Vet.* 91: 121–126.

Espeseth DA, Myers TJ, 1999. Authorities and procedures for licensing veterinary products in the United States. *Adv. in Vet. Med.* 41:585–593.

Office International Des Epizooties (OIE) 2000. Principles of vaccine production. In *Manual of Diagnostic Tests and Vaccines,* 6th ed., with annual updates Paris: OIE, pp. 489–492.

Pastoret PP, Blancou J, Vannier P, Verschueren C (eds.), 1999. *Veterinary Vaccinology.* Amsterdam: Elsevier Science Publishers. pp. 1–817.

Schultz RD, 1998. Effective immunization programs for cattle. *Proc. Am. Assoc. Bovine Practitioners* 31:110–112.

6

CLINICAL MANIFESTATIONS AND DIFFERENTIAL DIAGNOSIS

INTRODUCTION

In dealing with health problems, livestock owners see one or more animals with a principal complaint such as lameness or diarrhea. Veterinarians then formulate a list of diseases, the differential diagnosis, likely to cause that problem. Most differential diagnoses include viral infections that, along with other factors, can cause disease in fetuses, neonates, growing calves, and adult cattle.

Fetal infections are acquired from dams undergoing primary infections during pregnancy. These infections are manifested as abortion or congenital anomalies. In the neonate, viral infections are manifested principally as diarrhea or pneumonia.

In older cattle, primary infections are usually categorized by the anatomic system most obviously afflicted and are first recognized as respiratory disease, enteric disease, eye problems, neurologic disorders, lameness, skin lesions, or other principal complaints.

Several anatomic–pathologic disease groupings such as neonatal diarrhea, calf pneumonia, respiratory disease, mucosal diseases and vesicular diseases are entrenched in bovine diagnostic terminology. It is logical to preface disease-oriented chapters by discussing the differential diagnosis of these syndromes and the potential role of viruses in their etiology.

ABORTION

Diagnosing the cause of bovine abortions is complex and difficult. Aborted fetuses rarely have distinctive lesions to suggest a specific cause. The many non-viral abortifacient agents include brucella, salmonella and other bacteria, leptospira, protozoa, and fungi. These are more easily cultured from fetuses than are viruses, and a variety of bacteria may be present in fetal specimens as contaminants rather than etiologically significant organisms.

Abortions commonly occur as a result of foot-and-mouth disease (FMD), rinderpest, vesicular stomatitis (VS), infectious bovine rhinotracheitis (IBR), bovine viral diarrhea (BVD), bluetongue, and Akabane viruses. Most other bovine viruses have been isolated from fetuses and may cause abortion if primary infections occur during appropriate stages of pregnancy.

Isolation of viruses and identification of viral antigen or antibody in fetuses are diagnostic aids. These findings do not, however, always establish a cause-and-effect relationship between the virus and the abortion.

CONGENITAL ANOMALIES

Not only do BVD, bluetongue, Akabane, and probably other viruses cause abortion, they can also cause developmental anomalies in calves. Such conditions are hard to diagnose definitively and must be differentiated from hereditary defects and abnormalities caused by other agents.

NEONATAL DIARRHEA

Coronaviruses and rotaviruses are primary causes of neonatal diarrhea. Other viruses probably contribute to calf mortality by predisposing calves to infection with enteropathogenic bacteria. Management, nutrition, and colostrum deprivation are equally important factors to consider.

BVD virus, adenoviruses, rhinoviruses, and enteroviruses can be isolated from calves with diarrhea, but it is difficult to establish a clear-cut etiologic role for these viruses in specific outbreaks.

PNEUMOENTERITIS

In calves, diarrhea frequently occurs along with pneumonia or nasal catarrh. The term "pneumoenteritis" is used when calves with diarrhea also have respiratory signs such as excess nasal discharge or cough. The virologic literature abounds with reports of viruses of uncertain pathogenicity isolated from calves with pneumoenteritis. These include adenoviruses, enteroviruses, rhinoviruses, PI-3, BVD, bovine respiratory syncytial virus (BRSV), and IBR. The syndromes affecting calves yielding these isolates probably have multifactorial etiology, and the pathogenic significance of individual agents is hard to sort out.

CALF PNEUMONIA

Calf pneumonia has multifactorial etiology. Acute pneumonia has been associated with PI-3, adenoviruses, BRSV, IBR, respiratory coronaviruses, adenoviruses and others. Often, acute calf pneumonia progresses to a chronic debilitating condition usually referred to as enzootic calf pneumonia. This syndrome is characterized pathologically as a chronic bronchopneumonia and is usually most serious in the anteroventral portions of the lungs. The role of predisposing viral infections is varied but it is generally agreed that bacteria, principally *Pasteurella, Staphylococcus, Actinomyces,* and *Pseudomonas* species isolated from pneumonic lungs in fatal cases are secondary invaders opportunistically infecting tissues previously injured by viral infections, parasites, allergic reactions, or inhalation of foreign material.

Clinical diagnosis of calf pneumonia is easy, but specific etiologic diagnosis, particularly with respect to the role of viral infections, is difficult. Even if seroconversion or virus isolation is achieved, incrimination of specific viruses is difficult. The roles of management, diet, inhalation, and colostrally acquired antibody in calf pneumonia make the involvement of viruses even more difficult to evaluate.

BOVINE RESPIRATORY DISEASE (BRD)

Respiratory diseases are a significant cause of disease losses among cattle. In US feedlots, most respiratory disease fatalities result from terminal pulmonic pasteurellosis. Viruses contribute substantially to this syndrome. IBR, BRSV, parainfluenza-3 (PI-3), and BVD are common primary agents in clinical respiratory disease, but adenoviruses, enteroviruses, rhinoviruses, respiratory coronaviruses, and others may play an equal role.

Many diseases affecting bovine mucosa (DABM) are initially misdiagnosed as respiratory diseases if the oral mucosa is not examined carefully.

Distinctive lesions are rarely observed in bovine respiratory disease (BRD), and it is generally impossible to render an etiologic diagnosis solely on physical examination. Even when seroconversion is demonstrated or a virus is isolated from cattle with BRD, a simple causal relationship is frequently difficult to establish because of the complex nature of the syndrome and the high prevalence of inapparent viral infections.

The situation is further complicated by the ability of many viruses to establish persistent infections and the frequent use of live virus vaccines. The difficulty of experimentally producing disease, as is true of many viruses, is also a factor.

MUCOSAL DISEASES

Clinicians viewing cattle with ulcerations, erosions, or necrosis of the oral mucosa and muzzle frequently diagnose mucosal disease (MD), the chronic fatal syndrome appearing in young (and occasionally mature) cattle persistently infected with BVD virus. MD is characterized by unthriftiness, diarrhea, erosions in gastrointestinal mucosa, and death. When unspecified, the term MD suggests BVD virus is the etiologic agent, and it usually is in rinderpest-free areas.

The terminology becomes confused in some discussions, in which the plural terms "mucosal diseases" and the "mucosal disease complex" are used without specifying etiology to include malignant catarrhal fever (MCF), bluetongue, rinderpest, papular stomatitis, FMD, VS, and sometimes IBR.

To help clarify discussions of the differential diagnosis of the many so-called mucosal diseases, the ambiguous terms "mucosal diseases" and "bovine mucosal disease complex" will not be used in this book. Instead, the term "diseases affecting bovine mucosa" (DABM) will designate the collection of infections causing crusting of the muzzle and ulceration, erosion, vesiculation, necrosis, or hemorrhage in the bovine alimentary tract.

The viral-induced DABM must be differentiated from conditions such as mycotic stomatitis, photosensitization, contact allergies, ergot poisoning, and the ingestion of caustic or irritant substances that cause mucosal or skin sloughing. The differential diagnosis of DABM is discussed in Chapter 13.

VESICULAR DISEASES

Although vesicles may be a transient stage in development of lesions of other diseases, FMD and VS are the true vesicular diseases of cattle. The classic unruptured or recently broken vesicle (blister) or the adherent fragments of epithelium are easy to identify. They are not, however, always obvious and cattle are not always examined in the early stages of infection when these diseases are apparent.

In FMD and VS, vesicles occur in hairless areas (teats, mouth, and interdigital spaces) where contact pressure and sliding friction cause rapid rupture. The telltale fragments of epithelium slough promptly, leaving ulcers, which are difficult to distinguish from the lesions of other DABM, particularly when healing has started or secondary infections are present. Therefore the vesicular diseases must always be considered in the differential diagnosis of DABM and vice versa.

DIARRHEA IN ADULT CATTLE

After the neonatal period, cattle less frequently develop diarrhea. BVD and rinderpest are important viral causes of diarrhea in adult cattle, and cattle with MCF frequently have diarrhea.

In temperate climates, stabled cattle develop winter dysentery, which is usually self-limiting and not fatal and has been associated with several viruses, predominantly coronavirus.

Presence of blood in feces is common with winter dysentery, rinderpest, and arsenic toxicosis but uncommon with BVD and MCF.

Rinderpest and BVD may occur without perceptible diarrhea.

When point epidemics of gastroenteritis occur, food-borne or water-borne diseases such as salmonellosis must be considered. Also a possibility is that individuals may have ingested toxic substances such as organophosphate compounds or inorganic arsenicals.

Investigation of outbreaks of diarrhea in adult cattle should include thorough examination of the premises, careful examination of oral mucosa of affected and unaffected cattle for oral erosions, and fecal examination for coccidia and other intestinal parasites. Careful feeding history is needed to determine whether grain overload or sudden overeating of succulent materials like corn, legume hays, or fruit is involved.

The viral infections would be expected to produce a fever, but this symptom may be masked when diarrhea is present. Fever is not always apparent in the later stages of viral infections.

NEUROLOGIC DISEASE

Infections of the bovine brain and spinal cord received little attention prior to emergence of bovine spongiform encephalopathy (BSE). Now a significant problem in Europe, BSE (see Chapter 36) has caused a global revolution in the monitoring, surveillance, and reporting of bovine neurologic diseases that can result from several viral infections.

MCF is usually accompanied by fatal nonsuppurative encephalitis causing severe depression, head extension, and sometimes erratic and violent behavior.

Rarely, bovine herpesvirus-5, an IBR-like virus (see Chapter 18), localizes in the brain, causing opisthotonos, circling recumbency, and death.

Pseudorabies (Chapter 24), caused by porcine herpesvirus-1, occasionally results in fatal nonsuppurative encephalomyelitis in cattle that contact infected swine.

Bovine rabies (see Chapter 25) is usually acquired when cattle are bitten by wild animals. Skunks and foxes are the principal reservoirs in North America, while vampire bats are the principal source of bovine rabies in Central and South America.

As seen in North America, bovine rabies presents various signs from rumen atony, suggesting traumatic gastritis, or water deprivation to erratic, violent, aggressive behavior. Inconsistency of clinical signs is a hallmark of bovine rabies, but experienced diagnosticians become suspicious if pastured cattle in rabies-infected regions develop behavioral changes or vague signs of depression. The giveaway signs (a characteristic bellow, an alert "listening" ear position, and tenesmus) are regarded as almost pathognomonic, but few infected cattle manifest them.

Probably no two cases of bovine rabies present identical clinical signs. The encouragement to always examine oral mucosa for erosions must be prefaced by the warning that any unusual behavior of cattle in rabies-endemic areas signals extreme caution in examination of the mouth and mandatory use of gloves.

Any neurologic problem in cattle requires consideration of lead toxicosis, chlorinated hydrocarbon toxicosis, thromboembolic meningoencephalitis, and a variety of plant and chemical toxicoses, as well as viral diseases.

OCULAR DISEASE

When eye problems are the major clinical sign observed in cattle, the condition is usually infectious keratoconjunctivitis (pinkeye), caused by the bacterium *Moraxella bovis*. The conditions under which *M. bovis* is pathogenic vary, and isolation of IBR and other viruses from the eyes of affected cattle occasionally raises the possibility of a viral contribution to the condition. Best evidence, however, indicates that these are coincidental findings rather than etiologic agents. A similar situation exists for squamous cell carcinoma (cancer eye), a neoplasm common to white-faced cattle.

Conjunctivitis and Excessive Lacrimation

Pinkeye is a severe bacterial infection that spreads rapidly between cattle and causes lacrimation, reddened conjunctiva, photophobia manifested by squinting, and occasionally severe systemic manifestation. It sometimes progresses to blindness from orbital rupture or total opacity of the cornea of one or both eyes.

Conjunctivitis frequently accompanies respiratory infection with IBR virus. In the so-called conjunctival form of IBR, runny eyes are usually the principal complaint. Outbreaks of IBR conjunctivitis can be misdiagnosed as pinkeye, from which it can be distinguished if necrotic plaques are present on the conjunctivae.

Conjunctivitis sometimes accompanies adenoviral and BSRV infections. It is common with rinderpest, FMD, MCF, and BVD, all of which usually have other diagnostic signs and lesions occurring concurrently. The flow of lacrimal secretion anteroventrally over the face from the medial canthus is common in BVD infections but is not the sole criterion for diagnosis.

Corneal Opacity

Pinkeye is frequently accompanied by corneal opacities, which begin centrally. The peripheral opacity, rarely associated with IBR infections, originates at the corneoscleral junction and expands centrally.

Peripheral corneal opacity also occurs in MCF, where the opacity expands rapidly and the entire cornea usually becomes opaque. Severe panophthalmitis and systemic signs usually accompany MCF, so eye problems are usually not the principal complaint in MCF.

Peripheral corneal opacity, occasionally reported in association with BVD, may be an incidental finding. Most corneal opacities acquired postnatally in association with viral infections are peripheral, while pinkeye causes a central opacity.

Other Ocular Manifestations

Rabid cattle frequently have a strange, faraway staring look in their eyes. Cattle with lymphosarcoma frequently have exophthalmos due to postorbital tumors.

Congenital Ocular Disease

Calves are occasionally born with corneal opacities or cataracts resulting from numerous fetal conditions including BVD.

The bovine cornea becomes opaque as death approaches, particularly in neonates in freezing weather. Therefore, corneal opacities should not be designated congenital unless they were actually present at birth.

LAMENESS

The most common causes of bovine lameness are injuries; foot rot, a bacterial infection associated with *Fusobacterium necrophorum;* and papillomatous digital dermatitis, a lesion of questionable etiology involving spirochetes and possibly a virus. Lameness is a part of VS and FMD infection and is largely a result of secondary bacterial infection of ruptured vesicles or separation of the horny layers of the hooves from the sensitive underlying tissues. It also occurs in chronic BVD, acute bovine bluetongue, and occasionally MCF. Any cattle with mucosal or vesicular lesions should be examined for abnormalities of locomotion and lesions around the feet.

FMD must be considered when suspicious mouth lesions occur in lame cattle.

A characteristic transient lameness that is frequently one-legged occurs in ephemeral fever. Occasionally, individual cattle with lymphosarcoma are first observed as lame.

Rabid cattle may lift their feet unusually high and exhibit an unusual, exaggerated gait.

SKIN AND TEAT LESIONS

Skin lesions are most common on the teats where they result from bovine herpes mammillitis, FMD, VS, MCF, lumpy skin disease, papular stomatitis, cowpox, pseudocowpox (see Chapter 23), warts (see Chapter 16), and occasionally bluetongue and BVD.

When experimental infections are followed sequentially, each has unique characteristics. When viewed by clinicians, however, these infections are frequently similar, resembling scabs suggestive of healing injuries (FMD, VS, herpes mammillitis, and MCF) or pock-like lesions (cowpox, pseudocowpox, and papular stomatitis).

When they occur sporadically, virus-induced lesions of the teats are frequently passed off as injuries.

In lactating cows, teat lesions are frequently aggravated by milking, which causes bleeding. Likewise, they can be secondarily infected with bacteria and are frequently associated with mastitis, which is common in cattle with teat lesions.

Unless lameness is severe, lactating cattle with FMD or VS may be more seriously affected by secondary mastitis associated with teat lesions than with other signs of these diseases.

In addition to appearing on the teats, muzzle, and interdigital spaces, generalized nodular skin lesions occur in lumpy skin disease (Chapter 33), a poxvirus infection exotic to North America, and in a generalized form of bovine herpes mammillitis (Chapter 17) called pseudo lumpy skin disease. The skin form of lymphosarcoma is rare and resembles lumpy skin disease.

Occasionally cattle with bluetongue develop cracks in the skin (pityriasis), which can be confused with the dermal cracking and necrosis in nonpigmented areas caused by photosensitizing agents. Occasionally animals with MCF develop skin vesicles or papules that appear as tufting of hair and are hard to find or palpate. MD cases may present areas of hyperkeratosis, dandruff, and partial alopecia resembling that seen with chronic chlorinated hydrocarbon toxicosis.

CONCLUSIONS

The multiple clinical signs and lesions of bovine viral infections frequently overlap those of many common nonviral conditions. Experience, careful complete physical examination, and laboratory tests are essential to narrow the differential diagnosis and ultimately to determine true etiologies.

DISINFECTANTS AND DISINFECTION

INTRODUCTION

Disinfection is the process of eliminating infectious organisms by means of chemical or physical agents.

Disinfectants are relatively strong, usually toxic antimicrobial or biocidal chemicals applied to contaminated surfaces. Modern disinfectants are complex formulations of chemicals, soaps, detergents, and compounds that improve penetration of the active ingredients. They are sometimes used alternatively as sterilizing agents, sanitizers, or antiseptics on living tissues in more dilute, less irritating, and less toxic formulations.

Disinfectants are used in regulatory activities, research applications, and general disinfection of premises where cattle have been. Recommendations in this chapter address regulatory applications and exotic disease-eradication activities. These recommendations can be modified to apply to situations that call for routine general disinfection.

Effective disinfection requires thorough cleaning before application of chemicals. Prior cleaning is so important that cleaning and disinfection (C&D) are merged into one term with a singular meaning. Cleaning and disinfection (C&D) of surfaces of facilities and vehicles that have contacted cattle is crucial for controlling viral diseases on a local or national level and can be officially mandated in disease eradication efforts.

The thoroughness of predisinfection cleaning is the most important determinant of the effectiveness of disinfection processes.

Reviews of veterinary disinfection have been prepared by Linton et al. (1987), Quinn (1991), Kahrs (1995), and Blackwell (1998).

USE OF DISINFECTANTS IN CONTROLLING VIRAL DISEASES

People who use disinfectants must choose appropriate products, properly clean and prepare the site, and take precautions to ensure the safety of animals, other people, equipment, and the environment.

As applied in regulatory and on-the-farm animal disease control programs, disinfection is one way of limiting transmission of viral diseases. Disinfectants alone, however, will not eliminate infections if carrier animals are continually added to susceptible populations. Disinfection is most applicable as a control technique of diseases that are acquired by contact with bodily discharges or other materials found in yards, stalls, floors, and conveyances, or on equipment.

Viral diseases are controlled by limiting animal-to-animal contact or by vaccination. Disinfection, however, can play a major role in control of viral infections because most are inactivated by modern disinfectants. Surface disinfection is important in controlling viruses that survive in the environment after infected animals have been removed.

The development of new products and emergence of new infectious agents are continually changing disinfection science. Immunodeficiency viruses such as bovine lentivirus provide avenues for microorganisms that are normally considered saprophytic opportunists to become invasive. The prions identified with bovine spongiform encephalopathy are resistant to heat and disinfectants.

Advancing microbiologic and disinfection technology has combined with public interest in worker safety, food safety, and environmental preservation to produce major paradigm shifts in disinfection procedures. It becomes increasingly essential to train disinfection workers in safe application and storage procedures.

PLANS OF ACTION FOR DISINFECTION

Successful disinfection procedures, guidelines, or regulations require a clear, succinct plan of action for each disinfectant application. The plan should describe the objectives of the application, specific microorganisms to be eliminated, the predisinfection cleaning process, safety measures, and dilution and application instructions. It should also include the postdisinfection procedures by which the process will be measured and the documentation required to provide regulatory certification.

A checklist of factors for consideration in planning, implementing, and evaluating disinfection procedures should contain

- area, premises, and facility data
- legal considerations
- environmental factors
- objectives of disinfection
- predisinfection cleaning
- safety data for personnel and environmental protection

- disinfectant product data
- disinfectant application data
- postdisinfection data

Use of such a list will increase effectiveness and ensure compliance with health, safety, and environmental regulations and with current public concerns.

ANIMAL HEALTH APPLICATIONS OF DISINFECTANTS

Targeted disinfectant measures that permit selection of a disinfectant with a narrow but specific spectrum of activity against specific organisms are instituted at research facilities or during post-depopulation disinfection.

Routine disinfection, sometimes called general disinfection, requires a broad spectrum of antimicrobial activity to combat a wide array of unknown organisms. General disinfection is carried out on vehicles and equipment and at farms, sales barns, stockyards, exhibition grounds, quarantine stations, zoological parks, abattoirs, and processing plants.

The selection of disinfection strategies can be based on the disease-control scenario, the suspected microorganisms, or combinations thereof.

VIRAL SURVIVAL ON SURFACES

The potential for virus survival on contaminated surfaces depends on levels of contamination and their resistance to inactivating environmental conditions. While viruses replicate only in living cells, some are resistant to normal environmental conditions and can survive on inanimate objects. The virus of foot-and-mouth disease (FMD) survives for months under proper conditions, and poxviruses can survive for years if encased within desquamated scabs.

THE EFFICACY OF DISINFECTANTS

The effectiveness of disinfectants depends on the target viruses and their resistance to environmental conditions and chemicals. Usually enveloped viruses are more readily inactivated by disinfectants than are nonenveloped viruses. The concentration of the disinfectant and its time of contact with surfaces, the ambient temperature, and other factors are also involved (Kastenhuber 1991).

The amount of extraneous organic material is the paramount factor in the outcome of any disinfection operation because it dilutes and rapidly neutralizes biocidal chemicals. Therefore, vigorous scrubbing and voluminous water flushing must precede application of disinfectants. Neither large quantities of disinfectants nor high-pressure application can replace thorough predisinfection cleaning. Thus, preapplication cleaning is the most important part of C&D.

Testing disinfectants for virucidal properties is challenging because most disinfectants destroy reagents used in viral assays. Thus, few mutually acceptable methodologies have emerged (Cremieus and Fleurette 1991). Disinfectant efficacy determinations are made by postdisinfection virus-isolation procedures or observation of susceptible sentinel animals.

DISINFECTANTS USED IN ANIMAL DISEASE CONTROL PROGRAMS

The numbers of naturally occurring or synthetic disinfectant compounds, mixtures, and products are overwhelming. Approved disinfectant lists become obsolete as new products appear. Common disinfectants used in bovine health applications include hot water, bromides, chlorides, chlorhexidine, iodides, phenolic compounds, and quaternary ammonium compounds.

Water

While actually a cleaner rather than a disinfectant, water is the most important element in the C&D process. Hot water has major disinfecting applications and may be the main component of C&D where chemical residues must be avoided. Hot water under pressure cleans by flushing, scrubbing, and hydraulic impact. It dissolves inorganic salts, emulsifies fats, and washes away organic debris. When used for cleaning, sanitizing or disinfection, water must be of microbiologically acceptable quality, maintained at desirable temperatures, and applied in abundant quantities. Hot water must be used with caution to avoid scalding workers or bystanders. Under excessive pressure, water produces pockmarks in concrete and fractures mortar, tiles, and masonry grouting, permitting accumulation of organic material.

Calcium Oxide

Calcium oxide (quicklime) when mixed with water becomes lime wash, which has biocidal effects on some viruses but is not highly effective against FMD virus. Sometimes it is spread on the ground after depopulation of infected premises, but its value under these conditions has been questioned. Quicklime has also been used to retard putrefaction of buried carcasses after depopulation.

Chlorine Disinfectants

Chlorine has bleaching and germicidal properties and is commonly used in disinfection, sanitizing, and water purification. Chlorine disinfectants and sanitizers are readily available, inexpensive, have a broad antimicrobial spectrum, and present minimal environmental hazards. Aqueous chlorine solutions exert virucidal effects by mechanisms that are probably related to destruction of essential enzyme systems. Aqueous chlorine disinfectants have been replaced largely by organic chlorine compounds.

Viruses vary in their sensitivity to chlorine disinfectants (Chopra 1987). Chlorine disinfectants are effective in the absence of organic material. Other factors affecting the efficacy of chlorine-based disinfectants are the concentration, the pH, and the presence of natural proteins or ammonia, a major component of animal urine.

The hypochlorites, including sodium hypochlorite (chlorinated lime, bleaching powder, chloride of lime, or household bleach), are still commonly used in animal health programs (Blackwell 1998). They have broad antiviral spectrums of effectiveness, and are compatible with most detergents but are corrosive, easily neutralized by organic material, and decompose readily.

Chlorinated lime, a hygroscopic white powder containing a variety of calcium and chlorine compounds, is frequently sprinkled in barnyards and on manure piles, where the released chlorine serves as a general disinfectant.

Chlorhexidine

Chlorhexidine and its analogs are commonly used as skin cleaners, teat dips, and antiseptics. They are also used for cold sterilization of surgical instruments and for disinfecting milking equipment, barns, and buildings. Chlorhexidine is useful against fungi, gram-positive bacteria, and to an extent, against viruses. It retains some effectiveness in the presence of small amounts of clean organic material such as milk or serum but is ineffective when gross contamination is present. Its low toxicity makes it useful in combination with other disinfectants.

Iodine and Iodine-based Disinfectants

Many forms of iodine are used in animal health disinfection. Aqueous iodine (Lugol's solution) or alcoholic iodine (tinctures of iodine) are commonly used as antiseptics.

Iodophors are disinfectants formed by combination of iodine with various carrier compounds. These release iodine in an acid medium and have disinfectant properties that affect some viruses. Iodophors are used for general disinfection and cleaning, as bovine teat dips, and for surgical scrubs. Hard water and presence of large amounts of organic material reduce their effectiveness, but they can function effectively in the presence of traces of organic material.

Quaternary Ammonium Compounds

Quaternary ammonium compounds (QAC), also called quads, are natural biochemicals involved in transmission of neuromuscular impulses in mammals. Synthesized QAC act as one-step cleaner–sanitizers in aqueous solution or when combined with detergents. They are widely used in medical facilities and in food-processing establishments. While the QAC exert antiviral activity, their spectrum of effectiveness in agricultural settings is limited.

Sodium Hydroxide

In the 1930s, sodium hydroxide (lye, caustic soda, or soda ash) in a 2% solution was used to disinfect equipment, animal conveyances, surfaces, and water-resistant clothing when FMD was diagnosed. While also effective against other viruses, it has been largely replaced with less corrosive and less irritating modern disinfectants. In emergencies, however, it can still be an option because it is extremely effective and readily available because it is commonly used in the chemical and paper industries and as a septic line cleaner.

It should be used with extreme caution and under well-controlled conditions because of its corrosive and irritating properties and its potential dangers to the environment and workers. When applying lye, workers should wear raincoats, waterproof hats, boots, and goggles; they should avoid aluminum and be aware that lye will remove paint.

Phenolic Compounds

Although pure phenol (carbolic acid) is rarely used, related compounds are common components of general disinfectants. Some synthesized phenol compounds are odorless, but many have the characteristic odor traditionally associated with disinfectants. In some situations, such as in foot baths at the doorways of animal facilities heavily contaminated with manure in which bedding is not replenished regularly, they may be more effective as olfactory reminders that biosecurity is essential than as actual disinfectants. Most phenolic compounds in use today are synthesized and are purer and less pungent than earlier coal-tar distillates. They are effective against some viruses, but antiviral activity of the phenols varies among compounds. In general, enveloped and naked lipophilic viruses are more susceptible to the phenols.

Although their strong odor serves as warning of their deteriorating effects on plastics and rubber, and their irritating qualities and toxicity, it must be emphasized that they can be fatal if swallowed and that toxic doses can be absorbed through the skin. Swine and cats are particularly sensitive to phenols, and small doses can be fatal. Nonetheless, phenols are commonly used and highly effective general disinfectants.

Pine Oil

Pine oil, historically obtained by distillation of pitch-filled pinewood, cones, or needles is now prepared synthetically. Pine oil is a clear, colorless or amber-colored liquid with a characteristic odor that is more pleasant than that of coal tar–derived creosotes. If used alone, it is insoluble in water so it is usually emulsified with soaps, detergents, or other compounds. It is more effective as a general disinfectant when applied hot.

Today, wood-origin pine oils have largely been replaced by mixtures in which commercially synthesized chlorinated phenols provide the primary disinfectant activity, and pine oil is a relatively inactive ingredient contributing the disinfectant odor. There is a long-standing uncertainty over the antimicrobial efficacy of pure pine oil. In mixtures it may be of value if only for the warning created by its characteristic smell.

Inorganic Acids

Inorganic acids such as sulfuric acid and hydrochloric acid are used in very limited situations. Both are effective against FMD virus but are toxic if swallowed, highly irritating to the skin and eyes, and very corrosive to metals.

Organic Acids

Because they are less toxic and less corrosive than the inorganic (metallic) acids, a number of organic acids with mild viricidal properties are used in animal health and food processing. Acetic acid is readily available because it is present at a 4% level in vinegar. At 2% levels, acetic acid can significantly reduce levels of FMD virus on contaminated surfaces and is used to reduce bacterial levels in meat packing plants. Acetic, citric, lactic, formic, and propionic acids are sometimes used in meat and poultry packing plants and in calf barns.

Formaldehyde

Formaldehyde is a gas in its natural form but is more readily available as a 40% aqueous solution called formalin. Gaseous formaldehyde is used for fumigation when buildings, rooms, or conveyances can be sealed, and is effective against most viruses. Formaldehyde gas is relatively unstable and sometimes explodes.

It is difficult to get even distribution of the gas through buildings, and its effect is sometimes incomplete. For formaldehyde fumigation to be complete, the temperature must be above 55° F and the relative humidity above 70%. Spraying with hot water is sometimes necessary to achieve this goal. For fumigation purposes, formaldehyde gas can be produced by oxidizing formalin with potassium permanganate, by heating paraformaldehyde, by generating a mist of formalin mechanically, or by applying complex mixtures from which formaldehyde is slowly released after application. Formaldehyde fumigation is hazardous, and must be carefully supervised, but in some countries it is still used in disinfection of aircraft, ships, and livestock production facilities.

A 1% to 5% formalin solution is sometimes used to disinfect buildings or as a prophylactic and therapeutic footbath for foot rot of sheep and cattle. The use of formaldehyde in disinfectant situations is declining because of its strong irritating odor, its corrosiveness and fibrolytic properties, and its toxicity. The use of formaldehyde may be outlawed in some countries due to environmental concerns.

Sodium Carbonate

Sodium carbonate, also known as washing soda, has been used in a hot solution (180° F) for disinfection of buildings in which animals with FMD had been housed. It lacks effectiveness against some bacteria and most viruses and is more effective as a cleanser than as a disinfectant.

APPLICATION OF DISINFECTANTS

Appropriate disinfection procedures will vary in individual situations. Disinfection of animal quarters usually involves removing all animals, utensils and equipment, then scrubbing, scraping and flushing away all gross organic material with a cleaner–sanitizer or detergent compound, and rinsing thoroughly.

The chosen disinfectant is then applied and left in contact with the surface for as long as possible before rinsing thoroughly and leaving the facility free of animals for an effective interval.

Disinfectant Footbaths and Wheel Baths

Disinfectant footbaths are commonly placed at doorways of animal quarters, sale barns, quarantine stations, and research facilities to help exclude infectious agents and prevent exit of microorganisms. Footbaths are most effective when properly charged, when frequently replenished with appropriate products, and when users wear rubber footwear that can be soaked for several minutes. Otherwise, they probably serve more as biosecurity reminders than as effective disease-control mechanisms (Quinn 1991).

Disinfectant foot baths can be effective if refilled every two to three days, appropriately situated where rain or snow dilution cannot occur, and protected from freezing. In locations where footbaths freeze, they should be heated. Addition of antifreeze or salt may inactivate the disinfectant. If there is manure, bedding, mud or other debris on the feet of users, there should be a footbath for washing boots before soaking them in the disinfectant. These same guidelines apply to wheel baths that trucks are driven through when entering and leaving premises.

PREDISINFECTION CONSIDERATIONS

Before predisinfection cleaning is begun, the premises and its ownership should be identified. The goals of the operation and the plan of action must be written out. Then, based on the goals and consideration of the type of material being disinfected and the suspected organisms, a disinfectant can be chosen that best suits the situation while providing for optimum safety of animals, people, equipment, and the environment. The product chosen must be effective against the organism in question and approved for use by officials of the country.

In addition to choosing a disinfectant with an appropriate antimicrobial spectrum, the zoonotic potential of suspected organisms should be evaluated with respect to possible hazards to the disinfecting crew and other workers. Preplanning should also consider the toxic potential of the disinfectant and its irritating properties for skin and eyes, its corrosiveness and paint-removing capabilities, and what damaging effects it may have on wood, metal, fibers, concrete, rubber, or electrical outlets. If the organism is exotic, or has zoonotic potential, or if the disinfectant is toxic or irritating, corrosive protective clothing, masks, and rubber footwear must be worn.

The site drainage and disinfectant runoff must be considered with respect to the proximity to waterways and wells and possible contact with people, wildlife, livestock, or poultry. The local wildlife, bird, and rodent populations must be surveyed to determine if infection exists among susceptible species or if they can serve as mechanical or biological vectors of relevant pathogens. The disinfected area must be sealed to prevent wild creatures from entering. It must be determined if local ecosystems are amenable to carcass disposal by burning, burial, or composting.

DISINFECTION WHILE ANIMALS ARE PRESENT

If for some reason, animals must remain in the area to be disinfected, their presence will affect the predisinfection process, the product chosen, and the method of application. The presence of animals will cause loss of ability to completely clean prior to disinfection and will require use of a product that is nontoxic and has biocidal effects when applied as a mist or aerosol. Some chemicals that function well in this mode are the orthophenylphenols, hexylresorcinol, resorcinol, chloroxyphenol, propylene glycol, and trimethylene glycol. If at all possible, such applications should be avoided in favor of all-in-all-out practices with disinfection conducted when buildings are empty.

PREDISINFECTION CLEANING

Predisinfection cleaning is the most crucial part of the disinfection process. If well done, it will probably eliminate the majority of microorganisms. Predisinfection cleaning requires removal of all animals. Manure, litter, and bedding must be removed and buried, burned, or composted depending on the situation. Any movable equipment and utensils must be removed and individually cleaned, scrubbed, and rinsed.

The facility should be wet down to prevent excess dust from arising during the vigorous cleaning process. If zoonotic diseases are suspected, an appropriate disinfectant should be used for the predisinfection wetdown, and workers should be required to wear masks and protective clothing. All feces, dirt, dust, mud, or other material is removed by scraping, sweeping, scrubbing or power flushing. The facility is then hosed down with a detergent soap or sanitizer or a classic disinfectant–cleaner such as a 2% to 4% sodium carbonate solution, which must be completely flushed away so it cannot reduce the effectiveness of the disinfectants subsequently applied.

THE DISINFECTION PROCESS

Prior to application of the product, all traces of the material used in the predisinfection process must be flushed away with water to avoid diluting, neutralizing, or inactivating the chosen disinfectant. The applicators must read the entire product label and follow the dilution instructions explicitly to be sure the safest, most effective concentration is achieved. The disinfectant is then applied to every surface, nook, and cranny starting at the highest point and working downward.

While the disinfectant is being applied, there must be constant observation of the health status of the applicators and bystanders and there must be continual alertness for runoff heading in unexpected directions. The disinfectant must be left on surfaces as long as possible and at least as long as indicated in the instructions. It must then be thoroughly rinsed and the area left vacant as long as possible before postdisinfection samples are collected or sentinel animals are placed. Restocking with healthy uninfected animals occurs only when postdisinfection tests or sentinel-animal evaluations reveal that the premises have a low probability of harboring residual pathogens.

CAUSES OF DISINFECTION FAILURE

Some causes of disinfection failure are overdilution of disinfectant during premixing or application, incomplete or inadequate cleaning, poor disinfectant penetration or coverage, insufficient contact time on the surfaces, and inadequate temperature and humidity while the material is being applied. In addition, failure can result from inactivation or neutralization of disinfectant by residual cleaning liquids that have been inadequately removed before disinfectant application. A common mistake is selection of a product that is not effective against the organisms of concern.

The entire process must be repeated if examination of sentinel animals or laboratory tests on environmental samples indicate that pathogens have survived the procedure. A final frustrating cause of apparent disinfection failure is invalidation of the entire process by reintroduction of disease by restocking with infected animals.

DISINFECTANT STANDARDS, REQUIREMENTS, AND REGULATIONS

Regulations, requirements, and protocols for disinfection should be consistent with laws of promulgating nations. They require a sound technical basis and must be transparent and easily explained. They must be more than bureaucratic requirements put forward to demonstrate power or keep people busy. Under international trade agreements, sanitary requirements must have a true health basis and not serve as non-tariff trade barriers.

DISINFECTION CERTIFICATION

Certificates of disinfection required by regulatory agencies can take a variety of formats. The minimum required information includes

- identification of the location and ownership of the facility disinfected
- the date, the nature and extent of predisinfection cleaning
- the target microorganisms
- the name, active ingredients, and concentration (dilution) of the chemical used
- the ambient or surface temperature during application
- the length of time the product was in contact with treated surfaces
- the names of the applicators and inspectors.

REFERENCES

Blackwell JD, 1998. Cleaning and disinfection. In *Foreign Animal Diseases,* edited by WW Buisch, JL Hyde, CL Mebus. Richmond: U.S. Animal Health Assoc., pp. 445–448.

Chopra I, 1987. Microbial resistance to veterinary disinfectants and antiseptics. In *Disinfection in Veterinary and Farm Animal Practice,* edited by A Linton, W Hugo, A Russell. London: Blackwell, pp. 43-65

Cremieus A, Fleurette J, 1991. Methods of testing disinfectants. In *Disinfection, Sterilization, and Preservation,* 4th ed., edited by S Block. Philadelphia: Lea and Febiger, pp. 1009–1021.

Kahrs RF, 1995. General disinfection guidelines. *Rev. Sci. Tech. Off. Int. Epiz* 14(1):105–143.

Kastenhuber H, 1991. Physical factors influencing the activity of antimicrobial agents. In *Disinfection, Sterilization, and Preservation,* 4th ed., edited by S Block. Philadelphia: Lea and Febiger, pp. 59–72.

Linton A, Hugo W, Russell A, 1987. *Disinfection in Veterinary and Farm Animal Practice.* London: Blackwell, pp. 1–335.

Quinn P, 1991. Disinfection and disease prevention in veterinary medicine. In *Disinfection, Sterilization, and Preservation,* 4th ed., edited by S Block. Philadelphia: Lea and Febiger, pp. 846–870.

8

THE IMPACT OF BOVINE VIRAL DISEASES ON INTERNATIONAL TRADE

INTRODUCTION

If a nation's dairy and beef industries are to prosper they must be globally competitive and have sustained export markets for their products. Most countries impose sanitary (health) measures to prevent introduction of transmissible diseases through importation of live animals, animal products, or germ plasm. Animal health and food safety concerns of importing countries are based on scientific, economic, political, legal, and cultural considerations.

If a country's cattle industries are to be globally competitive, they must fulfill commitments to international trade agreements, conform to international standards, and meet legitimate requirements of trading partners.

The future portends exclusions of North American cattle, germ plasm, beef, and milk products due to lack of nationally endorsed monitoring, surveillance, and reporting (MS&R) systems, animal identification programs, and trace-back capacities.

Import requirements on North American live cattle and germ plasm are commonly imposed based on vesicular stomatitis and bluetongue (Kahrs 1998a). Bovine spongiform encephalopathy (BSE) requirements also include beef and beef byproducts. Less common but increasing requirements are being imposed for the control of bovine viral diarrhea (BVD), infectious bovine rhinotracheitis (IBR), and enzootic bovine leukemia (EBL) for which some nations are developing eradication programs (Kahrs and Morgan 1996). Thought must also be given to bovine lentivirus (see Chapter 11).

Meeting these ever-expanding requirements requires compliance with provisions of the World Trade Organization (WTO) Sanitary and Phytosanitary (SPS) agreement and conformity with disease reporting, testing, and trade standards of the Office International Des Epizooties (OIE). It also requires meeting animal disease MS&R, health certification requirements, and other expectations of trading partners.

Fulfillment of these expectations is essential for survival of national dairy and beef industries and will require new thought modes and concerted efforts on the part of veterinarians, farmers, and ranchers. It will also require enlightened cooperation between national animal health agencies and domestic beef and dairy industries so export certifications accurately reflect the animal disease situations and animal health infrastructures of countries or regions.

Appreciation of the impact of the global economy on domestic dairy and beef health systems impacts on how veterinarians, dairy farmers, and beef breeders address viral diseases in upcoming decades. Balanced perception of this impact requires understanding changes in international markets and global trade policies to which most countries are committed.

WTO EXPECTATIONS AND NATIONAL COMMITMENTS

Contemporary international trade expectations are outlined in the WTO SPS agreement that covers both animal health (sanitary) measures and plant health (phytosanitary) issues.

The principles of the WTO SPS agreement give countries the sovereign right to establish sanitary measures if they are scientifically sound, transparent, nondiscriminatory, equitably applied, in harmony with international standards, risk assessment based, and applicable on a regional basis. If those principles are fulfilled without discrimination or arbitrary and unjustified differences, nations may impose whatever sanitary requirements they deem necessary to protect their animal and human populations from disease. All WTO and OIE member countries are committed to those principles.

The WTO has a dispute resolution process but disagreements over sanitary measures are best resolved by amiable discussions among veterinary officials of involved countries.

PRINCIPLES OF THE WTO SPS AGREEMENT

International expectations are outlined in the WTO SPS agreement that was ratified by member countries and carries the force of international law.

The codified principles of this agreement reflect directions in which many countries have been moving independently for years as they have adapted to advancing animal health technology. Other areas of change are in the eradication and control of animal plagues, worldwide privatization of regulatory responsibilities, changing national boundaries, formation of trading blocs, and movement toward more open governments.

The principles of the WTO SPS agreement detailed below challenge governments and livestock interests to reevaluate the scientific, technical, and ethical basis of their sanitary policies from the perspective of both imports and exports.

Harmonization with International Standards

Under the WTO SPS agreement, nations are asked to strive cooperatively for international standardization of diagnostic tests, surveillance and reporting systems, import requirements, quarantine procedures, animal identification policies, vaccine standards, and risk-analysis systems.

The OIE, the WTO-designated international standards-setting organization for animal health, has over 150 member countries. It maintains a worldwide animal disease reporting system and recommends sanitary regulations, testing, quarantine, and health certification procedures to encourage world trade while minimizing the spread of animal diseases.

The OIE publishes the International Animal Health Code (the Code) that contains disease-by-disease and commodity-by-commodity guidelines for trade in animal products originating in infected or free countries. The OIE also publishes *Manual of Standards for Diagnostic Tests and Vaccines* (the Manual). These publications are updated regularly and provide standards that will usually go unchallenged if applied as import requirements.

Scientific Risk Assessments Using Regional Approaches

The requirement that sanitary measures more stringent than OIE standards be based upon scientific risk assessments using regional approaches caused many countries to change their import regulations. Because zero risk is unattainable, past strategies of attempting to eliminate all risk are being replaced by determinations of "acceptable levels" of disease-specific risks.

Risk assessment involves documentation that identifies diseases that could be introduced by a given commodity and estimates the probability of their entry and establishment in recipient countries under various risk management procedures such as processing, testing, or quarantine (see Chapter 3).

Country-by-country import requirements have been supplemented by regional approaches so that importation can be considered from parts of one or more countries, or groups of countries as long as there is an effective, responsible governmental infrastructure (Kahrs 1996).

Transparency

Transparency implies that importing countries clearly articulate the scientific basis of sanitary measures imposed upon animals or animal products entering their territory. It is accomplished by openly discussing the basis of import requirements; informing affected trading partners of new rules at least 60 days before enactment; promptly publishing regulatory changes; providing information, inspection privileges, and clear explanations of import requirements; and upon request, documenting that sanitary measures provide equal treatment to the exports of countries or regions with comparable animal health status.

National Treatment

The concept of national treatment requires that importing countries apply equal sanitary measures to exporting nations where similar conditions prevail and apply import requirements that are "no less favorable" than those applied to domestic movements, provided that equal conditions prevail.

Equivalency

Signatory countries must recognize similarities in animal health status and risks associated with specific diseases or commodities even if different methods are used to accomplish them.

Timetable for Universal Adoption of WTO SPS Principles

It will take decades before the international community unanimously understands and implements WTO SPS principles. During these years, national governments and domestic producers must face the reality that all nations may not be transparent and fair. Also, during this period, countries will be modifying their regulations to exclude diseases they consider threats to the health of their livestock.

OIE EXPECTATIONS

The OIE, the Global Organization for Animal Health, has about 150 member countries, each with one delegate and one vote. The OIE tries to collect and disseminate information about the global distribution of animal diseases and prevent spread of contagious animal diseases. It also seeks to improve animal production through animal health standards; encourage international cooperation among public and private veterinary authorities; and ensure that scientific measures govern international trade in animals and animal products by recognizing the disease-free status of countries. It categorizes diseases into List A, List B, and List C and sets standards for safe international movement of livestock and related products.

Member countries support OIE activities through financial contributions; attendance; active participation in policy discussions; offering technical assistance to developing nations; providing scientific input into proposed standards; and encouraging OIE efforts to report the global animal disease situation, establish standards for diagnostic tests, vaccines, and international trade, and offer member countries opportunity for declaration of disease-free status.

The OIE disease-reporting function requires the delegate of each member country to submit immediate reports of "significant epidemiological events," abbreviated monthly reports of national disease activity, and a detailed annual animal disease report. These are distributed worldwide in biweekly OIE Animal Disease Reports, Bimonthly OIE Bulletins, and in an annual review of the animal health situation worldwide prepared jointly by the Food and Agriculture Organization of the United Nations, the OIE, and the World Health Organization. These documents are distributed globally and used to develop protective import measures.

As the WTO-designated standards setting organization, the OIE develops, by consensus, disease-by-disease standards (guidelines) for safe international movement of animals, animal products, and germ plasm from disease-free and disease-affected countries or regions. These standards are detailed in the Code and the Manual.

OIE standards offer guidelines for importation from disease-free or disease-affected countries or regions. However, except for foot-and-mouth disease, for which OIE requires annual documentation supporting freedom, these self-proclaimed disease-free statuses of countries are unverified and not guaranteed. Thus, nations sometimes individually assess the animal health status of exporting countries using site visits to evaluate MS&R systems, diagnostic capacity, border security, and animal health infrastructure.

Despite occasional efforts to politicize them, OIE standards are usually based on sound science. The OIE uses regionally balanced expert working groups to develop draft standards, which are circulated to member countries for comment prior to adoption at annual general sessions. Comments are accepted only from delegates. Delegates best represent their countries if they involve the scientific, regulatory, practice, and agricultural communities in developing their comments.

Countries may apply import measures more stringent than OIE standards if they are transparent, science-based, nondiscriminatory, and founded on scientific risk analyses applied on a regional basis.

Import requirements based on OIE standards are exempt from requirements to conduct detailed risk assessments and to notify the WTO of regulation changes and cannot be challenged beyond consultation (a preliminary stage in the WTO dispute resolution process). These exemptions make OIE standards attractive and subject to abuse. Nations may review risk assessments, verify "disease-free" statuses and examine surveillance data, diagnostic facilities, and animal health infrastructures of other countries.

Most member countries support OIE initiatives and try to conform to its reporting requirements and international standards.

INTERNATIONAL DISEASE CATEGORIZATION AND CLASSIFICATION

Veterinarians and animal health officials need familiarity with the international classification of diseases to be aware of the relative urgency for diagnosis and reporting.

The OIE classifies and categorizes animal diseases with respect to international risk. This classification provides a basis for reporting country-by-country and region-by-region distribution of important animal diseases and for prioritizing control programs and sanitary measures imposed on importation of animals and animal products.

Current OIE categorizations place diseases in Lists A, B, or C based on epidemiologic factors, economic potential, public health importance, and urgency of reporting.

OIE List A Transmissible Diseases or Agents

List A diseases have the greatest potential for global spread, production losses, or public health impact. List A diseases require urgent extensive reporting, including monthly reports of their presence or absence and weekly status reports during new introductions or recurrences in regions considered free.

The OIE List A diseases of cattle are foot-and-mouth disease, vesicular stomatitis, rinderpest, contagious bovine pleuropneumonia, lumpy skin disease, Rift Valley fever, and bluetongue. Except for contagious bovine pleuropneumonia, they are all viral diseases addressed in separate chapters in this book.

Countries free of List A diseases take all possible precautions to exclude them and affected countries desiring competitive markets strive to eradicate them or confine them to certain areas, a process called regionalization.

OIE List B Transmissible Diseases or Agents

List B diseases have less serious potential for production losses and public health impact and are less urgently and extensively reported. Reporting of List B diseases is necessary when new epidemiologic findings are revealed or upon incursions into countries, regions, or zones previously considered free. National control measures for List B diseases usually command lower priority than for List A diseases.

Of 67 List B diseases, only IBR, EBL, and BSE are caused by viruses. Each of these is the object of eradication programs in some European nations that can legitimately impose import measures excluding bovine products from affected countries using requirements like those applied to exotic List B diseases by North American countries.

OIE List C Transmissible Diseases or Agents

List C diseases have the least serious potential for production losses and public health impact. They are not addressed in the code but appear on reporting forms sent by OIE to member countries. Reporting of List C diseases is optional and usually occurs when marked changes in geographic distribution, pathogenesis or epidemiologic characteristics are revealed or upon incursions into areas previously considered free.

List C diseases usually command lowest priority for national disease control programs. Except for countries with isolated ecosystems and extremely strong animal health infrastructures, national control measures for List C diseases are not generally instituted. BVD is a List C disease that some countries are attempting to eradicate (Kahrs and Morgan 1996).

EXPECTATIONS OF TRADING PARTNERS ARE BASED ON SCIENCE, POLITICS, AND CULTURE

Trading partners expect countries to comply with WTO/OIE policies, provide credible disease MS&R, and offer "equal national treatment" that ensures that import measures are nondiscriminatory, and (where comparable conditions prevail) "no less favorable" than domestic requirements.

It is the right of countries to establish their own import measures and appropriate levels of protection. Science, politics, and culture all contribute to import requirements and must be considered when dealing with trading partners.

The WTO SPS agreement indicates that import measures must be based on sound science. Science, however, is rapidly changing and is subject to variable interpretation. Data and publications can be distorted by economic objectives, political expediencies, and cultural influences. The dynamics of sound science are based on advancing diagnostic technology; advancing surveillance and investigative techniques; emergence of the science of risk analysis; emergence of the transmissible spongiform encephalopathies; emphasis on molecular biology; the global movement toward integrated production-management systems; and advancing marketing and transportation technologies.

While science is changing, the delicate interaction of science and politics is tilted toward protectionism and partnering with industry, a situation that can bias interpretations of scientific inquiries and risk analyses.

With respect to politics, animal health authorities and other officials with decision-making authority in trading countries must operate in a realistic domain that recognizes commitments to international trade agreements; the influence of multinational trading blocs; the limitations on preemptive regulatory authority of national governments over subnational units; and the global movement toward privatization of regulatory functions.

The worldwide emergence of politically influential activist groups has forced animal health regulators and politicians to think beyond the interests of traditional stakeholders (livestock producers and processors) and consider thoughtful input and public concerns raised by environmentalists; animal welfare groups; human rights groups; consumer interests; labor groups; traditional agricultural interests; national animal health groups; and the insistence by WTO, OIE, and most countries that sanitary issues be addressed on a government-to-government basis.

Unlike science, which is rapidly advancing, and political convictions, which can be ephemeral, values, ideals, attitudes, beliefs, and behavioral patterns (cultural traits) are a product of environments in which people grow up, are educated, and work. They are slow to change.

As regards international movement of animals and animal products, ethnic and religious traditions contribute to national animal health cultures that have a profound impact on import policies and requirements. Animal health cultures are easily institutionalized within regulatory agencies and adapt slowly to scientific advances and political or social pressures.

CREDIBLE ANIMAL HEALTH REPORTING

Accurate MS&R is the foundation of successful domestic animal health programs and the key to credibility in the international marketplace (Kahrs 1999). MS&R programs can exert both positive and negative effects on foreign markets.

Candid reporting of diseases raises questions of interpretation, proprietary confidentiality, potential use (or misuse) of information, and whether all countries openly report.

Countries asking trading partners to be transparent about their animal health status are obligated to reciprocate and willingly certify that their exports meet the standards imposed on their imports.

Developments in international law and information technology force national governments to upgrade their MS&R activities to preserve the competitiveness of their animal agriculture.

Under international law ratified by WTO member nations, importing countries can legally exclude exports from regions where the national veterinary service cannot provide credible certifications of its animal health status.

Unlike previous decades when animal health officials were bogged down by the logistics of animal disease reporting, electronic data gathering, analysis, and transmission now permit instantaneous global communication of animal health reports.

Some national animal health agencies are initiating MS&R systems and national animal identification programs. Under equivalency provisions of the WTO SPS agreement, they are preparing sanitary measures requiring that exporting countries have nationally verified animal health reporting systems and animal identification capacity capable of tracing (to farm of origin) carcasses showing signs of certain diseases.

In light of dependency on foreign markets for future expansion of animal agriculture and the expectations of the international community, nations should implement a nationally supervised, cooperative, veterinarian-based, animal disease MS&R system. This system must credibly reflect the animal health situation of the country and provide a scientific basis for national import measures.

Import measures should be limited to diseases that are truly exotic to the country, diseases for which there is a nationally supervised control or eradication program based on active surveillance, and diseases for which vaccines are neither produced nor legally used in the country.

IMPLICATIONS OF CHANGING TRADE PARADIGMS

Because of the importance of animal health issues in determining future markets, the cattle and dairy industries along with the national veterinary services of countries aspiring for world markets need to cooperate to ensure market niches in a dynamically competitive global economy (Kahrs 1998b).

Veterinary practitioners can assist their dairy, cow–calf, and feedlot industries in remaining competitive in the new global marketplace in several ways. They can create awareness of increased needs to exclude foreign animal diseases by constantly querying owners of cattle with DABM about visitors or other contact with foreign countries, and verify diagnoses by selected laboratory tests. They can upgrade reporting of existing diseases, and can work with state and federal colleagues to develop an industry, practitioner, diagnostic, research, and regulatory partnership to maintain and expand foreign markets for domestically produced bovine origin commodities.

REFERENCES

Kahrs RF, 1996. Applications of the concept of regionalization to domestic animal disease control and global market expansion. *Proc. U.S. Anim. Health Assoc.* 100:207–210.

Kahrs RF, 1998a. The impact of bluetongue on international trade. *Proc. U.S. Anim. Health Assoc.* 102:125–127.

Kahrs RF, 1998b. Effects of international standards and trade agreements on animal health programs and practices. In *Convention Notes 135th Annual Meeting, American Veterinary Medical Association,* Baltimore, pp. 301–304.

Kahrs RF, 1999. The international animal health community's expectations of the US national animal health reporting system (NAHRS). *Proc. U.S. Anim. Health Assoc.* 103:100–109.

Kahrs RF, Morgan AM, 1996. Changing world and European requirements for US exports of live cattle and bovine germ plasm. *Proc. U.S. Anim. Health Assoc.* 100:272–275.

9

ADENOVIRUSES

INTRODUCTION

The adenoviruses, so named because initial isolations were from human adenoids (Enders et al. 1956), are associated with human adenoconjunctival-pharyngeal fever and other infections. Over 100 distinct mammalian adenoviruses, mostly species specific, have been isolated. They are classified by species of origin and are differentiated immunologically. At least 10 serotypes of bovine adenoviruses (BAV) are presently recognized (Lehmkuhl et al. 1999) and are designated BAV types 1 through 10. New isolates are occasionally characterized and compared with recognized serotypes.

BAV infections are ubiquitous, easily transmitted, and frequently inapparent. They sometimes cause pneumonia, enteritis, and conjunctivitis. They are frequently found in association with other viruses or bacteria; laboratory tests are required for diagnosis.

The BAV have been reviewed by Mattson (1992), Burki (1990), and Thomson (1994).

ETIOLOGY

BAV are relatively stable, medium-sized, icosahedrally symmetrical DNA viruses of the genus *Mastadenovirus* in the family Adenoviridae. The first BAV isolates came from feces of cattle studied to evaluate a now debunked theory of bovine links to human poliomyelitis (Klein et al. 1959). BAV probably occur worldwide and have been isolated from both sick and apparently healthy cattle (Burki 1990 and Thomson 1994). Seroconversion or rising BAV titers have been observed in healthy cattle (Lehmkuhl et al. 1998).

BAV classification and typing methods include neutralization tests; complement fixation and immunodiffusion tests; hemagglutination procedures; fluorescent antibody assays; DNA restriction analysis; electron microscopy; and pathogenicity studies using calves, laboratory animals, and cell cultures.

Two antigenically distinct subgroups with slightly differing pathogenicity for animals and cell cultures have been identified. Subgroup 1 is more likely to produce respiratory disease and is more easily isolated in cell cultures than subgroup 2, which is more commonly associated with pneumoenteritis.

BAV selectively replicate in a variety of cell cultures and may contaminate bovine tissue cultures and sera used in cell culture media. Some BAV cause slowly developing cytopathology requiring two to eight blind passages before manifesting a characteristic rounding and clumping of cells. Other isolates cause more rapid changes (Coria and Lehmkuhl 1978). Most isolates produce intranuclear inclusions in cell cultures and tissues of infected animals.

BAV are resistant to environmental influences, most disinfectants, and stomach acidity to the extent that they survive and replicate in the bovine gastrointestinal tract.

An adenovirus closely related to BAV has been associated with an acute fatal disease in deer.

Adenovirus-associated viruses (AAV), incomplete parvoviruses that seem to require coinfection with adenoviruses or other helper viruses for replication, were found in association with some BAV (Coria and Lehmkuhl 1978), but they probably cause no disease (Thomson 1994).

CLINICAL SIGNS AND LESIONS

BAV contribute to respiratory and enteric syndromes, particularly in calves. Their clinical significance is obscured, however, by a multiplicity of serotypes, inapparent infections, and similarity of their signs and lesions to those of many other diseases. Nevertheless, observations on naturally and experimentally infected cattle indicate that BAV contribute to diarrhea, enteritis, pneumonia, conjunctivitis, and the so-called weak calf syndrome (Mattson 1992).

In clinically infected cattle, respiratory signs usually predominate, sometimes accompanied by diarrhea. Thus, diseases from which BAV isolates arise are often designated pneumoenteritis.

The role of BAV as a cause of pneumonia is supported by virus isolation from calves with pneumonia (Reed et al. 1978) and experimentally produced mild pneumonia (Mattson 1973). Establishing BAV as the primary etiologic agent in field cases of respiratory disease is complicated by the frequent presence of multiple infections with bacteria and other viruses. Nevertheless, BAV are considered among the many causes of bovine respiratory disease and may be the primary cause of some outbreaks of calf pneumonia (Lehmkuhl 1999).

Adenoviruses have been isolated from calves with naturally occurring (Reed et al. 1978) and experimentally induced diarrhea (McClurkin and Coria 1975).

When respiratory disease and enteritis occur simultaneously (pneumoenteritis), BAV should be considered a possible cause; this diagnosis, however, requires laboratory confirmation. Clinical signs associated with BAV-induced pneumoenteritis are fever, rapid respirations, coughing, conjunctivitis, lacrimal discharge, nasal discharge, and diarrhea. BAV isolates frequently come from calves with concomitant bacterial or viral infections.

Conjunctivitis is common in calves with pneumoenteritis and in cattle with respiratory disease. BAV have been isolated from the eyes of normal cattle, cattle with conjunctivitis, and cattle with keratoconjunctivitis.

Effects on the Developing Fetus

Widespread fetal infection is evidenced by isolations of BAV from normal fetal tissues harvested for cell cultures (Mohanty 1978) and the presence of neutralizing antibodies in fetal serum harvested as a tissue culture nutrient. Fetal infections with BAV probably can result in abortion under certain conditions. To date, BAV do not appear to be major causes of bovine abortion or fetal anomalies.

BAV have been isolated from synovial fluids of calves with weak calf syndrome (Cutlip and McClurkin 1975). Weak calf syndrome is characterized by joint stiffness noticed at birth or shortly thereafter, extreme weakness, recumbency, diarrhea, and death in a high percentage of cases. Typically the animal has polyarthritis, subcutaneous hemorrhage over the joints, bloody and fibrinous synovial fluid, and sometimes abomasal hemorrhages and ulcerations. The exact cause is undetermined. Several factors, including fetal hypoxia and preparturient maternal protein deficiency, may contribute to its etiology. The disease has also been associated with bovine viral diarrhea (BVD) virus.

NECROPSY FINDINGS

Cattle dying with clinical or experimental BAV infections have a variety of lesions, none of which is pathognomonic. Many lesions are attributable to concomitant infections.

The gross lesions of naturally occurring pneumoenteritis associated with BAV include enteritis, which varies from a mild catarrhal condition with a few petechial hemorrhages to severe hemorrhagic fibropurulent enteritis. BAV-associated pneumoenteritis has a wide variety of pulmonary lesions including reddening and consolidation of the lungs and fibrinous pneumonia that may result from secondary *Pasteurella* infection.

Experimental infections have been associated with lung consolidation, pulmonary edema, and hyperemia. They have also been associated with intralobular pulmonary edema with enlargement of mediastinal and bronchial lymph nodes (Mattson 1973).

A wide variety of nonspecific histopathologic lesions of the respiratory and gastrointestinal tracts and joints has been associated with pneumonia, enteritis, and joint involvement attributed to BAV.

Inconsistently present eosinophilic intranuclear inclusion bodies are diagnostically meaningful. These have been seen in lung, liver, kidney, adrenal, and gut tissues. Inclusion bodies are also common in cell cultures infected with BAV.

DIAGNOSIS

The diagnosis of BAV infections is difficult because of the multiple syndromes with which these agents have been associated, their nondescript signs and lesions that mimic those of many other infections, and the presence of multiple serotypes. Not all diagnostic laboratories have the reagents required for routine BAV diagnosis and subtype differentiation.

Although many other agents may be involved primarily or secondarily, BAV infection should be considered a possible contributing factor in calves that have pneumoenteritis, acute or chronic pneumonia, or weak calf syndrome, particularly if intranuclear inclusion bodies are found in lung tissue.

It is impossible to make a definitive diagnosis of BAV infection without laboratory tests.

Differential Diagnosis

Pneumoenteritis associated with BAV must be differentiated from BVD, infectious bovine rhinotracheitis, parainfluenza-3 virus, bovine respiratory syncytial virus, colibacillosis, and a host of other infectious, toxic, and allergic conditions. Most of these conditions are caused or complicated by multiple infections and environmental influences.

Laboratory Diagnosis

BAV can be identified by fluorescent antibody assays of tissue specimens and nasal and conjunctival swabs. The virus can be isolated in cultures inoculated with materials collected in the early stages of infection. In cell cultures these viruses are recognized by characteristic cytopathogenic changes, among which are intranuclear inclusion bodies.

The most appropriate specimen depends on the clinical signs and lesions, but nasal, conjunctival, and rectal swabs are good sources of BAV isolates.

Paired blood specimens for serology should be collected from each individual studied. These serums can be tested for BAV and other agents in the differential diagnosis.

For virus isolation, swabbings should be taken from the eyes and nasal passages as early as possible in the course of the disease. If the patient dies, tissues from lesions should be fixed for histopathologic study as well as frozen for virus isolation. In cases of weak calf syndrome, synovial fluid should be harvested.

Because of their ubiquity and the possibility of persistent BAV infections, caution is recommended in ascribing an etiologic role to isolated BAV unless seroconversion also occurs.

EPIDEMIOLOGY

BAV epizootiology, based on experimental infections and widespread seroconversion to multiple serotypes (some of which cross-react serologically and a few of which also infect sheep), is obscured by frequent complicating infections. Conclusions verified for one serotype are not necessarily applicable to all BAV.

The incubation period varies. Experimental intravenous injections, which vary by serotype, dose, and route of inoculation, produce fever in 2 to 3 days (McClurkin and Coria 1975). Field cases, however, may be unobserved for as long as two weeks' time after estimated exposure if secondary infections are required for severe signs to develop (Mattson 1973).

Although sheep can be infected with some BAV serotypes, it appears that cattle are the principal reservoir.

Most BAV infections probably are transmitted by direct calf-to-calf contact. The virus is present in nasal and lacrimal secretions and sometimes in feces. The route of entry is probably through the mouth and respiratory tract. Aerosol transmissions may occur.

Clinical disease associated with BAV infection is more common in calves and neonates than in adults, but infection occurs at all ages. It is probably non-clinical in adult cattle unless accompanied by severe stress or other infections.

THERAPY AND MANAGEMENT OF OUTBREAKS

There is no specific therapy for BAV-infected cattle. Treatment regimens are directed at controlling accompanying bacterial infections, diarrhea, and dehydration.

IMMUNITY

Following active infection, a humoral antibody response occurs. That virus-neutralizing activity can be detected in nasal and ocular secretions (Mattson 1973) suggests a role for local or secretary antibody in controlling infections.

Calves nursing during the first day of life may acquire type-specific antibody in colostrum. This colostrally acquired passive antibody remains in the serum for variable time periods and affords inconsistent protection against infection and clinical signs.

VIRUS PERSISTENCE

BAV have been recovered from urine 10 weeks after infection (Burki 1990) and from the respiratory tracts and conjunctiva of normal animals. Adeno-viruses have been found as persistent infections in human adenoids and ton-sils, and persistent bovine infections have been suggested but not definitely established.

PREVENTION AND CONTROL

Disease associated with BAV can be reduced by minimizing stress and judi-cious introduction of new cattle into herds. Management realities and the ubiquitousness of BAV have inspired research on live and inactivated vaccines (Mattson et al. 1987).

Inactivated BAV vaccines have been produced in Europe, but they have not gained enthusiastic acceptance. Their efficacy is variable, multiple repeated vaccinations are needed, and serotype variations exist (Burki 1990).

As the importance of the various BAV types in diseases of calves and feedlot cattle is sorted out, the need for vaccines may stimulate additional research and eventual production of improved BAV vaccines.

LIKELIHOOD OF ERADICATION

BAV infections are poor candidates for eradication because of the uncertainty of vaccine efficacy, multiplicity of serotypes, widespread distribution, and the possibility of persistent infections. The uncertainty of their pathogenesis complicates economic evaluation of their impact.

IMPACT ON INTERNATIONAL TRADE

BAV are not categorized as List A or List B diseases by the Office International Des Epizooties, and BAV-specific trade measures are usually not imposed.

PUBLIC RESPONSIBILITY

Human disease has not been associated with BAV, but anyone who works with sick cattle must avoid contact with other cattle. Likewise, cattle known to be experiencing respiratory, enteric, or conjunctival disease should not be allowed to contact healthy cattle.

Cattle undergoing clinical infection should not be transported or slaughtered until recovery is complete and all drug withdrawal times have been observed.

AREAS IN NEED OF RESEARCH

Further studies, using molecular technology, are needed to sort out the diagnostic challenges of type differentiation and pathogenicity of the various BAV types and the role of AAV (if any) in the effects of the virus on cattle. There is a need to develop rapid, simple diagnostic procedures. Development of new and improved vaccines may be needed.

REFERENCES

Burki F, 1990. Bovine adenoviruses. In *Infectious Diseases of Ruminants,* edited by Z Dinter, B Morein. Amsterdam: Elsevier Scientific Publishers, pp. 161–170.
Coria MF, Lehmkuhl HD, 1978. Isolation and identification of a bovine adenovirus type 3 with an adenovirus-associated virus. *Am. J. Vet. Res.* 39:1904–1906.

Cutlip RC, McClurkin AW, 1975. Lesions and pathogenesis in young calves experimentally induced by a bovine adenovirus type 5 isolated from a calf with weak calf syndrome. *Am. J. Vet. Res.* 36:1095–1098.

Enders JF, Bell JA, Dingle JH, Frances T, Hilleman MR, Huebner RJ, Payne AMM, 1956. Adenoviruses: Group name proposed for new respiratory tract viruses. *Science* 124:119–120.

Klein M, Early E, Zellat J, 1959. Isolation from cattle of a virus related to human adenoviruses. *Proc. Soc. Exp. Biol. Med.* 102:1–4.

Lehmkuhl HD, Briggs RE, Cutlip RC, 1998. Survey for antibodies to bovine adenoviruses in six to nine month old feedlot cattle. *Am. J. Vet. Res.* 59:1579–1580.

Lehmkuhl HD, Cutlip RC, DeBey BM, 1999. Isolation of a bovine adenovirus serotype 10 from a calf in the United States. *J. Vet. Diagn. Invest.* 11:485–490.

Mattson DE, 1973. Naturally occurring infection of calves with a bovine adenovirus. *Am. J. Vet. Res.* 34:623–629.

Mattson DE, 1992. Adenoviruses. In *Veterinary Diagnostic Virology: A Practitioners Guide,* edited by AE Castro, WP Heuschele. St. Louis: Mosby Yearbook, pp. 70–72.

Mattson DE, Wangelin JR, Sweat RI, 1987. Vaccination of dairy calves with bovine adenovirus type-3. *Cornell Vet* 77:351–361.

McClurkin AW, Coria MF, 1975. Infectivity of bovine adenovirus type 5 recovered from a polyarthritic calf with weak calf syndrome. *J. Am. Vet. Med. Assoc.* 167:139–141.

Mohanty SB, 1978. Adenoviruses. *Adv. Vet. Sci. Comp. Med.* 22:83–105.

Reed DE, Wheeler BA, Lupton HW, 1978. Isolation of bovine adenovirus type 7 from calves with pneumonia and enteritis. *Am. J. Vet. Res.* 39:1968–1971.

Thomson GR, 1994. Adenovirus infections. In *Infectious Diseases of Livestock With Special Reference to Southern Africa,* edited by JAW Coetzer, GR Thomson, RC Tustin. Capetown: Oxford University Press, pp. 901–908.

10

BLUETONGUE

INTRODUCTION

Bluetongue (BT) is an infectious but noncontagious vector-borne disease of sheep. The name comes from the swollen, cyanotic tongue sometimes observed in sheep.

Cattle are readily infected with BT virus (BTV). Bovine BTV infections are important because cattle serve briefly as sources of infection for midges that biologically transmit BTV to sheep and other ruminants and because BT-based sanitary measures restrict international trade in ruminants and germ plasm.

In cattle, most BTV infections are subclinical, although a rare, sporadic, sometimes fatal, syndrome may be associated with bovine BTV infection. It is included in the differential diagnosis of diseases affecting the bovine mucosa (DABM).

Control of BT is difficult because of its multiple serotypes and complex epidemiology.

BT has been reviewed by Verwoerd and Erasmus (1994), Stott (1998), Osburn (1998), and the Office International Des Epizooties (OIE)(1998).

ETIOLOGY

BTV, the prototype virus of the genus *Orbivirus* in the family Reoviridae, requires insect bites or direct experimental blood inoculations for transmission.

Twenty-four distinct serotypes of BTV, identified by serum neutralization tests, are known (OIE 1998). Of these, five have been found in the United States, where there are also two of nine serotypes of epizootic hemorrhagic disease (EHD), a closely related virus that cross-reacts with BTV (Mecham and Jochim 2000) and sometimes causes clinical disease in cattle (Abdy et al. 1999). Other closely related viruses are Ibaraki and Palyam viruses that have been identified in Japan and elsewhere.

Although best cultivated, passaged, and identified in sheep, BTV grows in chick embryos inoculated intravascularly via the yolk sac or allantoic vessels. Although BTV does not readily produce cytopathogenic changes on primary isolation, some isolates can be adapted to grow in cell cultures after isolation in other systems. With advancing technology enabling identification of strain-specific nucleic acid sequences, many of the difficulties involved in the study of BTV are being overcome.

CLINICAL SIGNS AND LESIONS

Bovine infection is usually inapparent, and few infected cattle demonstrate clinical signs.

When clinically observable signs occur, bovine BTV infection is characterized by fever, nasal discharge and encrustations of the muzzle, erosions and necrosis of the oral mucosa, and edema of the tongue. Pityriasis and sloughing of skin, swelling and cracking of the coronary band, and lameness resulting from laminitis or myositis may also occur.

Early clinical signs that may go unobserved in the field include hyperemia of mucous membranes and skin, particularly around the coronary band, udder, teats, and muzzle. Sometimes there is stiffness and lameness that appears to improve as the animal moves about. Fever and excess salivation may be observed, and the tongue may have hyperemia and edema that progresses to ulceration. Severe hyperemia or necrosis of the muzzle ("burnt muzzle") may be the first sign observed. Ulcerations or erosions of oral mucosa and dental pad may develop.

Pityriasis, skin sloughing, and scab formation may occur on the teats, coronary band, and occasionally on other skin areas, but widespread pityriasis rarely occurs.

Coronitis and lameness resembling laminitis may occur and may be followed by cracking or ulceration of skin around the coronary band. Rarely, the shell of the hoof sloughs. These lesions may become infected, and chronic lameness and debility can result.

Diarrhea is rare but is occasionally found in range cattle undergoing BT outbreaks. In most cases, the cattle survive with moderate debility.

These signs are unusual consequences of bovine BTV infection. It is usually inapparent.

BT is a serious disease of sheep. Deer and antelope infected with BTV may develop a hemorrhagic disease similar to EHD. In deer EHD is an acute, frequently fatal condition characterized by widely disseminated petechial and ecchymotic hemorrhages throughout the body.

Canine abortions due to vaccination of pregnant bitches with BTV-contaminated vaccines have been reported (Akita et al. 1994). In Africa, large carnivores have seroconverted to BTV, presumably as a result of eating the viscera of viremic ruminants.

EFFECTS ON THE DEVELOPING FETUS

Early reports (Barnard 1976 and Luedke et al. 1977) of BT-induced fetal wastage were not subsequently verified by experiments using BTV serotype 11 (Parsonson et al. 1994).

BTV was reported to be abortogenic and teratogenic (Luedke et al. 1977). Following experimental insect transmission of BTV to pregnant heifers, abortion, stillbirths, arthrogryposis (crooked leg syndrome), agnathia (tilted mandible), and prognathia with domed cranium were observed. Excessive gingival tissue with a red to purple discoloration was a common finding. In some cases two-thirds to three-fourths of each incisor tooth was covered with discolored viable gingival tissue (Barnard and Pienaar 1976).

Infection of pregnant cattle can also result in birth of calves with hydranencephaly and a dummy calf syndrome characterized by inactivity, dullness, and behavioral abnormalities (Richards et al. 1971). The stage of gestation at time of maternal infection, the serotype of virus, and multiple infections may be determinants of the outcome of pregnancies and the nature of fetal anomalies. This aspect of the disease requires further study.

NECROPSY FINDINGS

In rare fatal bovine cases, gross necropsy findings include ulcerations and necrosis of the oral mucosa and skin. Histopathologic lesions are principally those of vasculitis with degeneration of the intima of vessels. This finding may explain the necrosis and pityriasis.

Dummy calves with hydranencephaly resulting from in utero infection present a clearly visible gross necropsy finding (Barnard and Pienaar 1976).

DIAGNOSIS

The clinical diagnosis of bovine BT is difficult because it is usually an inapparent infection. Clinical cases are generally sporadic, and bovine BT is clinically similar to EHD and DABM.

The diagnostic profile of BT involves cattle in endemic areas, the majority of which appear perfectly healthy, and less than 2% to 10% demonstrate any combination of the clinical signs described above. Sick sheep may or may not be present. Midges of the genus *Culicoides* should be present. There may be abortions, stillbirths or dummy calves born with hydranencephaly. Clinical diagnosis is based on signs and sporadic cases in BT endemic areas where *Culicoides* are present. Some workers feel some so-called mycotic stomatitis is actually BT.

Differential Diagnosis

The differential diagnosis includes DABM including bovine viral diarrhea, rinderpest, malignant catarrhal fever, mycotic stomatitis, vesicular stomatitis, foot-and-mouth disease, and infectious bovine rhinotracheitis. If tongue protrusion is present, glossitis or botulism and other toxicoses should be considered. If pityriasis is present, photosensitization should be considered.

The congenital effects must be distinguished from those of Cache Valley virus, Polyam virus, Ibaraki virus, and Akabane virus. Abortions and stillbirths are always difficult to diagnose, and all abortifacient agents must be considered.

Laboratory Diagnosis

Detailed BTV testing procedures are outlined in the OIE *Manual of Standards for Diagnostic Tests and Vaccines* (the Manual) (OIE 2000). Paired serums may be used to demonstrate seroconversion using the agar gel immunodiffusion (AGID) or the enzyme-linked immunosorbent assay (ELISA) tests. Serotypes can be distinguished from one another and from strains of EHD by serum neutralization tests. Considerable cross-reactions occur, making serodiagnostic interpretations challenging.

Serologic tests can be used to determine suitability of cattle for export to countries that still require seronegative animals, but these requirements are becoming obsolete. Polymerase chain reaction (PCR)-based tests, however, can be used to determine the suitability of seropositive animals or their germ plasm for export (Miller and Mecham 1997).

Virus isolations from whole blood or serum samples have traditionally been attempted by sheep inoculations followed by serologic tests or intravenous inoculation of embryonating chicken eggs (ECE) followed by fluorescent antibody tests. These procedures are gradually being replaced by molecular technologies such as PCR and the capture ELISA test (Katz et al. 1994).

BTV is difficult to isolate from clinical material. The specialized techniques for BTV identification are available in only a few laboratories. BTV is usually isolated from the cell fraction of blood. Unlike many viruses, its infectivity can be maintained for prolonged periods in blood held at refrigerator or ambient temperatures in appropriate preservatives.

PCR technology permits identification of BTV nucleic acid in clinical samples and serotype differentiation of virus isolates (OIE 2000) in 3–5 days—much faster than ECE or sheep inoculation. BTV nucleic acids persist from 140 to 160 days after infection—more than twice the 60-day survival time of infective virus that is associated with red blood cells.

PCR-based tests are considered the best method of determining the suitability of seropositive animals for export (Miller and Mecham 1997).

Both intranuclear and intracytoplasmic inclusion bodies have been observed in BTV-infected cell cultures.

Early in the course of BT, the animal may have leukopenia, but with appearance of necrosis, leukocytosis may be observed.

Specimens for laboratory study include blood for serology and virus isolation, which should be collected aseptically.

Unless vaccination is practiced or major immigrations occur, serologic tests can establish the presence of BTV infection in regions.

The most suitable specimen for virus isolation is blood collected in an anticoagulant and refrigerated. It should not be frozen, and if it must be shipped, wet ice is the desired refrigerant. Spleen and lymph nodes can also be used.

Before collecting specimens, it is recommended that specific instructions be obtained from laboratories that have agreed to test them. In the United States, the National Veterinary Services Laboratories in Ames, Iowa, the USDA

Arthropod-borne Animal Disease Research Laboratory in Laramie, Wyoming, and several veterinary colleges work with BTV. Serologic tests are available in some state diagnostic laboratories.

EPIDEMIOLOGY

The seasonal and geographic distribution of competent vectors are key to the epidemiology of BTV. Cattle can serve as sources of infection from which *Culicoides* vectors acquire virus that is subsequently transmitted to sheep or other ruminants after a 6-to-8-day extrinsic incubation period, during which time BTV replicates in the insect's salivary glands. Only some 20 of approximately 1400 species of culicoids are competent BTV vectors (OIE 1998). Although *Culicoides* midges live only a few days to a month after feeding, they usually remain infective for life.

After years of vector, host, serotype, and environmental adaptations, assisted by unknown overwintering mechanisms in temperate climates, BTV circulates between mammalian hosts and specific species of night-feeding culicoids in serotype-specific foci between latitudes 35° South and 40° North. Although vectors may migrate beyond these latitudes causing seasonal infections, these foci are so stable that the geographic origin of BTVs can be identified by nucleic acid analysis of isolates.

Only a few species of culicoids have genetic capability to support replication of BTV as required for vector competence. Transmission capacity of competent vectors is determined by host preferences, biting rates, time intervals between feedings, extrinsic incubation periods, and daily survival probabilities, as well as environmental factors including the temperature at which they are reared. Probably less than one in 10,000 randomly tested culicoids is capable of transmitting BTV, but infective midges can cluster in time and space.

Experimentally, the incubation period is 6 to 8 days. The onset of new infections usually ceases within 2 weeks of a frost adequate to curtail *Culicoides* activity.

The nature of the lesions suggests that some clinical episodes may have complex etiologies, possibly due to hypersensitivity reactions involving sequential infection with different serotypes. Thus classic interpretation of incubation period data may not be apropos to clinical bovine BT.

Cattle and some wild ruminants probably serve briefly as inapparent reservoirs of BTV, providing a source of virus for biting culicoids. The midges become infective after an extrinsic incubation period of 6 to 8 days and usually remain infective for life.

Cattle are infected by the bite of infective *Culicoides*. Repeated exposures to heterologous serotypes may be needed to induce clinical disease in cattle.

In addition to biting insects, BTV may also be transmitted by blood transfusions or semen contaminated with blood from viremic bulls. Significant vertical transmission does not occur, and meat and dairy products are not risk factors (OIE 1998). Transmission by nonviremic seropositive bulls appears highly unlikely. Properly washed embryos present minimum risk. In utero infection may occur when cattle are infected during pregnancy.

Aside from the role of fetal infections and the possible role of colostrally acquired maternal antibody, age, sex, and breed do not appear to play a significant role in the distribution of clinical bovine BT cases.

As a vector-borne disease, BT in cattle generally appears toward the end of summer in temperate zones. BTV probably cycles year-round in the tropics.

IMMUNITY

Because immunity is serotype-specific, cattle immune to one serotype may be infected with others. It has been hypothesized that post-infection immunity prevents subsequent infection with homologous virus strains while it confers a sensitivity that may initiate a pathologic response upon infection by heterologous virus strains (Jochim et al. 1974).

Calves nursing seropositive cows acquire titers that decline progressively (Luedke et al. 1977). The protective value of this antibody is uncertain.

VIRUS PERSISTENCE

It was once thought that persistent infections and lifelong viremia occurred in some animals after prenatal or postnatal exposure (Luedke et al. 1977). Newer technology indicates that serotype-specific viremia lasts only 4 to 8 weeks (OIE 1998) and declines as antibody levels rise. Noninfective viral nucleic acids, detectable by PCR-based tests, persist in association with erythrocytes for longer periods than infective virus.

PREVENTION AND CONTROL

BT is difficult to control in cattle because of efficient transmission by *Culicoides* vectors, which are abundant throughout the world. Movement of cattle and wild ruminants in their natural habitats offers opportunities for viral perpetuation in stable ecosystems but provides minimal hazard of introduction of new serotypes into areas.

Modified live virus vaccines used successfully on sheep in southern Africa and elsewhere require serotype specificity for maximum efficiency. They should not be used for cattle because of the risk of transmitting vaccine strains that could interfere with diagnostic procedures. The danger exists as well of inducing serologic reactions, which could cause rejection of cattle for export.

THERAPY AND MANAGEMENT OF OUTBREAKS

Clinical BT is usually nonresponsive to therapy, but good nursing care, protection from sun, and provision of adequate food and water may expedite convalescence. Antibiotics may be used to control secondary bacterial infections.

Use of corticosteroids is contraindicated. Solar radiation is believed to be an exacerbating factor in production of skin necrosis. Cattle should be offered shade, adequate water, and soft food if there is mouth involvement.

BT in sheep or cattle is reportable in many countries. Where it is presently regarded as exotic, officials may initiate quarantine procedures. The appearance of positively diagnosed clinical cases in cattle usually indicates substantial inapparent infection and an epidemiological hazard to nearby ruminants.

Culicoides control measures include elimination of standing water and application of approved insecticides.

LIKELIHOOD OF ERADICATION

The likelihood of eradicating BT from cattle is small because of the multiple serotypes, wild ruminant carriers, and the ubiquity of the *Culicoides* vectors.

IMPACT ON INTERNATIONAL TRADE

BT is an OIE List A disease. Chapter 2.1.9 of the OIE International Animal Health Code indicates that countries or regions may claim freedom from BT if it is compulsorily reportable and appropriate surveillance indicates no evidence of BTV for two years.

Many sheep-producing countries with *Culicoides* populations restrict importation of ruminants and ruminant germ plasm from infected regions (Kahrs 1998) by imposing a variety of quarantine or testing requirements, including (and sometimes exceeding) those suggested in the OIE Code.

The United States Department of Agriculture conducts periodic ELISA test surveys of Northeastern and North Central states to establish a BT-free region with less than 2% seropositive cattle. Establishment of a BT-free region permits exports to some countries that claim freedom from US BTV serotypes.

BT-based import restrictions are controversial (Gibbs 1983) and will be subject to continuing discussion as technology advances and BT epidemiology is better understood.

PUBLIC RESPONSIBILITY

Little is known of the effects of BTV on humans, although laboratory infections can occur (Stott 1998). Nevertheless, its danger to sheep and its potential trade impact requires appropriate reporting and regulatory precautions when BT is diagnosed or suspected.

AREAS IN NEED OF RESEARCH

Future research on bovine BT should address diagnostic methodology, elaboration of epidemiologic details, effects of BT infection on developing fetuses, and vaccine research.

REFERENCES

Abdy MA, Howerth EA, Stallknecht DE, 1999. Experimental infection of calves with epizootic hemorrhagic disease virus. *Am. J. Vet. Res.* 60:621–626.

Akita GY, Ianescu M, MacLachin NJ, Osburn BI, 1994. Bluetongue disease in dogs associated with a contaminated vaccine. *Vet. Rec.* 135:283–284.

Barnard BJH, Pienaar JG, 1976. Bluetongue virus as a cause of hydranencephaly in cattle. *Onderstepoort J. Vet. Res.* 43:155–158.

Gibbs EPJ, 1983. Bluetongue—An analysis of current problems with particular reference to importation of ruminants into the United States. *J. Am. Vet. Med. Assoc.* 182:1190–1194.

Jochim MM, Luedke AJ, Chow TL, 1974. Bluetongue in cattle: Immunogenic and clinical responses in calves inoculated in utero and after birth. *Am. J. Vet. Res.* 35:517–522.

Kahrs RF, 1998. The impact of bluetongue on international trade. *Proc. U.S. Anim. Health Assoc.* 102:125–127.

Katz J, Alstad D, Gustafson G, Everman J, 1994. Diagnostic analysis of the prolonged bluetongue virus RNA presence found in the blood of naturally infected cattle and experimentally infected sheep. *J. Vet. Diagn. Invest.* 6:139–142.

Luedke AJ, Jochim MM, Jones RH, 1977. Bluetongue in cattle: Effects of *Culicoides varipennis* transmitted bluetongue virus on pregnant heifers and their calves. *Am. J. Vet. Res.* 38:1687–1695.

Mecham JO, and Jochim MM, 2000. Development of an enzyme-linked immunosorbent assay for epizootic hemorrhagic disease of deer virus. *J. Vet. Diagn. Inves.* 12:142–145.

Miller LD, Mecham JO, 1997. Report of the Committee on Bluetongue and Bovine Retroviruses. *Proc. U.S. Anim. Health Assoc.* 101:35–42.

Office International Des Epizooties (OIE) 1998. Supporting document for the OIE International Animal Health Code Chapter 2.1.9. (Bluetongue). Ad Hoc Working Group on Bluetongue. Paris: OIE, pp. 34.

Office International Des Epizooties (OIE) 2000. *Manual of Diagnostic Tests and Vaccines* (6th ed.) with annual updates. Paris: OIE, pp. 109–118.

Osburn BI, 1998. Bluetongue. In *The Merck Veterinary Manual, 8th* edition. Whitehouse Station, NJ: Merck and Company, pp. 520–521.

Parsonson, IA, Thompson, LH, Walton TE, 1994. Experimentally induced infection with bluetongue virus serotype 11 in cows. *Am. J. Vet. Res.* 55:1529–1534.

Richards WPC, Crenshaw, GL, Bushnell RB, 1971. Hydranencephaly of calves associated with natural bluetongue virus infection. *Cornell Vet* 61:336–348

Stott JL, 1998. Bluetongue and epizootic hemorrhagic disease. In *Foreign Animal Diseases,* edited by WW Buisch, JL Hyde, CL Mebus. Richmond: U.S. Animal Health Assoc., pp. 106–117.

Verwoerd D, Erasmus, BJ, 1994. Bluetongue. In *Infectious Diseases of Livestock With Special Reference to Southern Africa,* edited by JAW Coetzer, GR Thomson, RC Tustin. Capetown: Oxford University Press, pp. 443–459.

11

BOVINE IMMUNODEFICIENCY-LIKE VIRUS (BOVINE LENTIVIRUS)

INTRODUCTION

Bovine immunodeficiency-like virus (BIV), also called bovine immunodeficiency virus and bovine lentivirus, is widely distributed in cattle populations. It causes persistent, progressive infection of the lymphatic system with potential to induce immunologic deficits resulting in decreased resistance to bacterial infections and lowered productivity.

Animal health officials throughout the world are awaiting clarification of the significance of BIV to determine what actions (if any) are most appropriate.

The lentiviruses were reviewed by Campbell and Robinson (1998). BIV was summarized by St. Cyr Coats et al. (1995) and Jacobs et al. (1998).

ETIOLOGY

First isolated in 1969 (Van Der Maaten et al. 1972), BIV is a member of the genus *Lentivirus* in the family Retroviridae. Human immunodeficiency virus (HIV) is the best known of the lentiviruses.

Other Retroviridae of veterinary importance are bovine leukemia virus (BLV), feline immunodeficiency virus, equine infectious anemia virus, and Jembrana virus, which causes an acute, frequently fatal hemorrhagic lymphadenopathy in Bali cattle in Indonesia (Kertayadnya et al. 1993), but mild disease in other breeds.

Of the Retroviridae, BIV has the least clearly defined clinical, pathological, and immunological consequences. Because the classification and name suggest unrealistic similarities to HIV and the more dramatic immunodeficiency viruses, Campbell and Robinson (1998) suggest dropping the name "bovine immunodeficiency virus" and renaming the virus bovine lentivirus-1.

BIV infects and replicates in white blood cells (leukocytes) and other phagocytic cells. Viral replication probably occurs at low levels (Miller and Mecham 1998) and BIV is difficult to isolate (Suarez et al. 1994). BIV is often found in combination with other retroviruses (Jacobs et al. 1998) and there are indications that it has a high mutation rate (Suarez and Whetstone 1997).

The 1969 isolate, designated R29, upon which many preliminary conclusions were based, was maintained for years in the laboratory, possibly modified by passage in cell cultures, and at some point coinfected with bovine viral diarrhea virus. Experiments utilizing more recent isolates may clarify earlier questions about the pathogenicity and significance of BIV (Munro et al. 1998).

CLINICAL SIGNS AND LESIONS

Experimentally infected animals have had nonsuppurative encephalitis and lymphoid hyperplasia particularly in the hemal lymph nodes (Munro et al. 1998).

Encephalitis, lymphoid depletion, and secondary infection have been reported in a dairy herd (Snider et al. 1993 and 1996). It has been suggested that infected cattle may have reduced milk production (McNab et al. 1994) and lowered resistance to infection, and that they may suffer increased occurrences of mastitis, metritis, and foot infections. The clinical significance of BIV is frequently discussed by the Committee on Bluetongue and Bovine Retroviruses of the U.S. Animal Health Association (Miller and Mecham 1994 and 1998).

Much information about clinical effects of BIV infections is based on inferences about immunosuppression's permitting secondary infections that reduce productivity. Such conclusions are difficult to support or to refute. They are further complicated in the case of BIV because, in the field, it may be associated with coinfections with other viruses, including BLV.

EFFECTS ON THE DEVELOPING FETUS

As of this writing, clear effects of BIV have not been demonstrated.

NECROPSY FINDINGS

Naturally infected cattle often have lymphadenopathy and lymphoid depletion, and sometimes poor production, mastitis, and an array of nonspecific conditions. Because they are frequently coinfected with BLV or other agents, however, the actual cause of the lesions remains questionable.

Experimentally infected calves necropsied 12 months after infection had hyperplastic hemal lymph nodes and a nonsuppurative meningoencephalitis (Munro et al. 1998).

DIAGNOSIS

BIV cannot be diagnosed clinically.

Differential Diagnosis

BIV is distinct from bovine leukocyte adhesion deficiency (BLAD), a genetic defect of Holstein calves that renders them unable to resist common bacterial infections and leads to premature death unless the calves are maintained on antibiotics (Sipes et al. 1999). BIV must be differentiated from gross mismanagement.

Laboratory Diagnosis

Serologic tests including the indirect fluorescent antibody test, enzyme-linked immunosorbent assay, and western blot analysis are used to detect the presence of antibodies, which indicates previous infection and possibly active persistent infection. Virus isolation is a difficult and inconsistent method of determining the presence of infection and may be replaced by nested polymerase chain reaction tests or other genetic techniques (Suarez et al. 1995).

Both naturally and experimentally infected animals have transient and somewhat inconsistent lymphocytosis (St. Cyr Coats et al. 1995).

Development and validation of standardized tests will expedite diagnostic and research efforts.

EPIDEMIOLOGY

The mode of natural transmission of BIV is currently unclear, but BIV can be transmitted experimentally by blood inoculations. The virus has been detected, using molecular technology, in leukocytes in milk and blood (Nash et al. 1995a) and in semen (Nash et al. 1995b). Thus, transfer of these biologic materials from infected animals to susceptible individuals could possibly cause infection (St. Cyr Coats et al. 1995). The virus has been shown to experimentally infect sheep, goats, and rabbits.

BIV has global distribution (Zhang et al. 1997). It is widely distributed in many regions including the western hemisphere, Europe, the Pacific Rim and the United States, where surveys indicate it is more prevalent in southern states and more common in dairy cattle than in beef cattle.

IMMUNITY

Despite the lack of standardized tests and reagents, BIV infections appear to stimulate humoral antibody responses that persist for several years and then drop to undetectable levels (Suarez and Whetstone 1997).

VIRUS PERSISTENCE

Bovine infections are apparently persistent (Suarez and Whetstone 1997).

PREVENTION AND CONTROL

Transmission by blood inoculations can be reduced by use of individual needles for vaccinations and treatments and careful cleaning and disinfection of dehorners, castration equipment, and other surgical instruments.

Potential vertical transmission by colostrum is believed to be prevented by pasteurization.

When standardized tests are accepted and validated, prepurchase testing will be useful.

THERAPY AND MANAGEMENT OF OUTBREAKS

The pattern of BIV infection suggests economic losses are subtle and indirect; for this reason direct therapeutic procedures are not applicable.

The use of individual needles and sterile surgical equipment is essential to limiting spread.

LIKELIHOOD OF ERADICATION

Eradication is unlikely until sensitive, specific tests are developed and the impact (if any) of the disease on the economy or public health is clarified. At that point eradication may be feasible for countries with low infection rates and strong animal health infrastructures.

IMPACT ON INTERNATIONAL TRADE

Some European countries are considering BIV control or eradication programs. Such programs could improve foreign markets for bovine genetics, be used to establish barriers to imports from countries without surveillance or control programs, and proactively address any future efforts to dramatize the similarity and genetic relationship of BIV to the HIV.

PUBLIC RESPONSIBILITY

There is no evidence that human infections occur. Conscientious veterinarians should encourage use of individual needles and cleaning and disinfection of surgical equipment.

AREAS IN NEED OF RESEARCH

Research is needed to develop and standardize diagnostic tests to expedite pathogenicity studies that will help clarify the importance of BIV infection (Miller and Mecham 1998).

REFERENCES

Campbell, RSF, Robinson WF, 1998. The comparative pathology of the lentiviruses. *J Comp. Pathol.* 119:333–395.

Jacobs RM, Jefferson BJ, Suarez DL, 1998. Prevalence of bovine immunodeficiency-like virus in bulls as determined by serology and proviral detection. *Can. J. Vet. Res.* 62:231–233.

Kertayadnya G, Wilcox GF, Soeharsono S, Harganingsih N, Coelen RJ, Cood RG, Collines ME, Brownlie J, 1993. Characteristics of a retrovirus associated with Jembrana disease in Bali cattle. *J. Gen. Virol.* 74: 1765–1773.

McNab WB, Jacobs RM, Smith HE, 1994. A serological survey of bovine immuno-deficiency-like virus in Ontario cattle and associations between test results, production records, and management practices. *Can. J. Vet. Res.* 58:36–41.

Miller LD, Mecham JO, 1994. Report of the Committee on Bluetongue and Bovine Retroviruses. *Proc. U.S. Anim. Health Assoc.* 98:51–53.

Miller LD, Mecham JO, 1998. Report of the Committee on Bluetongue and Bovine Retroviruses. *Proc. U.S. Anim. Health Assoc.* 102:128–135.

Munro R, Lysons R, Venables C, Horigan M, Jeffrey M, Dawson M, 1998. Lymphadenopathy and non-suppurative meningo-encephalitis in calves experimentally infected with bovine immunodeficiency-like virus (FL112). *J. Comp. Pathol.* 119: 121–134.

Nash JW, Hanson LA, St. Cyr Coats, K, 1995a. Detection of bovine immunodeficiency virus in blood and milk derived leukocytes by use of polymerase chain reaction. *Am. J. Vet. Res.* 56:445–449.

Nash JW, Hanson LA, St. Cyr Coats K, 1995b. Bovine immunodeficiency virus in stud bull semen. *Am. J. Vet. Res.* 56:760–763.

Sipes KM, Edens HA, Kehrli ME, Miettinen HM, Cutler JE, Jutila MA, Quinn MT, 1999. Analysis of surface antigen expression and host defense function in leukocytes of calves heterozygous or homozygous for bovine leukocyte adhesion deficiency. *Am. J. Vet. Res.* 60:1255–1261.

Snider TG III, Luther DG, Gonda MA, 1993. Bovine immunodeficiency virus associated with encephalitis and secondary infections in Mississippi dairy cattle. *Vet. Pathol.* 30:478.

Snider TG III, Luther DG, Jenny BF, Hoyt PG, Battles JK, Ennis WH, Balady J, Blas-Machado U, Lemarchand TX, Gonda MA, 1996. Encephalitis, lymphoid tissue depletion, and secondary diseases associated with bovine immunodeficiency virus in a dairy herd. *Comp. Immun. Microbiol. Inf. Dis.* 19:117–131.

St. Cyr Coats K, Nash JW, Hanson LA, 1995. Bovine lentivirus (BIV) in peripheral blood, milk and seminal leukocytes of cattle: Implications for transmission. *Proc. U.S. Anim. Health Assoc.* 99:69–80.

Suarez DL, Van Der Maaten M, Whetstone CA, 1995. Improved early and long-term detection of bovine lentivirus by a nested polymerase chain reaction test in experimentally infected calves. *Am. J. Vet. Res.* 56:579–586.

Suarez DL, Whetstone. CA, 1997. Comparison of different PCR tests to detect bovine lentivirus in cell culture and experimentally infected cattle. *J. Vet. Diagn. Invest* .9:421–424.

Suarez DL, Whetstone, CA, Miller JA, Van Der Maaten MJ, 1994. Bovine lentivirus (BIV): diagnosis, prevalence and pathogenesis. *Proc. U.S. Anim. Health Assoc.* 98:33–42.

Van Der Maaten MJ, Boothe AD, Seger CL, 1972. Isolation of a virus from cattle with persistent lymphocytosis. *J. Natl. Cancer Inst.* 49: 1649–1657.

Zhang S, Wenzhi X, Wood C, Qi-min C, Kapil S, Minocha HC, 1997. Detection of bovine immunodeficiency virus antibodies in cattle by western blot assay with recombinant gag protein. *J. Vet. Diagn. Invest.* 9:347–351.

12

BOVINE LEUKEMIA VIRUS AND ENZOOTIC BOVINE LEUKOSIS

INTRODUCTION

Enzootic bovine leukosis (EBL), the usually persistent inapparent infection caused by bovine leukemia virus (BLV), is widely distributed in most cattle populations.

BLV is important because certain nations limit importation of cattle and germ plasm from infected areas or herds. In addition, some high-incidence herds have multiple animals with solid tumors and losses due to slaughter condemnations, some infected herds may have reduced productivity, and questions about interspecies transmission occasionally arise. Some countries have successfully controlled EBL.

EBL was reviewed by Van Der Maaten and Miller (1990), Evermann and DiGiacomo (1992), and Verwoerd and Tustin (1994).

ETIOLOGY

BLV is a single-stranded oncogenic RNA virus in the genus *Deltaretrovirus* of the family Retroviridae. BLV has biochemical, biophysical, and genetic similarities and some incomplete immunologic cross-reactivity with other mammalian leukemia viruses. They all have C-type characteristics featuring a spherical nucleoid centrally located in an enveloped particle. These similarities suggest common evolutionary ancestors.

The early identification of BLV resulted from electron microscopic (EM) visualization of C-type particles in cultured lymphocytes from cattle with lymphocytosis (Miller et al. 1969).

BLV persists and replicates largely in lymphocytes. It also replicates in bovine or ovine cell cultures with syncytium formation and can replicate and induce solid tumors in sheep.

Infection with BLV is usually inapparent, persistent, and accompanied by serum antibodies whose presence is considered evidence of infection.

BLV is readily inactivated by organic solvents, disinfectants, and heat, including pasteurization of milk, and does not survive well in environments outside of living cells. It requires transfer of blood or leukocytes for transmission (Van Der Maaten and Miller 1990).

CLINICAL SIGNS AND LESIONS

Bovine lymphocytic tumors are classified by age of occurrence (adult, juvenile, or calf), anatomic location (thymic, skin, or multicentric), pattern of distribution in populations (enzootic or sporadic), and etiologic relationship to BLV.

In addition to widespread lifelong persistent inapparent infections accompanied by antibodies, BLV causes rare but ultimately fatal adult lymphosarcoma (AL) and benign persistent lymphocytosis (PL), a usually nonclinical hematologic finding that sometimes precedes tumor development.

Persistent inapparent infections are accompanied by lifelong serum antibody levels that may decline markedly at parturition because of a shift of immunoglobulins from serum to colostrum.

Herds with high antibody prevalences sometimes have reduced production efficiency, increased culling rates, and higher incidence of clinical lymphosarcoma than uninfected herds.

PL (abnormally high blood lymphocyte levels demonstrable in at least two blood samples collected 3 months apart) is commonly found in enzootic leukosis herds. Early European control programs were based on this finding. Cattle can, however, be infected with BLV and develop tumors without the presence of lymphocytosis (Van Der Maaten and Miller 1990).

Enzootic AL, the adult multicentric form that occurs in cattle over 3-5 years of age, is caused by BLV, probably acting in concert with multiple etiologic factors. Clinical cases are most common in "enzootic leukosis herds" characterized by high antibody prevalence. Even in these herds, it is unusual if more than 3% of cattle develop clinically recognizable lymphosarcoma annually. Once infected herds are identified, increased case-finding activity sometimes results in identification of lymphadenopathy in ever-increasing numbers of cattle.

Typical AL cases have enlarged superficial lymph nodes and a wide variety of clinical signs, depending on location of the tumor masses and the bodily functions affected. Occasionally, owners observe swollen prefemoral, supramammary, prescapular, or mandibular lymph nodes on otherwise healthy cattle that later develop clinical signs. Sometimes the first sign seen is a "popped eye," resulting from a tumor behind the eyeball.

Generally, however, superficial lymphadenopathy is first observed when cattle are examined because they are ill. The size and distribution of enlarged lymph nodes sometimes explains the observed signs but clinical manifestations cannot always be correlated with lesions.

Anorexia of unknown origin, indigestion, and chronic bloat are common principal complaints in AL cases. Many cases are diagnosed following parturition and owners suspect common postpartum diseases like metritis, mastitis, ketosis, or milk fever. Occasionally, lameness, unusual gait, or paralysis resulting from epidural tumors that impinge on nerves are the first signs observed. Some cases with extensive uterine involvement are first detected during routine pregnancy or fertility examination,

Most AL cases follow a chronic course with progressive debility, weakness, gradual emaciation, and varying degrees of anorexia preceding death or slaughter for humane reasons. Many cases are first recognized at slaughter, where the animals may have been sent because they were "poor doers" and condemned as unfit for human consumption. Occasionally, peracute death occurs, particularly if lymphocytic infiltration of heart muscles has occurred or if splenic rupture causes exsanguination. In a minority of cases, AL is accompanied by lymphocytosis.

EFFECTS ON THE DEVELOPING FETUS

In utero transmission resulting in congenital BLV infection occurs in a small percentage of births. Abortions or congenital anomalies have not been associated with in utero infection but such calves may be carriers for life and can develop tumors if appropriate genetic and supportive factors are present.

NECROPSY FINDINGS

Gross pathologic findings of AL include enlargement of lymph nodes, discrete tumor masses, or diffuse lymphocytic infiltration of vital organs. The lung is rarely involved, but the liver, spleen, heart, kidney, intestines, abomasum, spinal cord, and retrobulbar tissue are commonly infiltrated.

Histologically, there is proliferation of mitotic cells of the lymphocytic series and massive widely distributed lymphocytic infiltration of areas usually devoid of lymphocytes.

DIAGNOSIS

Diagnosis involves clinical and pathologic confirmation of malignant lymphomas; determination of the presence of BLV infection serologically by AGID or C-ELISA tests on cattle over 6 months old, the usual age of loss of colostrally acquired maternal antibody; or identification of the virus.

BLV-infected herds have antibody prevalence varying from 5% to 90%. Infected herds may have no clinical disease, or they may have single cases or multiple cases of clinical lymphosarcoma.

Each clinical case follows a slightly different course depending on the nature and distribution of tumors. Except for atypical cases, external tumors and lymph node enlargement or tumors identifiable on palpation per anum are the keys to clinical diagnosis of lymphosarcoma.

Differential Diagnosis

There is no consistent clinical pattern of enzootic AL, and the differential diagnosis includes most conditions affecting the involved anatomic system. Since the respiratory system and mucosa are seldom involved and most cases are afebrile, lymphosarcoma is rarely misdiagnosed as a respiratory disease or disease affecting the bovine mucosa (DABM).

Uterine lymphosarcoma or tumors in the abdominal cavity that are detectable on palpation per anum must be differentiated from normal pregnancy, mummified and macerated fetuses, fat necrosis, and ovarian cysts or granuloma cell tumors.

When AL affects the alimentary tract, it must be differentiated from traumatic gastritis. If diarrhea is present, it must be distinguished from other causes of enteritis. Eye involvement must be distinguished from ocular squamous cell carcinoma. Heart-base tumors may resemble endocarditis or pericarditis.

It is important to distinguish between EBL, the usually inapparent infection, which is common, BLV-induced disease, which is rare, and in between, lymphosarcomas caused by BLV and those of other etiology.

Diagnostically important sporadic noninfectious bovine lymphoid tumors that are unrelated to BLV are calf, thymic, and skin lymphosarcomas.

Unlike AL and PL, which seem to cluster in BLV-infected herds, the calf, thymic, and skin forms have a more sporadic distribution (Crocker and Rings 1998). They are assumed to be noncontagious and unrelated to BLV (Van Der Maaten and Miller 1990).

Multicentric calf lymphosarcoma is unrelated to BLV but could be confused with AL. It is occasionally present at birth and is recognized most often in calves under 6 months old, but may be seen in calves up 3 years of age. There is generalized and frequently symmetric enlargement of most lymph nodes and lymphocytic infiltration of bone marrow and internal organs.

Clinical signs vary, depending on which vital organs are the first infiltrated or subject to pressure from space-occupying lymphosarcomas. Sometimes the calf is alert and apparently normal, but the owner observes swollen superficial lymph nodes that are firm, smooth, mobile, painless, and not hot to the touch. Such calves usually sicken as the condition progresses and eventually succumb. Other cases are identified because the calf has anorexia, rapid respiration, or difficulty in walking. Not infrequently, the onset is sudden and the calf is treated for pneumonia prior to recognition of lymphomas.

Occasionally, ventral edema or precocious development of the udder is the principal complaint. At necropsy, the calf usually has generalized enlargement of lymph nodes and lymphocytic infiltration of most major organs.

Thymic lymphosarcoma, also not associated with BLV, could be confused with severe parasitism, which causes dependent edema of the brisket, dewlap, and submandibular region; traumatic pericarditis; and high-altitude disease.

Thymic lymphosarcoma usually occurs in cattle from 6 to 24 months of age. It is characterized by massive lymphocytic infiltration of the thymus, and thoracic lymph nodes may also be involved. It is frequently characterized by dyspnea, rapid respiration, distension of the jugular veins, muffled heart sound, ruminal tympany, cough, and subcutaneous edema in the brisket and dewlap, and sometimes the forelimbs and ventral abdominal walls.

Skin lymphosarcoma, which is also not a BLV infection, must be differentiated from insect bites, urticaria, mange, lumpy skin and pseudo lumpy skin disease, generalized papillomatosis, and hyperkeratosis.

Skin lymphosarcoma, one of the rarest of the bovine lymphosarcomas, usually appears in cattle 18 to 30 months of age. It is characterized by grayish-white, raised, circular nodules or plaques that are widely distributed over the entire body of the animal. The lesions may be observed first as slight hives over the neck and back. When numerous, they coalesce. They may be largely subcutaneous and smooth, or they may be irregularly shaped and protrude. The lesions tend to form scabs, are frequently friable, and tend to bleed easily. There may be generalized enlargement of superficial, and some internal, lymph nodes. Subcutaneous edema frequently develops.

The skin tumors may regress spontaneously but sometimes reappear or persist and affected cattle develop swellings of major lymph nodes, lymphocytosis, and lymphocytic infiltration of internal organs.

Laboratory Diagnosis

Laboratory diagnosis of AL is contingent upon histopathologic determination that tumor masses are indeed lymphosarcomas and that diffuse tissue changes are actually the result of lymphocytic infiltration. Determination of the lymphocytic nature of disease is aided by finding abnormally high total lymphocyte counts in blood, but this sign is frequently absent in histopathologically confirmed cases.

Identification of PL in individual cattle or herds suggests infection with BLV, but its absence does not indicate freedom from infection. Infection with BLV is best ascertained by serologic and virologic procedures.

Lymphocytosis may be transient or absent in BLV infections and is not a consistent diagnostic indicator. Thus absolute lymphocyte counts have limited diagnostic value. Almost all cattle with PL will be positive to serologic tests, but only approximately 30% of serologically positive cattle will have PL.

Animals with AL may have depressed enzyme levels and if there is bone marrow involvement (which is rare), they may be anemic.

Serologic tests including the virus neutralization, complement fixation, indirect fluorescent antibody assay, radioimmunoassay, and agar gel immunodiffusion tests were adapted for detecting BLV antibody during the 1970s. Although the radioimmunoassay system appears most sensitive, the agar gel immunodiffusion test with a glycoprotein portion of the viral envelope as the antigen (AGIDgp) is less expensive and is the most practical screening test. The AGIDgp test is used as a basis for cattle and semen to meet importation requirements. Test kits are commercially available.

The European Economic Community recommended that all laboratories studying BLV adopt the AGIDgp test for uniformity in discussions of antibody prevalence and its significance to control measures (Van Der Maaten and Miller 1979).

A positive serologic (AGIDgp) reaction indicates that the animal is persistently infected with BLV. It does not, however, imply that the animal is actively shedding BLV or that it has clinical disease. Because of the widespread prevalence of BLV infection detectable by AGIDgp tests, it is necessary to exercise caution in interpreting test results. On the other hand, when classic AL is diagnosed clinically and histopathologically, the affected animal is invariably AGIDgp positive. The vast majority of AGIDgp-positive cattle can be shown to be infected by virus isolation procedures.

BLV was first identified by EM visualization of type-C particles in cultured lymphocytes from lymphosarcomatous cattle (Miller et al. 1969). Since that first identification, a variety of techniques have evolved for identifying virus, which include syncytia-infectivity assay, immunofluorescence, and competitive radioimmunoassay. They require tissue culture techniques or elaborate labeling procedures and are superb research tools.

However, the high correlation between serology and infection suggests serologic procedures are practical and adequate under most circumstances. The Office International Des Epizooties (OIE) publishes the *Manual of Diagnostic Tests and Vaccines,* which details laboratory techniques for BLV (OIE 2000).

As regards specimens for the laboratory, serologic procedures require only clotted blood. Virus isolation and identification require buffy coat cells or other sources of lymphocytes. Persons anticipating virus isolation should contact the cooperating laboratory for specific instructions on the specimen and its collection, preservation, and transportation.

EPIDEMIOLOGY

The epidemiology involves assumptions that detectable antibody represents infection that is persistent, lifelong, and transmissible by blood; that AL and PL are uncommon consequences of BLV infection; and that calf, skin, and thymic forms are probably noncontagious and unrelated to BLV. The likelihood of exposure to BLV, the susceptibility to infection, and the nature of the consequences of infection are influenced by a variety of immunologic and environmental factors as well as the peculiarities of individual hosts. In addition, there may be some degree of genetic control over the susceptibility to BLV infection and the development of PL and AL.

The incubation period between exposure and appearance of detectable antibody usually ranges from 3 to 16 weeks (OIE 1996) depending on the test used and the inoculating dose.

Cattle are the natural reservoir of BLV and serve as the immediate source of infection for other susceptible cattle. Following infection, both virus and antibody without tumor-inhibiting or protective effects persist for prolonged periods and probably for life (Van Der Maaten and Miller 1990). Thus, equilibrium between BLV and cattle seems to be struck. If this equilibrium is upset, as manifested by tumor formation or lymphoproliferative activity, it probably represents intervention on the part of genetic, immunologic, or environmental determinants.

Sheep and goats can be infected naturally and experimentally with development of tumors. Significant transmission from these species to cattle is probably rare but could become a factor in countries that eradicate EBL from their cattle populations.

Transmission seems to require parenteral injection of lymphocytes, which are the host cells of BLV. Thus, mechanical transmission by insects, blood transfusion, and the use of common needles or surgical instruments can play a role (Van Der Maaten and Miller 1990). Clusters of cases among cattle vaccinated against cattle fever (piroplasmosis) by transfer of blood from donor cattle have been reported. Vertical transmission from dam to offspring has been demonstrated and may account for something less than 20% of new infections. BLV-infected leukocytes have been found in milk and colostrum, but nursing infected cows does not appear to be a major means of transmission, possibly because of interference by neutralizing antibody in colostrum. Semen does not appear to be a major means of transmission (Mecham and Monke 1999), although cattle can be infected by experimental uterine infusion of infected lymphocytes.

It appears that in dairy cattle, the prevalence of infection increases with age, and contact with infected adult cattle seems to be the major influencing factor. Infection rates are higher in dairy cattle than in beef cattle (Dargatz et al. 1998). This higher incidence may reflect opportunities for exposure rather than specific breed susceptibilities. The prevalence of infection varies tremendously between herds. In the United States, probably more than 20% of dairy cattle and around 10% of beef cattle are infected.

In the United States, antibody prevalences are higher in southern regions. Globally, prevalence of infection is usually higher in tropical than in temperate regions.

Transmission occurs slowly within herds unless there are vaccinations with common needles or other practices that transfer blood to susceptible cattle.

IMMUNITY

Almost all infected cattle develop antibody detectable within 3 to 9 weeks postinfection. The simultaneous presence of BLV and its antibody suggests that incomplete protection (if any) results. On the other hand, colostral antibody transferred to susceptible calves may confer a degree of resistance to infection for several months or as long as 9 months in extreme cases.

VIRUS PERSISTENCE

Persistent infection of blood leukocytes occurs in the presence of circulating antibody; once infected, cattle should be regarded as lifelong carriers.

PREVENTION AND CONTROL

For EBL, the usual management practices for controlling infectious diseases must be expanded beyond sanitation and extreme care in introducing cattle. Controlling BLV requires limitations on use of common needles for vaccination, and particularly for blood sampling. It also requires careful sterilization of surgical equipment (Roenfeldt 1997). Insect control may be of some value.

The problems inherent in introduction can be minimized by requiring all herd additions to be negative to two AGIDgp tests 16 weeks apart. Test-and-slaughter, test-and-segregate, and test-and-manage procedures are feasible options for control or eradication efforts (Evermann and DiGiacomo 1992).

Some degree of control can be achieved by restricting introductions to cattle from AGIDgp-negative herds and requiring certification thereof. Certification criteria for BLV-free herds include testing and segregation in addition to insect control and steps to prevent blood transfer (Miller and Mecham 1998). These steps include use of individual sterile needles, individual disposable obstetrical sleeves for pregnancy examinations and obstetrical procedures, and electrical rather than surgical dehorning procedures (Lein et al. 1996).

Currently no vaccines for BLV are available.

THERAPY AND MANAGEMENT OF OUTBREAKS

Lymphosarcomas are malignant, progressively fatal neoplasms for which no specific therapy is available. Affected cattle can be kept alive for short periods by good nursing care or surgery to relieve pressures of space-occupying lesions. Cows pregnant with valuable calves may be delivered by cesarean section, but the genetic aspects of BLV infection suggest that salvaging such calves may merely propagate genes determining susceptibility to both the infection and its clinical manifestations.

Once the infection is identified in a herd, it is necessary to undertake precautions against transmission via needles, surgical instruments, and hemorrhage-inducing pregnancy examination per rectum.

Vaccine studies indicate that successful vaccines may be forthcoming (Verwoerd and Tustin 1994).

LIKELIHOOD OF ERADICATION

Denmark, Germany and other European countries are attempting EBL control or eradication by slaughtering herds with infected animals and restricting import of cattle from such herds.

If nations judge BLV to be of adequate importance to indemnify owners, eradication could be achieved in temperate climates where insect populations are minimal and where cattle are housed in winter and available for testing with individual sterile needles. Eradication is feasible in such well-controlled areas by AGIDgp testing and immediate slaughter of infected herds. The lack of sensitivity of AGIDgp may require that other tests be employed as eradication is approached. In tropical regions with vast inaccessible cattle populations and uncontrolled cattle movement, such programs may not be economically and logistically feasible.

Standards for certification of BLV-free herds based on serologic testing and isolation procedures are outlined by the Committee on Bluetongue and Bovine Retroviruses of the United States Animal Health Association (Miller and Mecham 1998).

IMPACT ON INTERNATIONAL TRADE

EBL is an OIE List B disease. The International Animal Health Code (OIE 1997) states that countries or zones can be considered EBL-free if all lymphosarcoma-like tumors are reported and examined in approved laboratories, and if all herds of origin are tested and 99.8% of these herds are EBL free. To maintain EBL-free status, statistically based annual national serosurveys must reveal seroprevalences not greater than 0.2%. Importing EBL-free countries should accept cattle only from EBL-free areas or from EBL-free herds.

Several Scandinavian and western European nations are successfully eradicating EBL, and reject importation of cattle and bovine germ plasm from EBL-infected countries, including the United States. About 50 countries, some without infrastructure adequate to detect endemic BLV, impose EBL-based restrictions on US cattle.

There have been instances where US cattle met BLV seronegativity requirements of importing countries on departure and tested positive after arrival in the recipient territory. If tests on both ends were valid, such an event could be explained by TB or blood testing of assembled export candidates with common needles, rejecting BLV positives, and shipping seronegative animals, which became infected by blood inoculation and subsequently seroconverted.

PUBLIC RESPONSIBILITY

Cattle in known infected herds should be sold only with knowledge of the purchaser. Transmission of BLV, anaplasmosis, piroplasmosis, bovine immunodeficiency virus, and other diseases by blood transfer indicates new education programs are needed to reduce use of common needles, dehorners, and surgical instruments on cattle.

Despite common distant evolutionary ancestry for cattle and human cancer viruses, current information suggests that BLV is not oncogenic for humans (Van Der Maaten and Miller 1990). As new information on interspecies transmission of mammalian oncogenic viruses emerges, this contention must be reevaluated periodically.

AREAS IN NEED OF RESEARCH

Many questions regarding epidemiology, pathogenesis, and control require answers and complete understanding.

REFERENCES

Crocker BC, Rings DM, 1998. Lymphosarcoma of the frontal sinus and nasal passage in a cow. *J. Am. Vet. Med. Assoc.* 213:276–280.

Dargatz DA, Johnson R, Wells SJ, Kopral CA, 1998. Descriptive epidemiology of bovine leukosis virus in U.S. beef and dairy Cattle. *Proc. U.S. Anim. Health Assoc.* 102:120–123.

Evermann JF, DiGiacomo RF, 1992. Perspectives on the recognition and control of bovine leukemia virus infection. *Proc. U.S. Anim. Health Assoc.* 96:197–206.

Lein DH, Brunner MA, Dubovi EJ, 1996. Experiences with the New York State Bovine Leukosis Certification Plan. *Proc. U.S. Anim. Health Assoc.* 100:63–66.

Mecham JO, Monke DR, 1999. Report of the Committe on Bluetongue and Bovine Retroviruses. *Proc. U.S. Anim. Health Assoc.* 103:137–143.

Miller LD, Mecham JO, 1998. Report of the Committee on Bluetongue and Bovine Retroviruses. *Proc. U.S. Anim. Health Assoc.* 102:134–136.

Miller JM, Miller LD, Olson C, Gillette KG, 1969. Virus-like particles in phytohemagglutinin stimulated lymphocyte cultures with reference to bovine lymphosarcoma. *J. Natl. Cancer Inst.* 43:1297–1305.

OIE 2000. Enzootic bovine leukosis. Office International Des Epizooties (OIE) 2000. In *International Animal Health Code,* 8th ed. with annual updates. Paris: OIE, pp. 1–452.

Roenfeldt S, 1997. Stop BLV. *Dairy Herd Management.* August: 42–44.

Van Der Maaten MJ, Miller JM, 1990. Bovine leukosis virus. In *Infectious Diseases of Ruminants,* edited by Z Dinter, B Morein. Amsterdam: Elsevier Scientific Publishers, pp. 419–429.

Van Der Maaten MJ, Miller JM, 1979. Appraisal of control measures for bovine leukosis. J Am Vet Med. Assoc. 175:1287–1290.

Verwoerd DW, Tustin RC, 1994. Enzootic bovine leukosis. In *Infectious Diseases of Livestock With Special Reference to Southern Africa,* edited by JAW Coetzer, GR Thomson, RC Tustin. Capetown: Oxford University Press, pp. 778–792.

13

BOVINE VIRAL DIARRHEA

INTRODUCTION

Bovine viral diarrhea (BVD), caused by the bovine viral diarrhea virus (BVDV), a ubiquitous, easily transmitted pestivirus with worldwide distribution, was first recognized in the United States in herds with acute, sometimes fatal diarrhea and ulcerations of the alimentary mucosa (Olafson et al. 1946). Chronic cases were named mucosal disease (MD) and both terms were adopted and used interchangeably.

Over the years, extensive research has clarified some details about BVD and BVDV. Many questions remain, however, about the diversity of virulence and tissue trophisms among genotypes, biotypes, subtypes and strains and the pathogenesis and immunopathogenic pathways of the multiple associated clinical syndromes.

Until terminology changes, BVDV infections can be considered to cause two biologically distinct syndromes called acute BVD (ABVD) and MD. They may occur simultaneously in herds and can be difficult to distinguish clinically in individual animals.

ABVD results from primary BVDV infections of susceptible cattle. It is frequently nonclinical and usually mild but sometimes manifests as serious respiratory, intestinal, or thrombocytopenic disease and occasionally as fatal peracute cases. A significant consequence of ABVD is fetal infection, which causes abortions, congenital anomalies, and birth of persistently infected (PI) calves that perpetuate the disease by shedding large amounts of virus and that may eventually develop MD.

MD is the chronic usually fatal clinical syndrome appearing in young (and occasionally mature) PI cattle. It is characterized by fever, diarrhea, erosions in gastrointestinal mucosa, and death.

To help clarify discussions of the differential diagnosis of ABVD and MD the now defunct ambiguous collective terms "the mucosal diseases" and "the bovine mucosal disease complex" will not be used in this book. Instead, the term "diseases affecting bovine mucosa (DABM)" will designate the collection of infections that cause crusting of the muzzle and ulceration, erosion, vesiculation, necrosis, or hemorrhage in the bovine alimentary tract.

Although some countries are attempting eradication, in most places control is attempted by elimination of PI animals and vaccination.

BVD has been reviewed by Liess (1990), Bolin et al. (1996), and Murphy et al. (1999).

ETIOLOGY

BVDV, a small single-stranded RNA virus of the genus *Pestivirus* of the family Flaviviridae, occurs in two genotypes (BVDV-1 and BVDV-2) and in cytopathic and noncytopathic biotypes.

BVDV-1 and BVDV-2 can be distinguished by genetic analyses and have subtle immunological differences. BVD-1, the most studied genotype, was used in vaccines prior to application of gene-sequencing techniques. These techniques demonstrated the existence of virulent BVDV-2 strains that were associated with major bovine epizootics in the 1990s (Carman et al. 1998). Genetic analyses have demonstrated the tendency of BVDV subtypes and strains to mutate and recombine causing emergence of antigenically variant viruses.

The production of cytopathic effects (CPE) in cell cultures is a valuable laboratory marker that makes cytopathic BVDV (CBVDV) biotypes useful in diagnosis, research, or vaccine production. Noncytopathic BVDV (NCBVDV) biotypes are more common and give rise to CBVDV strains by mutation. NCBVDV requires indirect immunologic or genetic techniques for identification, sometimes coexists with CBVDV in animals and cultures, and has been incriminated in producing persistent infections and major ABVD outbreaks.

BVDV is antigenically related to the pestiviruses that cause hog cholera and border disease (hairy shaker disease) of sheep. It grows in swine, causing problems in hog cholera diagnosis and in sheep, goats, and deer, where it is of questionable clinical or epidemiological significance.

BVDV is present in high quantities in secretions and excretions of PI animals and to a lesser extent in discharges from acutely infected animals.

BVDV is a common contaminant of bovine fetal serums used in cell culture media and pharmaceutical and biological manufacture (Bolin and Ridpath 1998). Also, fetal serums frequently contain BVDV antibody.

BVDV is relatively unstable in the environment and has little resistance to disinfectants.

CLINICAL SIGNS AND LESIONS

In addition to MD, BVDV infections cause a wide range of manifestations including inapparent nonclinical infection or mild febrile disease with biphasic temperature elevation and leukopenia, and other syndromes including acute fatal hemorrhagic thrombocytopenia. Prenatal infections cause abortion and a variety of fetal disorders. Most postnatal infections with BVDV are nonclinical and unless they occur in epizootics, losses from them are usually sporadic.

When virulent BVDV strains infect totally susceptible or improperly immunized populations, however, the morbidity and mortality can be staggering (Carman et al. 1998). BVDV is also associated with bovine respiratory disease (Grooms 1998), and subclinical BVDV infections in feedlots may predispose to pulmonic pasteurellosis.

The clinical signs and lesions caused by BVDV will be discussed as syndromes that frequently coexist in nature and have overlapping diagnostic features.

Most primary BVDV infections of susceptible cattle are inapparent or mild and undiagnosed. When diagnostic efforts are initiated after clinical cases have been recognized in a herd, it sometimes becomes evident that normal-appearing herdmates are undergoing mild BVDV infections characterized by fever, leukopenia, and cough. They may also have sparsely scattered erosions of oral mucosa that may be unnoticed because they are small and few in number and because of the difficulty in examining the mouths of active cattle.

Inapparent infections or mild cases may be followed by abortions, birth of calves with congenital anomalies, or birth of PI animals.

Acute or peracute BVD resulting from primary BVDV infection is characterized by fever; leukopenia; diarrhea, which may be intractable; cough; rapid respirations; nasal and ocular discharge; oral erosions; and frequently death, which may be signaled by severe dehydration. There may be erosion and ulceration of the oral mucosa with gingivitis and salivation. Sometimes ulcers and erosions are widespread, coalescing to produce vast red areas devoid of superficial epithelium; they may also be sparse and unrecognized or appear as slight reddening of the tips of cheek papillae. Diarrhea is not always present. In totally susceptible populations, young and adult cattle can manifest similar syndromes. Clinical cases are frequently accompanied by milder cases or inapparent infections among contact cattle.

In the 1990s, there was renewed interest in ABVD when major outbreaks accompanied by respiratory signs, diarrhea, and abortions occurred in Canada and the United States due to primary infections with highly virulent BVDV-2 strains (Carman et al. 1998).

An acute or peracute fatal hemorrhagic thrombocytopenic syndrome characterized by fever, diarrhea, mucosal erosions, and petechial hemorrhages in the esophagus, rumen, and abomasum has occurred in naturally infected calves and mature cattle and was reproduced experimentally with BVDV-2 (Walz et al. 1999).

It has long been believed that BVDV plays a role in some (but not all) bovine respiratory disease (BRD) outbreaks. In some ABVD outbreaks—in which diarrhea and mucosal erosions are absent or unobserved, but in which fever, excessive nasal discharge, and rapid respirations are present—it appears to be a respiratory disease. When BVDV appears as a coinfection with other bovine viruses, including infectious bovine rhinotracheitis (IBR) and bovine respiratory syncytial virus (BRSV) with which it has a synergistic effect (Brodersen and Kelling 1998), it contributes to BRD. In feedlots and veal calf operations, immunosuppressive effects of BVDV may predispose to pulmonic pasteurellosis (Grooms 1998).

Classic systemic BVD can occur in calves exposed postnatally and in calves from dams exposed in late gestation (Lambert et al. 1969).

PI cattle with chronic BVD (also called MD) usually have a viremia acquired in utero and fail to develop detectable circulating antibody. This antibody deficit is due to specific immune tolerance; the animal's system fails to treat BVDV antigens as foreign because they were present and identified as self during development of the fetal immune system in midgestation. PI cattle excrete large quantities of virus and the early detection and removal of these cattle is crucial to control efforts.

Usually chronic PI animals are eventually recognized as "poor doers," with an unthrifty hair coat and a generally run-down appearance. Most eventually die or are culled from herds.

PI animals develop classical MD when they are superinfected with other BVDV biotypes (Bolin et al. 1985) and possibly via other mechanisms. MD may also develop as a sequel to subclinical or mild primary BVDV infections but current thinking tends to diminish this definition in favor of that of superinfection of PI animals.

MD cases may have continuous or intermittent diarrhea, nasal discharge, and sometimes a severely crusted muzzle. They frequently have excessive, persistent, clear ocular discharge, which drains anteroventrally from the medial canthus of each eye, forming a channel of cracked skin. If examined repeatedly, chronic MD cases can be seen to have oral necrosis and ulcerations, which heal rapidly and can recur.

Animals with MD may be lame because of chronic laminitis or severe interdigital necrosis with secondary bacterial infections. There is frequently reddening, swelling, and erosions or ulcerations of the skin around the coronary band. Hyperkeratosis and alopecia may be present, particularly on the neck.

ABVD, mild subclinical BVD, or MD occasionally follows vaccination. When these syndromes appear within a month of vaccination, modified live virus (MLV) vaccines may be blamed. The blame may or may not be justified because the problems may be preexistent but MLV may cause superinfection of PI animals with resultant MD (Bolin et al. 1985).

EFFECTS ON THE DEVELOPING FETUS

Insemination during BVDV viremia results in reduced conception rates (Dubovi 1994).

BVDV infection of pregnant susceptible cattle can be followed by birth of normal offspring or a wide range of abnormal pregnancy outcomes including abortion, stillbirths, mummified fetuses, calves born with various congenital defects, and PI calves that excrete BVDV for most of their lives.

Different BVDV strains may affect fetuses differently but the gestational age at the time of fetal infection and the virulence of infecting BVDV strains largely determine the pregnancy outcome. NCBVDV strains are more common and possibly more abortifacient; they are believed to be the major cause of PI animals.

In order for fetal infection to occur, the cow or heifer should be both pregnant and susceptible at the time she is infected. Vaccination does not ensure protection from fetal damage (Dubovi 1994). Fetal infection can occur in herds in which ABVD or MD is not recognized because maternal infections can be mild or undiagnosed and parturition can occur months after maternal exposure, infection, and antibody response.

The etiologic diagnosis of BVDV-induced fetal disease is retrospective and challenging. Abortion is more likely to occur if the dam is infected in the first trimester of gestation; it can probably result from some second-trimester infections as well.

BVDV-induced congenital defects can result from second-trimester fetal infections. They may include ocular disorders such as microphthalmia, cataracts, optic neuritis, and retinal degeneration. Neurologic defects are also possible, such as microencephaly, cerebellar hypoplasia, hydrocephalus, and hypomyelinogenesis. An array of other teratogenic defects including brachygnathia, thymic aplasia, alopecia, and pulmonary hypoplasia can occur as well (Dubovi 1994).

Experimentally BVDV causes a variety of congenital anomalies in lambs (Ward 1971).

NECROPSY FINDINGS

Cattle dead of MD are usually thin, severely dehydrated, and anemic. There is usually (but not always) evidence of severe diarrhea, and the animal frequently has a scruffy hair coat. The vulvar mucosa occasionally has erosions, and healing sores may be present at the mucocutaneous junction of the vulva. There is generally encrustation of the nasal orifices and evidence of persistent excessive lacrimation.

Although not always present, cardinal lesions include ulceration or erosion of the mucosa of the oral cavity and erosions arranged in linear arrays in the esophagus. Some cattle have erosions throughout the rumen, particularly on the mucosa of the rumen pillars. There is usually hemorrhage, necrosis, or lymphoid depletion of Peyer's patches. All these lesions may be absent, healed, or merely overlooked if small and few in number.

Aborted fetuses rarely have significant lesions, although the oral mucosa may have erosions.

Histopathologic lesions confirm the gross impressions of ulcerative lesions in the upper gastrointestinal tract, of hyperemia, erosion, ulceration, crypt epithelial necrosis in the intestines, and of lymphoid depletion in Peyer's patches.

Cattle dead from acute or peracute BVDV infections present similar lesions, but mucosal and intestinal lesions are less common in animals younger than 6 months old (Carman et al. 1998).

DIAGNOSIS

Clinical diagnosis, based on history, signs, and external lesions, should be supported by necropsy findings, testing of paired serums for neutralizing antibody, and viral isolation and identification.

ABVD usually produces mild or subclinical infections but may induce diarrhea, mucosal lesions, and death. Unless populations are totally susceptible to virulent BVDV strains, outbreaks usually involve a small percentage of animals in affected herds.

Herdmates may undergo mild infections characterized by coughing, fever, and leukopenia. Seroconversion usually results, and abortions or birth defects and birth of PI animals may result. A few animals survive ABVD to become chronically affected, but most chronic BVD and MD cases are probably PI animals.

BVDV-induced abortions are not diagnostically distinctive. Prenatal BVDV infections are suggested when the virus is isolated from fetal materials or when individual calves are born near term with developmental defects and pre-nursing serum antibody. Sometimes retrospective diagnoses of BVD are based on histories of undiagnosed illness in herds during the period when cows subsequently aborting or delivering anomalous calves would have been in midgestation.

A common cause of diagnostic error is failure to search the oral cavity for erosions that may be absent in sick cattle but present in the mouths of apparently healthy herdmates.

Clinicians should inquire about introduction of new cattle, which could be PI animals or possible contacts with Africa and Asia where rinderpest, which resembles acute BVD, exists.

Differential Diagnosis

When excess nasal and ocular discharge, crusted muzzle, or ulcers or erosions of the oral mucosa are observed, the differential diagnosis should include ingestion of caustic substances and all DABM. These DABM include diseases caused by BVDV (ABVD and MD), as well as malignant catarrhal fever (MCF), rinderpest, bovine papular stomatitis (BPS), IBR, bluetongue (BT), vesicular stomatitis (VS), and foot-and-mouth disease (FMD). Necropsy, virus isolations, and serology are necessary for definitive diagnoses.

Bovine MCF causes crusting of the muzzle and oral erosions. Although it may occur in multiple-case outbreaks, MCF is usually sporadic. It occurs in association with sheep or wild ruminants and is characterized by hyperemia of the oral and nasal mucosa, severe panophthalmia, and behavioral changes due to fatal encephalitis. Vasculitis and perivascular cuffing are seen on histologic examination of the brain.

Papular stomatitis, a mild poxvirus infection usually seen in calves, causes mouth lesions containing characteristic brown streaks and irregular edges that help distinguish them from BVD erosions. Occasionally these lesions are depressed but they are usually level or slightly elevated above the mucosal surface and have a sandpaper-like consistency when palpated. Papular stomatitis can be confirmed histologically by finding intracytoplasmic poxvirus inclusions. Papular stomatitis infections are usually nonclinical, and the lesions are noticed only if the oral mucosa is examined.

Rinderpest is enzootic in parts of Africa and Asia but exotic to North America, South America, and Europe. Although it is caused by an unrelated virus, this acute, devastating disease can be considered an exotic counterpart to ABVD because identical lesions occur.

Introduction of rinderpest virus into immunologically naive populations would be expected to result in high attack rates and rapid transmission. Rinderpest must be ruled out when diagnosing BVD because variations in virulence can occur with both viruses.

VS, which also affects swine and horses, causes rapidly rupturing vesicles on the oral mucosa, teats, and coronary bands. In cattle, these lesions may resemble the erosions of BVD, particularly if epithelial tags remaining from the vesicles have disappeared. When VS or FMD is suspected, it should be investigated by regulatory officials.

Bovine BT infections are usually inapparent but may rarely produce a clinical syndrome with symptoms similar to those of MD, with necrosis of the oral mucosa, crusting of the muzzle, and lameness. In these cases, diffuse necrosis of the oral mucosa and dental pad and drying and cracking of the skin suggestive of photosensitization may serve as clues for differentiating bovine BT from MD.

Acute *Salmonella* infections may cause profuse, intractable diarrhea in cattle. They can be differentiated from BVD by the lack of the characteristic oral lesions and the isolation of Salmonella from feces or tissues of infected animals.

Acute arsenic poisoning causes severe gastroenteritis and diarrhea and must be differentiated from ABVD.

Toxic indigestion and concomitant diarrhea resulting from rumen overload can be distinguished from ABVD by evidence of ingestion of large quantities of succulent feeds and the lack of such symptoms as mucosal erosions, fever, conjunctivitis, and nasal discharge.

ABVD can be diagnosed as a respiratory disease on the basis of elevated temperatures, nasal discharge, increased respiratory rate, and cough. Uncomplicated ABVD usually is not accompanied by pneumonia and pulmonic rales. If rales are heard, pulmonic pasteurellosis should be considered.

When ABVD manifests as a respiratory disorder, careful examination of the oral mucosa, gums, tongue, and hard palate of affected cattle and healthy herdmates may reveal oral erosions. The nasal mucosa must be carefully examined for the white fibrinous plaques of IBR. Paired serum specimens should be tested for antibody to BVD, IBR, VS, parainfluenza-3 (PI-3), BRSV, adeno-viruses, and respiratory coronaviruses.

Diagnosing BVDV as the cause of abortions is difficult. Abortions occur several weeks to several months after BVDV infections of pregnant cattle. By the time abortion occurs, serologic titers have stabilized and further rise cannot be detected. Serologic tests on aborted fetus sometimes reveal BVDV antibody indicating prenatal infection and suggesting BVD as a cause of abortion.

Diagnosis of congenital defects caused by infection of pregnant cattle around midgestation is less problematic, particularly if pre-nursing serum specimens are available. BVDV antibody in serums of calves that have not suckled indicates prenatal infection and a presumptive, but not guaranteed, diagnosis of BVDV as the etiologic agent of observed teratologic defects.

Laboratory Diagnosis

A profound leukopenia may be present in the early stages of infection. Total white blood cell counts return to normal levels several weeks after exposure. This event may occur before the illness is recognized, so normal levels or even leukocytosis may be present at the height of clinical signs. Profound leukopenia in early cases or in clinically normal herdmates helps support the diagnosis.

Other laboratory procedures include isolation of virus by inoculation of specimens into cell cultures and observation for cytopathic changes or procedures for identification of viral antigen. These involve staining suspect cultures or fixed tissues with fluorescein-conjugated antibody to detect the presence of BVDV antigen. Immunologic reagents developed for BVDV-1 are adequate to detect BVDV-2. Viral RNA can be detected using reverse transcriptase polymerase chain reactions (PCR).

Serologic diagnosis of BVD usually requires paired serum specimens. Because the prevalence of BVDV antibody in many bovine populations exceeds 50%, the detection of BVDV antibody in single serum specimens indicates only that the animal has been exposed or vaccinated. In most cases of fatal BVD, the animal dies before a second specimen is collected.

When patients survive or paired serums are available from herdmates, the detection of BVDV antibody in serum of cattle that were seronegative 3 weeks earlier is convincing evidence of BVDV infection. Significant rises in titer in a number of cattle in herds also suggest active BVDV infection, but serologic diagnosis is more convincing if changes from negative to positive between acute and convalescent serums are demonstrated. In cases of the respiratory form of the disease, concomitant serologic tests for other respiratory viruses should be done.

Serologic diagnosis is complicated by failure of PI animals to develop detectable serum antibody. Thus, the animals with the greatest epidemiologic significance are seronegative and can be identified only by virus isolation from serum or leukocyte suspensions. False-negative virus isolation attempts can occur in PI calves with colostrally acquired antibody or the rare PI animal that develops serum titers sufficient to neutralize virus in the specimen (Brock et al. 1998).

BVDV strains can be detected in tissue cultures inoculated with nasal discharge, ocular discharge, or the blood of sick animals or with specimens of spleen, lymph nodes, lungs, liver, or other tissues collected at necropsy. These procedures all require the prompt shipment of fresh, sterile specimens to laboratories that have agreed to study them.

Serums should be collected as aseptically and early as possible from suspected cases and some apparently normal contact cattle. A second serum specimen collected 2 to 3 weeks later is needed to demonstrate seroconversion.

EPIDEMIOLOGY

BVDV is endemic globally. Its ease of transmission, high antibody prevalence, irregular incubation periods, frequency of inapparent or undiagnosed infections, and the presence of PI animals make it an epidemiologically complex virus.

Experimentally, the first evidence of infection occurs within a few days of primary exposure when the first of two febrile peaks and leukopenia occur. Mucosal erosions or diarrhea may occur within 3 to 8 days of exposure, but frequently they are not evident for several weeks. In the field, there may be an interval of several weeks to several months between the observed onset of disease among cattle in close contact. This pattern suggests unique transmission requirements or prolonged incubation periods or that some signs and lesions may require superinfections or immunopathogenic mechanisms.

PI cattle, which excrete virus in high concentrations and acutely infected cattle (which excrete smaller amounts) are principal reservoirs and major sources of infection. While BVDV also infects swine, sheep, deer, and other wild ruminants, these hosts are probably less significant than PI cattle in transmission and perpetuation of BVDV.

Cow-to-cow contact probably explains most transmission. Infection can be carried from farm to farm by people directly contacting infected cattle, but it is more likely to be introduced by PI cattle that are efficient spreaders.

When susceptible populations are initially exposed to virulent BVDV strains, animals of all ages become infected and may develop clinical disease, the severity of which is modulated by serum antibody.

In endemic areas, the preponderance of clinical cases among young cattle (between 4 and 24 months of age) probably reflects high antibody prevalences among adult cattle and temporary benefits of colostrally acquired antibody in young calves rather than actual age-related susceptibilities.

There does not appear to be any unique distribution of BVDV infection or clinical manifestations between breeds and sexes except that fetal infections occur only from exposure of pregnant females.

Infection spreads quickly among susceptible cattle in close contact, but the appearance of clinical signs is protracted by the irregular incubation period and the variable intervals between maternal infection and abortion or birth of anomalous or PI calves.

IMMUNITY

Questions remain about the role of immunity in controlling BVDV infections and the potential contributions of immune responses to the pathogenesis of its syndromes and lesions. These questions involve the solidarity and duration of natural, vaccine-induced and colostrally acquired strain-specific immunity and cross protection and the roles of BVDV-induced immune tolerance and immunosuppression.

A simplified summary of BVDV immunology suggests the following. Unexposed and unvaccinated susceptible cattle usually develop BVDV strain-specific serum antibody that is detectable by numerous tests within 8 to 10 days of primary infection whether clinical signs are evident or not. Although they do not protect against infection, circulating actively induced antibody levels probably afford protection against serious clinical manifestations from homologous and antigenically related BVDV strains.

Although they are usually protected from clinical disease, actively immunized animals can become infected and, if pregnant, fetal infections and their numerous sequelae may follow. Depending on the gestational age at exposure, fetuses infected in utero can be born as antibody-negative PI animals with strain-specific immune tolerance (Liess 1990) or with strain-specific active immunity that is detectable by tests on serums collected before nursing.

Colostrally acquired passive antibody capable of modulating the outcome of exposure or vaccination appears in the serum of calves that absorb strain-specific immunoglobulins in colostrum on the first day of life. These passive antibody levels decline because of metabolic degradation and are undetectable by 2 to 11 months of age.

The rate of disappearance of colostrally acquired passive antibody is consistent. The age at which depletion occurs, however, varies from calf to calf depending on initial serum levels. Colostrally acquired antibody levels in calves are determined by the titer in the dam's colostrum, the amount of colostrum ingested, and the efficiency of absorption of each calf's digestive tract. In most calves it has probably dissipated by 6 months of age.

Humoral neutralizing antibody, whether actively or passively acquired, affords variable protection from disease caused by antigenically related strains and is a major factor in limiting the spread of BVDV within herds; this protective value is probably less upon exposure to antigenically heterogeneous strains. Cattle with low levels of humoral antibody (particularly colostrally acquired antibody levels approaching extinction) can be infected and stimulated to produce active antibody. Low antibody levels can be overcome by challenge with virulent virus strains and some vaccines. High levels of serum antibody generally indicate protection against homologous virus strains and possibly neutralize the effects of MLV vaccines.

Lack of detectable antibody in infected cattle has been associated with PI, prolonged viremia, chronic unthriftiness, and altered responsiveness of humoral lymphocytes. Failure of individual susceptible cattle to produce antibody when infected may result from fetally acquired immune tolerance or from immune suppression.

The presence of PI cattle and immigration of new susceptibles perpetuates the virus in populations and stimulates herd immunity.

VIRUS PERSISTENCE

PI animals resulting from in utero infections play a major role in the epidemiology and clinical manifestations of BVDV.

PREVENTION AND CONTROL

Under most farm conditions, attempts to maintain a "closed herd" have proven inadequate to prevent infection with BVDV. Thus preventive measures are largely based on identification and removal of PI animals or vaccines.

Identification of PI animals can be based on clinical suggestions that are usually not evident until the entire herd is infected. Thus, additions should be screened by virus isolation procedures before they are commingled with herds. Virus isolation from entire herds becomes impractical so a sample of blood specimens or bulk tank milk samples (Renshaw et al. 2000) can be screened for virus as an initial herd strategy.

MLV vaccines for BVD were first introduced in the late 1950s and have undergone numerous modifications over the years. They are widely used in combination with other vaccines.

Successful immunization requires that vaccinated cattle be infected with vaccine virus and respond with production of humoral antibody. Because of their abortifacient properties, many MLV vaccines are not approved for pregnant animals. If used prior to pregnancy, some may induce resistance adequate to prevent fetal infection and BVD-associated abortion in cattle exposed during pregnancy.

To avoid interference by colostrally acquired antibody, the MLV vaccine should be administered after 6 months of age. Although vaccine administered before that age can successfully immunize seronegative calves and some calves with waning antibody titers, animals initially vaccinated before 6 months should be revaccinated.

The duration-of-immunity issue is clouded by the frequent natural infection of both vaccinated and unvaccinated cattle.

Aside from contraindications for pregnant cattle, another safety concern associated with MLV BVD vaccines has been the development of postvaccination MD. This condition, resembling either ABVD or MD, appears within weeks of vaccination and is frequently blamed on vaccines. Some so-called postvaccination disease is probably natural disease occurring in cattle already infected at the time of vaccination or superinfection of PI animals with MLV vaccine viruses.

A suggested conservative approach to BVD vaccination is that MLV vaccination should be reserved for healthy, unstressed cattle with the intent of providing protection against future catastrophic episodes. This approach cautions against use of MLV vaccine in pregnant, sick, exposed, recently assembled, or stressed cattle. For breeding herds, heifers can be vaccinated after 6 months of age and before the first breeding.

Inactivated vaccines are safer but necessitate two initial doses; revaccination is required at least annually.

All vaccines should be used strictly according to the manufacturer's instructions.

THERAPY AND MANAGEMENT OF OUTBREAKS

Once overt clinical signs or fetal wastage is observed, the infection is usually well established in individuals and herds. MD cases usually succumb. Although fluid therapy, antibiotics, and antidiarrheals are used, fatal outcomes are not greatly influenced by therapy or supportive measures. Blood transfusions from seropositive cattle may produce temporary improvement but when they are discontinued, transfused patients often relapse and die.

Mild ABVD cases may appear to be helped by antibiotics to control secondary infection.

When BVD is recognized in herds, owners should be apprised of the grim prognosis. The outlook should include predictions that pregnant animals may abort or produce calves with congenital anomalies. Owners should be made aware that intervals between the appearance of new cases is sometimes several months, that severely affected cattle frequently die regardless of therapy, and that recovered cattle may be unthrifty and unprofitable.

The question of vaccination after a diagnosis is established in herds or feedlots must be evaluated in light of several considerations. These factors include the fact that vaccine use is contraindicated for pregnant cattle, that there may be diagnostic uncertainties, and the likelihood that entire herds are already exposed and incubating the infection. Also important to consider are existing stress levels, the effects of restraint, the cost of vaccine and vaccination, and the fact that introduction of vaccine viruses may preclude the opportunity to make a diagnosis. These considerations must be balanced with herd health philosophies of veterinarians and herders and people's tendency to regard diseases occurring after vaccination as iatrogenic.

LIKELIHOOD OF ERADICATION

Several factors complicate the possibility of eradicating BVDV: the virus is ubiquitous and easily transmitted. Also, the fact that the infection is frequently inapparent and the presence of PI animals and nonbovine hosts make BVDV eradication feasible only for regions with well-financed national animal health infrastructures. Such regions must have strict border controls, outstanding diagnostic capacity, effective monitoring surveillance and reporting systems, and accessible cattle populations.

IMPACT ON INTERNATIONAL TRADE

BVD is categorized as a List B disease by the Office International Des Epizooties (OIE). Because it is regarded as globally ubiquitous, countries imposing BVD-based trade measures should be prepared to demonstrate the presence of nationally controlled bona fide eradication programs.

PUBLIC RESPONSIBILITY

As far as is known, human infection does not occur. Clinicians suspecting BVD are obligated to consider the possibility of rinderpest, to use professional judgment in vaccination decisions, and to present a thoughtful, candid prognosis.

AREAS IN NEED OF RESEARCH

Details about BVD and BVDV are gradually emerging, but there are gaps in understanding of the pathogenesis of the multiple clinical syndromes BVDV appears to cause. Also in need of further study are the complex immunopathogenic pathways by which these syndromes are manifested. There is also need to understand, through genetic characterization, the basis of the diversity of virulence and tissue trophisms among genotypes, biotypes, subtypes, and strains of BVDV and how they emerge, coexist, combine, recombine, and mutate under environmental and immunologic pressures.

In addition, the names of the disease and its etiological agent need revision to conform to current viral nomenclature and to properly emphasize the multitude of syndromes BVDV causes in addition to diarrhea and mucosal erosions. There is need to elaborate the immunosuppressive effects (if any) of field and vaccine BVDV strains and the immunologic responses of cattle to the virus.

REFERENCES

Bolin SR, Ridpath JF, 1998. Presence of bovine viral diarrhea virus genotypes and antibody against those viral genotypes in fetal bovine serum. *J. Diag. Invest.* 10:135–139.

Bolin S, Brownlie J, Donis R, Dubovi E, Tremblay R, 1996. Proceedings of an international symposium. *Bovine Viral Diarrhea Virus: A 50-Year Review.* Ithaca, NY: Cornell University College of Veterinary Medicine. June 23–25 1996, pp. 1–210.

Bolin SR, McClurkin AW, Cutlip RC, Coria MF, 1985. Severe clinical disease induced in cattle persistently infected with noncytopathic bovine virus diarrhea virus by superinfection with cytopathic bovine virus diarrhea virus. *Am. J. Vet. Res.* 46: 573–576.

Brock KV, Grooms DL, Ridpath J, Bolin SR, 1998. Changes in levels of viremia in cattle persistently infected with bovine viral diarrhea virus. *J. Vet. Diagn. Invest.* 10:22–26.

Brodersen BW, Kelling CL, 1998. Effect of concurrent experimentally induced bovine respiratory syncytial virus and bovine viral diarrhea virus infection on respiratory and enteric diseases in calves. *Am. J. Vet. Res.* 59:1423–1430.

Carman S, van Dreumel T, Ridpath J, Hazlett M, Alves D, Dubovi E, Tremblay R, Bolin S, Godkin A, Anderson N, 1998. Severe acute bovine viral diarrhea in Ontario, 1993–1995. *J. Diagn. Invest.* 10:27–35.

Dubovi EJ, 1994. Impact of bovine viral diarrhea virus on reproductive performance in cattle. *Vet. Clin. North. Am.: Food Animal Practice.* 10(3):503–514.

Grooms, DL, 1998. Role of bovine viral diarrhea virus in the bovine respiratory disease complex. *Bovine Practitioner* May (32):7–12.

Lambert G, Fernelius AL, Cheville NF, 1969. Experimental bovine viral diarrhea in neonatal calves. *J. Am. Vet. Med. Assoc.* 154:181–189.

Liess B, 1990. Bovine viral diarrhea virus. In *Infectious Diseases of Ruminants,* edited by Z Dinter, B Morein. Amsterdam: Elsevier Scientific Publishers, pp. 247–256.

Murphy FA, Gibbs EPJ, Horzinek MC, Studdert MJ, 1999. Bovine viral diarrhea. In *Veterinary Virology,* 3rd ed. San Diego: Academic Press, PP. 563–566.

Olafson P, MacCullum, AD, Fox FH, 1946. An apparently new transmissible disease of cattle. *Cornell Vet* 36:205–213.

Renshaw R, Ray R, Dubovi EJ, 2000. Comparison of virus isolation and reverse transcriptase polymerase chain reaction assay for detection of bovine viral diarrhea virus in bulk milk tank samples. *J. Diagn. Invest.* 12:184–186.

Walz PH, Bell TG, Steficek BA, Kaiser L, Maes RK, Baker JC, 1999. Experimental model of type II bovine viral diarrhea virus-induced thrombocytopenia in neonatal calves. *J. Vet. Diagn. Invest.* 11:505–514.

Ward GM, 1971. Experimental infection of pregnant sheep with bovine viral diarrhea-mucosal disease. *Cornell Vet* 61:179–191.

14

CORONAVIRUSES

INTRODUCTION

Bovine coronaviruses (BCV) have been associated with neonatal calf diarrhea (NCD), bovine winter dysentery (BWD), and bovine respiratory disease (BRD).

While subtle antigenic differences occur among isolates, the BCV associated with various clinical syndromes are virtually identical.

BCV are globally ubiquitous and present in feces and nasal discharges of acutely infected animals and possibly some carrier cattle. Isolates are sometimes identified by the anatomic system of their origin, as enteric BCV (EBCV) or respiratory BCV (RBCV) (Lin et al. 1997).

BCV have been reviewed by Pensaert and Callebaut (1994) and Mebus (1990).

ETIOLOGY

BCV, first isolated in 1971 (Mebus et al. 1973) and once called the Nebraska calf diarrhea virus, is now known to have global distribution (Espinasse et al. 1990). BCV are classified in the genus *Coronavirus* in the family Coronaviridae.

Coronaviruses occur in a variety of avian and mammalian species and are abundant in nature.

The crown-like appearance of the organism gives coronavirus its name. Its form derives from club-like, pear-shaped, or petal-shaped projections that radiate outward from the lipid-containing envelope; the result is a halo surrounding the central RNA core.

BCV replicate, after adaptation, in the cytoplasm of a number of cell lines and organ cultures (Pensaert and Callebaut 1994). Their cytopathic effect (CPE) is largely syncytial in nature; it is inconsistent and frequently not evident on primary isolation. Most BCV require adaptation to a given cell line before CPE is a useful marker. A human rectal tumor cell line, which is highly susceptible to RBCV infection, may expedite studies to further elaborate their role in bovine respiratory disease (BRD) (Storz et al. 2000).

Viral antigen can be identified immunologically, by electron microscopy (EM), or by the appearance of syncytia in cultures.

Bovine isolates cause hemagglutination and hemadsorption of red blood cells of chickens and rodents. Most BCV are closely related antigenically (Hasoksuz et al. 1999).

BCV have been convincingly implicated in NCD, and strongly associated with BRD and BWD (Smith et al. 1998).

While strong evidence implicates EBCV as a primary cause of BWD, there remain lingering beliefs that *Campylobacter jejuni,* enteroviruses, adenoviruses, reoviruses, chlamydia, bovine viral diarrhea (BVD), Bredavirus, parainfluenza-3 virus, and perhaps other agents may play a role in its etiology (Espinasse et al. 1990).

CLINICAL SIGNS AND LESIONS

NCD of various etiologies causes high mortality on dairy farms, cow-calf ranches, and veal-raising operations. EBCV infect the absorptive epithelium of the gut and contribute to these losses. After a two- to three-day incubation period, calves develop acute diarrhea with normal or slightly elevated temperatures. The feces may be liquid in consistency and may contain coagulated milk or mucus.

The diarrhea may persist for 5 or 6 days, and affected calves may remain alert or they may die (Mebus 1978). Weakness, depression, lethargy, severe dehydration, and hypovolemic shock precede death. The diarrhea probably results from villous atrophy in small-intestine mucosa and consequent malabsorption and loss of intestinal activity (Mebus 1978).

Clinically, BCV infection cannot be distinguished from other causes of neonatal diarrhea. A laboratory diagnosis can be obtained by identifying the virus in feces or tissue sections using electron microscopy or various virologic procedures.

Immunodeficiency, failure to ingest colostrum, secondary bacterial infection, and multiple viruses and parasites undoubtedly contribute to the NCD syndrome. These influences are not always essential to the pathogenesis of NCD, because EBCV can produce diarrhea experimentally without presence of bacteria.

BCV have been isolated from the feces of cattle with BWD (Benefield and Saif 1990). BWD is an acute diarrhea characterized by loose, occasionally bloody feces with a characteristic fetid or musty odor. The infection occurs in closely housed, immature and adult cattle. Affected cattle may occasionally cough, causing forceful expulsion of feces.

As the name implies, BWD usually occurs in late fall, winter, or early spring, frequently after abrupt weather changes. It spreads rapidly from animal to animal with a 2- to 6-day incubation period and from farm to farm frequently in association with movement of people or use of common equipment for handling feed and manure.

Recovery usually occurs within three to six days, and abortion is not a sequel. Although temporary weight loss may occur, deaths are rare and usually attributable to concomitant or preexisting life-threatening conditions. Major losses arise from decreased milk production. BWD is usually diagnosed clinically by this classic profile.

When appropriate cell cultures are used, BCV can be isolated from feedlot cattle with mild or moderate BRD (Storz et al. 1996). Thus, RBCV must be considered in the multifactorial etiology of BRD (Storz et al. 2000).

EFFECTS ON THE DEVELOPING FETUS

To date, BCV infection of pregnant cattle and its effect (if any) on the developing fetus have not been elucidated.

NECROPSY FINDINGS

Necropsy findings in BCV infections are generally limited, nonspecific, and of minimal value in determining a specific etiologic diagnosis.

In studies on NCD, no gross lesions except for a bowel and small intestine distended with liquid feces, were usually found in experimental infections (Mebus 1978). In the field, calves dying with NCD and its complications may show signs of severe dehydration, and their rear parts may be splattered with feces. They are usually emaciated, and there is serious atrophy of depot fat. The intestine may be distended with liquid, and mucoid fecal casts may be present in the colon. There may be pulmonary congestion and pneumonia, but these findings are usually considered secondary.

Histopathologic lesions consist of severe shortening and atrophy of villi in the small intestine. This effect results from degeneration and detachment of villous epithelium and its replacement with immature epithelial cells.

Electron microscopic examination of experimentally infected calves indicates that virus replication occurs in the cytoplasm of the adsorptive intestinal epithelial cells and in some cells in the lamina propria (Storz et al. 1978).

Unless the disease is complicated by other life-threatening conditions, deaths from BWD are rare and patients are usually not necropsied.

Fatal BRD cases have variable lesions depending on the nature of the primary and secondary infections involved. RBCV infections may cause necrosis of nasal and tracheal epithelium.

DIAGNOSIS

BCV must be considered in the differential diagnosis of NCD, BWD, and BRD. The role of BCV in these syndromes must be confirmed by laboratory tests.

DIFFERENTIAL DIAGNOSIS

A diagnosis of undifferentiated NCD can be based on clinical signs. A specific etiologic diagnosis of EBCV infection requires laboratory procedures. The differential diagnosis of BCV-induced NCD includes dietary gastroenteritis, bacterial diarrhea, rotaviral diarrhea, bovine viral diarrhea (BVD), and many other infections. Most cases probably have multifactorial etiology.

The differential diagnosis of BWD in adult cattle includes BVD, acute salmonellosis, and various toxic and dietary disorders. Determining the specific etiology of outbreaks requires virologic and bacteriologic studies. Unless research or foreign animal disease investigations are involved, laboratory work is rarely undertaken. The mildness of the condition and its classic clinical profile usually make it unnecessary.

BCV should be included in the differential diagnosis of BRD along with infectious bovine rhinotracheitis, BVD, bovine respiratory syncytial virus, bovine parainfluenza-3 virus, and pasteurellosis. Like NCD and BWD, the determination of the role of BCV in BRD requires laboratory confirmation.

Laboratory Diagnosis

RBCV can be isolated from nasal swabs from cattle with BRD.

BCV can be identified in specimens of gut wall by immunofluorescent microscopy or thin-section immunoelectron microscopy. The small intestine or midsection of the spiral colon is frequently chosen for examination.

In feces, virus can be detected by immunoelectron microscopy and enzyme-linked immunsorbent assay (ELISA) (Pensaert and Callebaut 1994).

Humoral serum antibody is detectable by serum neutralization tests in cell cultures or hemagglutination inhibition tests. Rising titers are, however, difficult to detect in field cases.

Specimens for detection of BCV or their antigens include nasal, colonic, or small intestinal epithelium.

BCV can be found in feces by electron microscopy and special concentration procedures on fresh frozen feces collected immediately after onset of diarrhea. Carcasses necropsied within 4 hours of death are useful for fecal examination or for viewing gut sections by immunofluorescent microscopy.

The principal clinicopathologic finding in NCD is dehydration resulting from loss of water, bicarbonate, sodium chloride, and potassium in feces. The dehydration causes hemoconcentration, acidosis, serious electrolyte imbalance, and sometimes hypoglycemia.

EPIDEMIOLOGY

BCV have worldwide distribution in cattle and water buffalo (Pensaert and Callebaut 1994).

It appears that infected cows and calves are the reservoir and immediate source of infection, that virus escapes in feces and nasal secretions, and that infection occurs via ingestion.

The exact influence of age on the outcome of infections remains to be elaborated, but it appears that primary infection of neonates is most significant clinically, and infection of mature animals is frequently nonclinical except when conditions favor BCV-induced BWD.

IMMUNITY

The nature of the bovine immune response to BCV infections and the role of immunity in preventing disease need further study. In the case of NCD, humoral antibody does not necessarily protect against infection of the intestinal epithelium, but colostrally acquired antibody in the gut may afford partial protection for a few days (Mebus 1978). Animals infected as neonates may be reinfected later in life, and such reinfections may partly explain viral persistence in herds.

VIRUS PERSISTENCE

Recurrent infections occur, (Heckert et al. 1990) and some carrier animals may exist (Mebus 1990).

PREVENTION AND CONTROL

Prevention of all NCD, BWD, or BRD will probably never be accomplished. For NCD, the role of management and sanitation cannot be overemphasized, but even the best-managed calving operations can have serious outbreaks with high mortality. Calves have the best chance of survival if parturition occurs in clean areas, the cow's vulva and udder are scrubbed and disinfected, and colostrum is provided immediately.

If it is determined that BCV is present in a herd, cows should be vaccinated during pregnancy, and oral vaccination of newborn calves with modified live rotavirus-coronavirus vaccine should be initiated.

Calfhood vaccination, which should be accomplished immediately after birth to ensure maximum vaccine effectiveness, is sometimes difficult logistically. The presence of an attendant at birth can increase survival rates by instituting hygienic measures for the cow, the calf, and the premises. The benefits of clearing the calf's airways, disinfecting its navel, and ensuring intake of colostrum can be great.

Prevention of winter dysentery requires biosecurity measures that exclude visitors from contact with cattle and their feed and demands strict sanitary practices by inseminators and veterinarians who must contact animals in their work. Manure-handling equipment must not contact feed. While inconsistent, observations indicate a degree of herd immunity lasting two to three years follows BWD outbreaks.

Prevention of RBCV infections requires cautious addition of new cattle and isolation of purchased additions for three to four weeks prior to contact with the herd.

A modified live virus (MLV) vaccine, propagated in bovine kidney cells and administered orally to calves as soon as possible after birth, can successfully reduce morbidity and mortality in herds infected with BCV.

The combined rotavirus-coronavirus vaccine may be used on pregnant cattle to stimulate colostral antibody levels. If possible, the calf should nurse or be force-fed colostrum; its presence in the gut lumen can have considerable protective effect. Because of the multifactorial etiology of neonatal diarrhea, the vaccine cannot be regarded as a panacea.

THERAPY AND MANAGEMENT OF OUTBREAKS

Therapy for BCV infections is based on the clinical syndrome present. Therapy for BWD and BRD is less crucial than treatment for NCD, which requires prompt initiation of measures to control dehydration and secondary bacterial infections and maintain normal electrolyte balance.

Prevention requires a combination of hygienic calving conditions, assurance that newborn calves receive first-day colostrum, sanitary calf-rearing practices, and use of a modified live virus (MLV) vaccine on pregnant cattle and newborn calves.

Participating variables important in neonatal calf diarrhea include diet, management, sanitation, environmental temperature and humidity, stress, bacteria, and viruses. Different cases probably result from differing etiologic combinations of these factors.

Therapy of calf diarrhea and concomitant bacterial infections is usually similar, regardless of the etiology. These measures must be instituted before laboratory diagnosis is available. Dehydration should be corrected, milk feeding replaced with electrolyte solution, and antidiarrheal drugs and antibiotics administered orally and systemically.

The wisdom of indiscriminate antibiotic therapy is questioned on the basis of cost effectiveness and the fact that antibiotics need to be specific to the bacteria contributing to the disease. Also of concern are antibiotic residues in veal, the possible development of antibiotic-resistant bacterial strains, alteration of normal intestinal bacterial flora, and possible negative effects on the outcome of the disease. When severe dehydration and depression are present, intravenous fluid therapy is required.

Successful treatment requires early recognition of diarrhea and prompt initiation of electrolyte transfusions, correcting management deficiencies that permit transmission of infection to stressed or colostrum-deprived calves, and initiation of prompt, successful therapeutic and preventive measures including vaccination.

A specific etiologic diagnosis of EBCV-induced NCD or even the suspicion of one in a herd is an indication to immediately initiate programs for hygienic calving and collection and delivery of colostrum on the day of parturition. Extreme sanitary measures for rearing calves should be instituted, and vaccination of newborn calves and pregnant cattle should be considered. Vaccination, however, is no panacea and will not replace good management practices.

LIKELIHOOD OF ERADICATION

The ubiquitousness of BCV in cattle populations suggests that eradication is unlikely. Thus, BCV-induced NCD, BWD, and BRD, and their complications will continue to plague dairy and cattle farmers.

IMPACT ON INTERNATIONAL TRADE

BCV infections are not categorized as List A or List B diseases by the Office International Des Epizooties, and countries do not impose BCV-based import measures.

PUBLIC RESPONSIBILITY

Individuals addressing NCD and other BCV-induced diseases should make all possible efforts to obtain laboratory assistance in determining the specific etiology of the problem. Also, owners must be advised of the role of biosecurity in controlling BWD and BRD. For NCD control, stress control, sanitation, good management, and colostrum feeding are essential for minimizing calf losses. Vaccination should be employed where indicated, but there is an obligation to point out that vaccine alone will not eliminate all NCD and BWD.

AREAS IN NEED OF RESEARCH

Epidemiologic and laboratory research is needed to clarify the mechanisms of immunity and resistance to BCV infections and to explore possibilities of carrier states or persistent latent infections.

REFERENCES

Benefield DA, Saif LJ, 1990. Cell culture propagation of a coronavirus isolated from cows with winter dysentery. *J Clinical Microbiol* 28:1454–1457.

Espinasse J, Savey M, Viso M, 1990. Winter dysentery of adult cattle. In *Infectious Diseases of Ruminants,* edited by Z Dinter, B Morein. Amsterdam: Elsevier Scientific Publishers, pp. 301–307.

Hasoksuz M, Lathrop SL, Gadfield KL, Saif LJ, 1999. Isolation of bovine respiratory coronaviruses from feedlot cattle and comparison of their biological and antigenic properties with bovine enteric coronaviruses. *Am J Vet Res* 60:1227–1233.

Heckert RA, Saif LJ, Hoblet KH, Agnes AG, 1990. A longitudinal study of bovine coronavirus enteric and respiratory infections in two dairy herds in Ohio. *Vet Microbiol* 22:187–201.

Lin X, O'Reilly KL, Storz J, 1997. Infection of polarized epithelial cells with enteric and respiratory tract bovine coronaviruses and release of viral progeny. *Am J Vet Res* 58:1120–1124.

Mebus CA, 1978. Pathogenesis of coronaviral infection in calves. *J Am Vet Med Assoc* 173:631–632.

Mebus CA, 1990. Neonatal calf diarrhea virus. In *Infectious Diseases of Ruminants,* edited by Z Dinter, B Morein. Amsterdam: Elsevier Scientific Publishers, pp. 297–300.

Mebus, CA, Newman, LE, and Stair, EL. 1975. Scanning electron, light, and immuno-fluorescent microscopy of intestine of a gnotobiotic calf infected with calf diar-rheal coronavirus. *Am J Vet Res* 36:1719–1725.

Mebus CA, Stair EL, Rhodes MB, Tweihaus MJ, 1973. Neonatal calf diarrhea: propa-gation, attenuation, and characteristics of a coronavirus-like agent. *Am J Vet Res* 34:145–150.

Pensaert MB, Callebaut P, 1994. Bovine coronavirus infection. In *Infectious Diseases of Livestock With Special Reference to Southern Africa,* edited by JAW Coetzer, GR Thomson, RC Tustin. Capetown: Oxford University Press. pp. 878–883.

Smith DR, Fedorka-Gray PJ, Mohan R, Brock KV, Wittum TE, Morely PS, Hoblet KH, Saif LJ, 1998. Epidemiologic herd-level agents and risk factors for winter dysen-tery in dairy cattle. *Am J Vet Res* 59:994–1001.

Storz J, Doughri AM, Hajer I, 1978. Coronaviral morphogenesis and ultrastructural changes in intestinal infections of calves. *J Am Vet Med Assoc* 173:633–635.

Storz J, Stine L, Liem A, Anderson GA, 1996. Coronavirus isolation from nasal swab samples from cattle with signs of respiratory tract disease after shipping. *J Am Vet Med Assoc* 208:1452–1455.

Storz J, Purdy CW, Lin X, Burrell M, Traux RE, Briggs RE, Frank GH, Loan RW, 2000. Isolation of respiratory coronavirus, other cytocidal viruses, and *Pasteurella* spp from cattle involved in two natural outbreaks of shipping fever. *J Am Vet Med Assoc* 216:1599–1604.

15

ENTEROVIRUSES

INTRODUCTION

The emergence of cell culture technology in the 1940s and 1950s led to isolation of hundreds of antigenically variable cytopathogenic bovine enteroviruses (BEV) from the gastrointestinal, respiratory, and reproductive tracts of both healthy and sick cattle and aborted fetuses. Occasional evidence suggests that certain BEV serotypes may be pathogenic.

Despite their ability to cause systemic and gastrointestinal infections of cattle, however, they rarely produce overt clinical disease. The large variety of BEV isolates and the difficulty of experimentally producing clinical disease have discouraged detailed study of their pathogenesis, epidemiology, and control.

BEV have worldwide distribution and are ubiquitous among cattle populations. The importance of BEV hinges on questions about their possible role (if any) in the etiology of idiopathic abortion, infertility, respiratory disease, and neonatal and adult diarrhea. Isolation of BEV can cause confusion in diagnosis of other conditions, and there is always a possibility (however remote) of emergence of pathogenic variants. BEV have been reviewed by Knowles and Mann (1990).

ETIOLOGY

Members of the genus *Enterovirus* are small RNA viruses in the family Picornaviridae that contain some important animal viruses including foot-and-mouth disease and swine vesicular disease. Enteroviruses have worldwide distribution and infect most animal species.

The genus *Enterovirus* is subdivided serologically and by species of origin. Among human enteroviruses, poliovirus, coxsackieviruses, and echoviruses are pathogens. BEV by comparison, are relatively nonpathogenic and may lack nucleotide sequences essential for pathogenicity.

Enteroviruses are resistant to ether, chloroform, and many common disinfectants. They are distinguished from *Rhinoviruses* (another genus of Picornaviridae) by their acid resistance, which permits them to survive in the gastrointestinal tract and in frozen and refrigerated meats.

Enteroviruses are readily isolated from feces and bodily secretions. They are easily identified in a variety of cell cultures by their rapidly developing cytopathic effects (CPE), which can be neutralized by virus-specific antiserums.

Early efforts to classify enteroviruses by neutralization tests were complicated by serologic cross-reactions between viruses and by acquisition of antigenic characteristics of cell cultures in which the viruses were grown. The fact that aggregation of viral particles provides protection from antibodies was another complication (Melnick 1996). Ultimately the genus *Enterovirus* and the family Picornaviridae may be completely reclassified on genetic data derived from amino acid sequencing (Rodrigo and Dopazo 1995).

Over the years, hundreds of BEV, probably all of common ancestry (Urakawa and Shingu 1987), have been isolated from sick and healthy cattle.

Neutralization and hemagglutination tests with antiserums raised in different species of laboratory animals have been used to distinguish among BEV isolates (Dunne et al. 1974). These tests provided the basis for several proposed classification schemes suggesting slightly conflicting BEV serogroups (Knowles and Barnett 1985; Knowles and Mann 1990; and Urakawa and Shingu 1987).

Some isolates were designated enteric cytopathogenic bovine orphan (ECBO) viruses (Klein and Early 1957), because they appeared to be viruses in search of a parent disease. This name has lost favor.

CLINICAL SIGNS AND LESIONS

Most BEV isolates come from feces, pharyngeal washings, or nasal secretions of normal cattle. Many BEV, however, have been isolated from cattle experiencing a gamut of clinical signs including respiratory signs, enteric signs (Andersen and Scott 1976), ocular signs, and reproductive signs (Huck and Cartwright 1964).

Experimental BEV infections produced variable results. A few strains appear to cause mild clinical signs, but most cause only seroconversion indicating infection. A few experimental BEV inoculations have resulted in diarrhea. However, most indications suggest BEV are fellow travelers rather than causes of disease.

EFFECTS ON THE DEVELOPING FETUS

BEV have been isolated from aborted fetuses and antibodies against several BEV serotypes have been found in aborted fetuses (Dunne et al. 1973). While this finding indicates fetal infection and suggests a possible role in fetal disease, BEV have not achieved status as important causes of bovine abortion.

NECROPSY FINDINGS

No specific necropsy findings are associated with BEV.

DIAGNOSIS

Without clearly delineated clinical signs, there is no distinct diagnostic profile, and clinical diagnosis of BEV infections is not possible. These agents are sometimes incriminated etiologically if they are the only microorganisms recovered from sick cattle. They have been found, however, in association with such a wide variety of conditions and other disease-producing agents that they are generally regarded as incidental findings.

Differential Diagnosis

In animals the lack of disease manifestations precludes development of a differential diagnosis. In cell cultures, where BEV are commonly observed, they must be differentiated from a variety of cytopathogenic agents. Differentiation is accomplished by neutralization tests and other immunological procedures.

Laboratory Diagnosis

Infection with BEV is diagnosed by isolation of viruses from fecal material, rectal swabs, nasal swabs, esophageal-pharyngeal fluids, or other specimens. Isolations are conducted in cell cultures, and CPE is the initial indicator of the presence of virus. Cytopathogenic agents replicating on subsequent cell culture passages are identified as BEV by neutralization tests with specific antiserums.

EPIDEMIOLOGY

BEV are globally ubiquitous in normal, healthy animals. They are acquired by ingestion, survive and multiply in the gastrointestinal tract, and are excreted in feces and in nasal and ocular discharges.

There is high prevalence of BEV-neutralizing antibodies in healthy cattle, and antibodies that cross-react with BEV are found in a variety of domestic and wild ruminants, equines, monkeys, and dogs (Knowles and Mann 1990). This evidence suggests inter-and-intra-species transmission, which is probably assisted by the survival of the viruses in manure, their resistance to acid conditions in the gastrointestinal tract, and their stability in the presence of environmental influences that inactivate less vigorous viruses.

IMMUNITY

Infection is usually inapparent and is followed by production of specific neutralizing antibodies that probably vary in duration, quality, and in their roles in resistance and recovery from infection. When maternal infection is systemic, BEV can infect fetuses, which, if immunocompetent, produce serum antibodies that can be detected before nursing.

Because BEV antibodies are present in the serum and colostrum of many healthy cows, antibody is found in the serum of many newborn calves that have nursed. The protective value of colostrally acquired antibody is uncertain.

The dependence upon neutralization tests for identification and classification of BEV causes some confusion because some BEV-neutralizing activity can be found in the serums of most animal species. Cattle infected with some BEV serotypes have neutralizing antibodies that can cross-react with some serotypes of foot-and-mouth disease virus (Scott and Cottral 1967; Andersen 1978).

Conversely cattle serums sometimes contain neutralizing activity against human coxsackieviruses, enteroviruses, and poliovirus (Rovozzo et al. 1965). Human enteroviruses contain nucleotide sequences different from those of BEV (McNally et al. 1994). At one time BEV were hypothesized to have a role in the epidemiology of human poliomyelitis, but that theory did not survive vigorous investigation and has been discarded.

VIRUS PERSISTENCE

The frequent isolation of BEV from feces of normal cattle suggests that BEV may be normal, persistent resident flora of the bovine alimentary tract. They are invasive enough to access the immune system and stimulate production of circulating antibodies, but they lack the pathogenic capacity to produce significant disease.

PREVENTION AND CONTROL

Aside from hygienic measures and precautions against introduction of new cattle into herds, there are no specific preventive measures for BEV.

Nonetheless, despite their questionable economic significance, BEV must be kept in mind because they are frequent contaminants of cell cultures used for diagnostic purposes or vaccine development. In addition, their rapidly developing CPE results in frequent isolations that can confuse diagnostic procedures. Furthermore, with the pressures of changing ecosystems, some BEV could ultimately emerge as pathogens. Vaccine development has not been initiated to date.

THERAPY AND MANAGEMENT OF OUTBREAKS

BEV infections are largely inapparent and unrecognized. Other than symptomatic treatment and good nursing care, no specific recommendations for handling individual cattle or herds infected with BEV can be presented. Because of the uncertainty of the pathogenic potential of BEV, all efforts should be made to determine the actual etiology of clinical episodes before incriminating BEV as causative factors.

LIKELIHOOD OF ERADICATION

Attempts to eradicate BEV are unlikely because of the multiplicity of serotypes, their global ubiquitousness, their questionable pathogenicity, and the sparse knowledge about their epidemiology.

IMPACT ON INTERNATIONAL TRADE

BEV are not considered important enough to be categorized as a List A or List B disease by the Office International Des Epizooties and are unlikely to impact international trade.

PUBLIC RESPONSIBILITY

There is no evidence that BEV are pathogenic to humans. There are no precautions or actions in the public interest that are unique to BEV.

AREAS IN NEED OF RESEARCH

Research on BEV is hindered by the multiplicity of cross-reacting serotypes found in cattle and other species. Nevertheless, much research is needed to clarify the taxonomy, epidemiology, and immunology of BEV and to develop improved procedures to study their pathogenic potential.

REFERENCES

Andersen AA, 1978. Cross-reaction between bovine enterovirus and South African territories foot-and-mouth disease virus. *Am. J. Vet. Res.* 39:59–63.

Andersen AA, Scott FW, 1976. Serological comparison of French WD-42 enterovirus isolate with bovine winter dysentery in New York State. *Cornell Vet* 66:232–239.

Dunne HW, Ajinkya SM, Bubash GR, Griel LC Jr, 1973. Parainfluenza-3 and bovine enteroviruses as possible important causative factors in bovine abortion. *Am. J. Vet. Res.* 34:1121–1126.

Dunne HW, Huang CM, Lin WJ, 1974. Bovine enteroviruses. *J. Am. Vet. Med. Assoc.* 164:290.

Huck RA, Cartwright SF, 1964. Isolation and classification of viruses from cattle during outbreaks of mucosal or respiratory disease and from herds with reproductive disorders. *J. Comp. Pathol.* 74:346–365.

Klein M, Early E, 1957. The isolation of enteric cytopathogenic bovine orphan (ECBO) viruses from calves. *Bacteriol. Proc.* 57:73.

Knowles NJ, Barnett ITR, 1985. A serological classification of bovine enteroviruses. *Arch. Virol.* 83:141–155.

Knowles NJ, Mann JA, 1990. Bovine Enteroviruses In *Infectious Diseases of Ruminants,* edited by Z Dinter, B Morein. Amsterdam: Elsevier Scientific Publishers, pp. 513–516.

McNally RMP, Earle JAP, McIlhatton M, Hoey EM, Martin SJ, 1994. The nucleotide sequence of the 5' non-coding and capsid coding genomic regions of two bovine enterovirus strains. *Arch. Viro.* 139:287–299.

Melnick, JL, 1996. My role in the discovery and classification of the enteroviruses. *Ann. Rev. Microbiol.* 50:1–24.

Rodrigo MJ, Dopazo J, 1995. Evolutionary analysis of the picornavirus family. *J. Mol. Evol.* 40:362–371.

Rovozzo GC, Luginbuhl RE, Helmboldt CF, 1965. Bovine enteric cytopathogenic viruses. I. Characteristics of three prototype strains. *Cornell Vet* 55:121–130.

Scott FW, Cottral GE, 1967. Comparison of strains of bovine enterovirus with foot-and-mouth disease virus. *Am. J. Vet. Res.* 28:1597–1600.

Urakawa T, Shingu M, 1987. Studies on the classification of bovine enteroviruses. *Microbiol. Immunol.* 31:771–778.

16

FIBROPAPILLOMATOSIS (WARTS) AND PAPILLOMAVIRUSES

INTRODUCTION

Cutaneous fibropapillomas (cattle warts) are benign, self-limiting, hairless cutaneous neoplasms caused by bovine papillomaviruses (BPV). They are transmitted by direct or indirect contact and are ubiquitous in cattle populations throughout the world. In addition to causing fibropapillomas that involve fibrinous tissue, BPV are also involved in malignant transformations by cellular and biochemical cofactors to produce carcinomas of the skin, reproductive or urinary tract mucosa, and possibly the cornea.

Because of their viral etiology, warts are an infectious disease subject to regulatory measures; their presence may cause rejection of cattle proposed for show or export. Their spread can be minimized by management practices and to some extent by vaccines.

Bovine papillomaviruses and the syndromes they cause have been summarized by Olson (1990), Bastianello and Thomson (1994) and Campo (1997).

ETIOLOGY

BPV, DNA viruses of the genus *Papillomavirus* in the family Papovaviridae have long been known to cause cattle warts. Their study has been hindered by their failure to grow in cell cultures. Viral assays usually have required animal inoculations. With advancing molecular technology, an ever-increasing array of clinical syndromes have been associated with BPV infections.

The papillomaviruses are highly resistant to desiccation, disinfectants, and environmental influences. They are relatively host-specific and designated according to their natural host species in which they produce tumors in both cutaneous and mucosal epithelium. Some intraspecies transmission can be accomplished experimentally.

BPV are immunologically distinct from the papillomaviruses of other species. While over 70 types of human papillomaviruses are associated with various human neoplasms, only six distinct BPV have been identified to date. Most BPV strains are similar antigenically but they can be distinguished by molecular technologies.

BPV are tentatively classified into two major groups on the basis of genomic similarities and standard taxonomic properties of isolates and biologic characteristics of the tumors induced.

Group A viruses (bovine fibropapillomaviruses) are somewhat larger than group B BPV and induce neoplasms of both connective tissue and epithelium. Group B (epitheliotropic bovine papillomaviruses) induce epithelial neoplasms (papillomas) without fibroblast proliferation. BPV are further differentiated serologically and by DNA hybridization into six types with distinct characteristics (Jarrett et al. 1980). Over time, more types may be identified. Multiple BPV types can be present in the same animal and sometimes in the same lesion.

Group A BPV, which includes BPV-1, BPV-2 (frequently discussed together), and BPV-5, are fibroblast transformers producing usually benign, self-limiting cutaneous lesions. BPV-1 produces classic self-limiting pedunculated warts on the teats and penile fibropapillomas. BPV-2 produces pedunculated warts on both hair-covered body parts and on the teats and has been associated with enzootic bovine hematuria and equine sarcoid. BPV-5 causes rice-grain warts of the teats and udder.

Group B BPV produce mucosal lesions without fibroblast involvement; they have the potential to evolve into malignant tumors of epithelium (carcinomas) if appropriate carcinogens and immunosuppressive factors are present. Group B includes BPV-3, BPV-4, and BPV-6.

BPV-3 was first described in Australia. It is immunologically distinct from BPV-1 and BPV-2 and induces persistent nonpedunculated, flat, nonregressive warts, which lack a fibromatous component and affect adult as well as young cattle.

BPV-4 is associated with papillomas and sarcomas of the mouth, esophagus, and upper and lower gastrointestinal tract among cattle grazing on bracken fern.

BPV-6 causes nonpedunculated branch-like frond teat lesions. It is genetically distinct from BPV-1 and BPV-2 and more closely related to BPV-3 and BPV-4.

CLINICAL SIGNS AND LESIONS

In addition to classic bovine skin warts and several types of warts on bovine teats, BPV have been linked etiologically with other syndromes.

Classic cattle warts are transmissible fibropapillomatous growths, usually hairless and gray colored, that generally appear on the skin of young cattle several months after entrance of BPV-1 or BPV-2, through abrasions. They usually regress in several months without impairing function. They vary from pinhead size to several inches in diameter. They are generally narrower at the base (pedunculated) and may have a horny consistency. They vary in number from single growths to several hundred per animal. They occur most commonly around the face (sometimes on the eyelids), head, and neck. Sometimes they persist for a year or more but rarely progress to malignancy and rarely cause significant economic losses.

Persistent cutaneous papillomas are nonfibrinous squamous wart-like lesions that are nonpedunculated, flatter than classic warts, and may coalesce to cover large areas of skin on any part of the body. They develop in occasional individual animals in certain herds, particularly those infected with BPV-3. These lesions can become generalized and cover much of the body, and they may persist into adulthood. They cause economic loss due to hide damage and exclusion from sale, shows or export. When extensive, they usually result in culling of affected animals.

Bovine teat warts, caused by BPV-1, BPV-2, BPV-5, or BPV-6, occur on the teats of milking cattle, which may be infected simultaneously with several BPV types. Teat warts usually differ in shape and appearance from those seen on hair-covered areas of the skin. They can be nonpedunculated, whitish-colored benign nodules called rice-grain warts due to BPV-5, long filamentous frond warts due to BPV-6, or pedunculated warts associated with BPV-1 and BPV-2.

Teat warts are usually innocuous unless they are unusually large, cause bleeding, or are associated with secondary infection with bacteria or other viruses such as pseudocowpox or bovine herpes mammillitis. Lesions on the teat ends can injure the teat canal and predispose to mastitis.

Penile fibropapillomas are classic bovine warts caused by BPV-1 that attach to the penile mucosa and can be transmitted to vulvar skin or vaginal mucosa during breeding. They can cause problems in young bulls on range or in bull studs. They are difficult to manage because of the vascularity of the glans penis where they usually attach (McEntee 1950) and sometimes they interfere with breeding or semen collection. Spread to females does not occur in herds using artificial insemination.

Warts occasionally appear on the eyelids or corneoscleral junction and may serve as one precursor of squamous cell carcinomas of the eye (cancer eye). However, to date extensive efforts have failed to establish firm etiologic links between BPV and cancer eye (Rutten et al. 1992)

Enzootic hematuria, accompanied by BPV-2-induced carcinoma of the bladder, occurs in specific ecosystems in western Scotland and Brazil and has been reported in Colombia, Japan, Turkey, India, Kenya, the United States, and elsewhere. It is associated with prolonged grazing on bracken fern (*Pteridum aquilinum*), which apparently contains immunosuppressive and carcinogenic factors. Affected animals lose blood through hemorrhage into the urinary bladder and may also have carcinomas of the esophagus, rumen, and intestines associated with BPV-4. They become anorexic, lose weight and condition, and may succumb. Enzootic hematuria probably results from chronic consumption of low levels of bracken fern, as ingestion of massive amounts can produce acute bracken fern toxicosis.

BPV-1 and BPV-2 genomes are found in lesions of equine cutaneous sarcoid. They appear to have an etiologic role in this nonregressive, invasive, ulcerous neoplasm of horses that often resembles proud flesh, the exuberant granulation tissue that appears at equine wound sites. Currently this is the sole example of apparent trans-species transmission of BPV.

Bovine fibropapillomatous digital dermatitis (foot warts) has yet to be convincingly associated with BPV. This disease, so named because of a histologic resemblance to viral papillomas, produces a painful interdigital lesion and lameness. It is an ever-increasing problem in large dairies worldwide.

It appears to have multifactorial etiology with bacteria and spirochetes playing a major role. Read and Walker (1998) suggested renaming it papillomatous digital dermatitis to reflect its infectious nature as well as its papillomatous (but not fibropapillomatous) appearance. The necrotic nature of this lesion and the highly contaminated environment in which it thrives, along with the medicines and disinfectants applied to it, tend to reduce the diagnostic value of specimens and confuse efforts to elaborate its etiology. Nonetheless, molecular studies may eventually identify BPV genetic material in these lesions.

EFFECTS ON THE DEVELOPING FETUS

BPV are not generally regarded as causing fetal infections.

NECROPSY FINDINGS

Warts are nonfatal and necropsy is rarely done. Wart-like growths are occasionally found in the esophagus, rumen, and bladder. They should be examined histologically for similarities to BPV-4-induced lesions to distinguish from papular stomatitis or lesions of other diseases affecting bovine mucosa (DABM).

Histopathologically, bovine warts differ from infectious cutaneous papillomas of most species, which are generally solely a hyperplasia of dermal epithelium. In cattle, BPV involves a connective-tissue response and a dermal fibroplasia. Thus, bovine warts are correctly named fibropapillomas (Cheville and Olson 1964). The fibromatous component is more prominent in lesions of the reproductive tract and in the lesions seen following intradermal inoculation (Pulley et al. 1974). It is less prominent or absent in atypical and persistent lesions.

Inclusion bodies are absent in fibropapillomas. This helps distinguish fibropapillomas from bovine papular stomatitis or pseudocowpox lesions.

Viral particles can be seen by electron microscopy in the nucleus of cells in the stratum corneum, stratum spinosum, and stratum granulosum (Pulley et al. 1974).

DIAGNOSIS

Classic cases are readily diagnosed clinically by their characteristic appearance and location. Atypical lesions, persistent lesions, or unusual situations may require histopathologic examination and may be of suitable interest to warrant serologic or virologic studies.

Differential Diagnosis

BPV infections of the teats must be distinguished from the poxvirus infections of the teats (Chapter 23) and from trauma, photosensitization, bluetongue, malignant catarrhal fever, cowpox and pseudocowpox, foot-and-mouth disease, and vesicular stomatitis. Careful physical examination and thorough history together with histopathologic examinations of specimens taken for biopsy and virologic and serologic tests are usually needed for an etiologic diagnosis.

BPV infections of the skin must be distinguished from pseudo lumpy skin disease, true lumpy skin disease, malignant catarrhal fever, sporotrichosis, the skin form of lymphosarcoma, mange, insect bites, and urticaria of allergic origin.

When the oral mucosa of nursing calves or growing cattle is involved, DABM (see Chapter 13) must be considered.

Laboratory Diagnosis

Serology for BPV is used mainly as a research tool or used for investigation of unusual cases. Variable results have been experienced with neutralization, complement fixation, and agar gel precipitin tests. These tests are not done routinely in diagnostic laboratories, and special arrangements must be made.

For histopathologic examination, a lesion fixed in Bouin's fixative, 10% formalin, or the fixative of the pathologist's choice is appropriate. If possible, normal surrounding tissue should be included with specimens collected for biopsy.

EPIDEMIOLOGY

The distribution of the infection and lesions in populations resembles that of an easily transmitted infection with a long incubation period and a moderate degree of immunity.

The interval between exposure and appearance of observable lesions depends on the method, dosage, and route of exposure. Under natural conditions, the incubation period can range from 1 to 6 months.

Cattle are regarded as the reservoir and usual source of infection. A variety of fomites, however, can serve as intermediate sources of infection for cutaneous lesions. The likelihood of transmission is increased if contaminated objects have sharp edges capable of causing abrasions.

Transmission of BPV occurs via direct contact with infected animals or via indirect contact with contaminated tack, fences, stall boards, and stanchions. Hypodermic needles, dehorning, tagging, tattooing, or other instruments can also transmit the BPV (Pulley et al. 1974). In nature, the virus enters through skin, and most successful transmissions require an abrasion at the site of exposure that subsequently becomes the site of the lesion.

Transmission to nursing calves via teat lesions and transmission via breeding and rectal exams can also occur (Bastianello and Thomson 1994). Congenital cutaneous papillomatosis has been reported (Desrochers et al. 1994). Transmission by biting insects may occur rarely.

Cutaneous fibropapillomatosis is most common in calves. Lesions are rarely seen before 3 months of age and are usually gone by the time cattle are two years old. Persistent cutaneous papillomas occur in cattle of all ages, as do most other conditions associated with BPV.

Warts and other BPV infections occur in both sexes and all breeds.

IMMUNITY

Cattle respond immunologically to infection with BPV. The humoral component of this response is measured by serological tests in cattle and laboratory animals. Repeated inoculations of BPV result in resistance to infection. Occasionally, infected cattle experience reinfection. Precipitating antibody can be found in the serum of most naturally occurring and experimental cases (Koller and Olson 1972).

It is speculated that immune reactions are implicated in rejection of warts; rejection probably involves mechanisms different from those involved in protection against infection. Duncan et al. (1975) suggested that a deficiency in the cell-mediated component of the immune system may be associated with some cases of generalized persistent papillomatosis.

VIRUS PERSISTENCE

Viral particles are present in papillomas and both persistent and latent BPV infections probably occur (Campo et al. 1994). The mechanisms of viral persistence or of latent infections, which can be reactivated by immunosuppressive factors, stress, or physical trauma, are unknown.

PREVENTION AND CONTROL

Although enzootic hematuria, penile fibropapillomatosis, and foot warts are serious problems, the usually benign nature of most uncomplicated BPV infections precludes major concern over their prevention and control. There is some disagreement over the practicality of excluding cattle with a few warts from shows, because BPV are regarded as ubiquitous.

Spread can be minimized by isolation of affected calves, by management procedures that minimize opportunities for direct and indirect transmission, and by excluding carcinogenic cofactors such as bracken fern.

Commercial wart vaccines used repeatedly as directed yield variable results possibly due to BPV type specificity and probably have little value for cattle that are already affected. Because of the self-limiting nature of the lesions, however, the therapeutic value of vaccines in inducing tumor rejection is difficult to evaluate. Clinical studies with sub-unit BPV vaccines that may eventually have application in both human and veterinary medicine are underway (Campo 1997).

THERAPY AND MANAGEMENT OF OUTBREAKS

Therapy and outbreak management depends on the clinical signs and location of BPV-induced lesions.

In simple, uncomplicated cutaneous fibropapillomatosis (classic warts), the lesions regress spontaneously and no treatment is required. The self-limiting nature of human warts has promulgated the myth that certain mystically endowed individuals (wart-witches) can cast a curative spell, the occasional failure of which is attributed to the nonbelieving nature of skeptical patients.

In cattle, castor oil, cod liver oil, olive oil, or healing and soothing ointments or lotions are sometimes used. Surgical removal can be achieved with pedunculated warts, and many times hemorrhage is minimized by rapidly twisting them off rather than using cutting instruments. There is an old adage that surgical removal of one cutaneous wart stimulates rejection of others on the same animal. This and other treatments are difficult to evaluate with a self-limiting disease.

When cutaneous warts are observed, any sharp edges in the environment should be eliminated to minimize transmission, and care should be taken to avoid common use of ropes, tack, needles and surgical equipment. Commercial wart vaccines or autogenous bacterins prepared from suspensions of ground warts taken from affected animals on the same premises may have some prophylactic utility.

Most cattle owners regard conventional warts as a nuisance but of little economic significance. In show herds or in cattle with great value for sale or export, they can be a concern. In such situations, affected animals can be separated, efforts can be made to reduce direct and indirect transmission, and unaffected stock can be vaccinated.

Generalized and persistent cutaneous papillomas usually fail to respond to treatment. Surgical removal of multiple or flat, broad-based lesions is possible with exceptionally valuable cattle (Desrochers et al. 1994) but is usually impractical.

Enzootic hematuria can be minimized by excluding cattle from bracken fern infested pastures or by pasture improvements to eliminate bracken fern.

LIKELIHOOD OF ERADICATION

The ubiquitousness and multiplicity of BPV virus types as well as the lack of a simple test to detect asymptomatic infected cattle makes eradication appear unreasonable at this time.

IMPACT ON INTERNATIONAL TRADE

The Office International Des Epizooties (OIE) has not categorized BPV as List A or List B diseases, and freedom from BPV is rarely specified in certifications for international exchange of cattle. Most health certificates, however, require certification that transported animals are free of infectious or contagious diseases. Thus, cattle with warts are best not shipped or sent to livestock shows without special permission.

PUBLIC RESPONSIBILITY

Transmission to humans has not been demonstrated. Nevertheless, people with AIDS, chronic skin problems, or those undergoing immunosuppressive therapeutic regimens should probably avoid direct contact with warts or other bovine skin lesions. Introduction of affected cattle into herds that have never had warts should be avoided.

AREAS IN NEED OF RESEARCH

Further studies are needed on immunity to BPV. There is also need to elaborate the immunologic or other factors associated with persistent and generalized distribution of lesions. Molecular research on the relationship of papillomaviruses to neoplasms of all species will continue to elucidate the mechanisms of cancer and aid efforts to develop effective preventive and therapeutic vaccines to assist in the rejection of human papillomavirus-induced neoplasms (Campo 1997).

REFERENCES

Bastianello SS, Thomson GR, 1994. Papillomavirus infections. In *Infectious Diseases of Livestock With Special Reference to Southern Africa,* edited by JAW Coetzer, GR Thomson, RC Tustin. Capetown: Oxford University Press, pp. 804–809.

Campo MS, 1997. Review: Bovine papillomaviruses and cancer. *Vet. J.* 154:175–188.

Campo MS, Jarrett WFH, O'Neil W, Barron RJ, 1994. Latent bovine papillomavirus infection in cattle. *Res. Vet. Science* 56:151–157.

Cheville NF, Olson C, 1964. Epithelial and fibroblastic proliferation in bovine cutaneous papillomatosis. *Pathol. Vet.* 1:248–257.

Desrochers A, St-Jean G, Kennedy GA, 1994. Congenital cutaneous papillomatous in a one-year-old Holstein. *Can. Vet. J.* 35:646–647.

Duncan JR, Corbeil LB, Davies DH, Schultz RD, Whitlock RH, 1975. Persistent papillomatosis associated with immunodeficiency. *Cornell Vet* 65:205–211.

Jarrett WHF, McNeal PE, Laird HM, O'Neal J, Murphy J, Campo MS, and Moar MH, 1980. Papilloma viruses in benign and malignant tumors of cattle. *Proc. Cold Spring Harbor Conference on Cell Proliferation* 7:215–222.

Koller LD, Olson C, 1972. Observations on antigen-antibody complex in bovine papillomatosis. *Am. J. Vet. Res.* 33:317–321.

McEntee K, 1950. Fibropapillomas on the external genitalia of cattle. *Cornell Vet* 40:304–312.

Olson C, 1990. Papillomaviruses. In *Infectious Diseases of Ruminants,* edited by Z Dinter, B Morein. Amsterdam: Elsevier Scientific Publishers, pp. 189–200.

Pulley LT, Shively JN, Pawlicki JJ, 1974. An outbreak of cutaneous fibropapillomas following dehorning. *Cornell Vet* 64:427–434.

Read DH, Walker RL, 1998. Papillomatous digital dermatitis in California dairy cattle: clinical and gross pathologic findings. *J. Vet. Diagn. Invest.* 10:67–76.

Rutten VPMG, Klein WR, De Jong MAC, Quint W, Den Otter W, Ruitenberg EJ, Melchers WJG, 1992. Search for bovine papilloma virus DNA in bovine ocular squamous cell carcinoma (BOSCC) and BOSCC-derived cell lines. *Am. J. Vet. Res.* 53: 1477–1481.

17

HERPES MAMMILLITIS AND PSEUDO LUMPY SKIN DISEASE

INTRODUCTION

Bovine herpes mammillitis (BHM) and pseudo lumpy skin disease (PLSD) are syndromes produced by bovine herpesvirus-2 (BHV-2). They differ in severity, geographic distribution, probable mode of transmission, as well as location of lesions on individual animals.

BHM is manifested clinically as ulceration of the skin of the teats and udder and PLSD is a generalized skin disease.

BHM and PLSD were reviewed by Barnard (1994) and Martin (1990).

ETIOLOGY

The etiologic agent, BHV-2, is classified in the genus *Simplexvirus* in the family Herpetoviridae. BHV-2 was first isolated in Africa (Anderson et al. 1953). Antigenically and genetically, it is more closely related to herpes simplex, the human cold sore virus, than are the other herpesviruses that infect cattle. It has been speculated that BHV-2 may have descended from primates rather than from ungulates (Ehlers et al. 1999).

Over the years, BHV-2 and the diseases it causes have had other names. Today it is assumed that the Allerton virus causing pseudo lumpy skin disease in South Africa; the bovine dermatotrophic herpesvirus studied in the United States (Dardiri and Stone 1972); and the virus causing skin gangrene of the bovine udder, bovine ulcerative mammillitis and herpes mammillitis in Britain (Martin 1973) are similar and probably identical.

Serologic surveys indicate widespread inapparent infections in Europe, North America, Africa, and Australia (Gibbs and Rweyemamu 1977).

Many questions remain about pathogenesis and transmission but it is known that in vivo replication of BHV-2 is enhanced by lowered temperatures (Letchworth and Carmicheal 1984).

Many cell cultures support replication of BHV-2, which induces cytopathic effects (CPE), with foci of degenerative rounded and clumped cells, syncytia, and intranuclear inclusion bodies. Primary isolation may require 2 to 3 blind passages, but once adapted to cell cultures, BHV-2 causes rapid CPE, which can be neutralized by convalescent serums.

BHV-2 is sensitive to organic solvents, and iodophor (and to a lesser extent chlorine-based) disinfectants, but it is somewhat resistant to environmental influences.

CLINICAL SIGNS AND LESIONS

BHM and PLSD occasionally occur simultaneously but for the most part they can be regarded as separate syndromes resulting from the interaction of BHV-2 with different ecosystems. BHM is usually localized to the teats and udder and PLSD is a generalized skin condition.

BHM is a BHV-2 infection manifested clinically as ulceration of the skin of the teats and udder; it does not produce serious signs of systemic illness. Occasionally, lesions develop on the mouth and muzzle of calves nursing affected dams. BHM occurs in scattered herd outbreaks in temperate climates causing a nuisance for milkers and losses through discarded milk and mastitis.

Infection of the udder and teats may be observed initially as scabs, ulcers, or pox-like lesions. If solitary lesions occur, they may be considered traumatic in origin, but frequently multiple lesions occur in several cows. The onset is frequently sudden, and careful observation may reveal edema of the teats and vesicle formation that precedes epithelial rupture, serum exudation, and scab formation.

These lesions are painful, and cows often kick at milking machines or their operators. Mastitis is a common sequel, particularly when the teat ends are involved. Milk from infected cows may be discarded on account of mastitis or contamination with blood or medications. The disease is self-limiting in individual cattle and the lesions heal without scarring in several weeks (Gibbs and Rweyemamu 1977). When lesions are widespread or complicated by mastitis or secondary infections, healing is prolonged, and some affected cattle may be culled.

Similar lesions may appear on the skin of the udder and perineum, areas of skin may slough, and some affected animals may have a febrile reaction, but generally there are few systemic manifestations (Martin 1973).

Involvement of the udder and teats generally occurs in the absence of generalized skin lesions, but in some herds both BHV and PLSD appear.

PLSD, a generalized skin condition, occurs mostly in Africa but has appeared in Europe (Woods et al. 1996) and in the United States where it occurs sporadically.

In the first outbreak of PLSD in the United States, the index case was a lame cow with edema of the front legs and raised nodules the size of pencil erasers all over the body. In this 17-cow herd, 6 cows had generalized skin lesions and 2 had pox-like teat lesions (Yedloutschnig et al. 1970).

PLSD was originally recognized and named in South Africa, where it was confused with true lumpy skin disease (a poxvirus infection described in Chapter 33). PLSD is characterized by the sudden appearance of firm, round, raised nodules that develop a characteristic flat surface and slightly depressed center (Gibbs and Rweyemamu 1977). These lesions occur anywhere on the body but are most prevalent on the head, neck, back, and perineum. After about 2 weeks, they dry up and eventually slough, taking superficial skin layers and hair, which regrow in a few weeks. Calves nursing affected cows may develop ulcers of the oral mucosa or muzzle.

PLSD was produced experimentally by intravenous inoculation of viral cultures (Castrucci et al. 1978).

EFFECTS ON THE DEVELOPING FETUS

To date, no fetal infections have been documented.

NECROPSY FINDINGS

The gross lesions were described under Clinical Signs and Lesions. The disease is not fatal and necropsy is rare.

Histopathologic lesions are usually confined to the epidermis and consist of intracellular edema, cellular infiltration, and formation of syncytia with intranuclear inclusion bodies.

DIAGNOSIS

Diagnosis, based on clinical and virologic findings, is not always simple. When first confronted, clinical cases rarely present a textbook array of signs and lesions. Laboratory tests may be required to distinguish BHM from the many conditions causing vesicles or ulceration of the teats and udder (see Chapter 23) and there are other conditions resembling PLSD.

Classic outbreaks of mammillitis are characterized by edema, vesiculation that may be imperceptible, ulceration, and the formation of scabs on the teats and udders of milking cows and sometimes on nonlactating heifers. Skin may slough from udders and teats of more seriously affected cattle. Mildly affected cases may have only a few discrete lesions.

PLSD is characterized by nodules on the skin throughout the body. It may occur separately or in herds with cases of mammillitis.

Spread of both conditions will appear to occur within the herd and area, but obvious sources of infection and modes of transmission may not be evident.

Differential Diagnosis

Teat and udder lesions must be distinguished from trauma, photosensitization, bluetongue, malignant catarrhal fever (MCF), cowpox and pseudocowpox, foot-and-mouth disease (FMD), and vesicular stomatitis (VS). Careful physical examination and thorough history, together with histopathologic examinations of specimens taken for biopsy and virologic and serologic tests, are usually needed for an etiologic diagnosis.

PLSD must be differentiated from true lumpy skin disease, MCF, sporotrichosis, the skin form of lymphosarcoma, mange, insect bites, and urticaria of allergic origin.

When the oral mucosa of nursing calves is involved, the diseases affecting the bovine mucosa (DABM) (see Chapters 6 and 13) must be considered.

Laboratory Diagnosis

Serology, virus isolation, immunofluorescent assay, and histopathology are all useful in the hands of experienced workers if they possess the required reagents.

Virus neutralization or agar gel immunodiffusion and indirect fluorescent antibody tests can be used to detect seroconversion or rising titers.

Virus can be isolated from fresh lesions by cell culture inoculations. The CPE produced is similar to that of other herpesviruses, and isolates should be identified by neutralization tests with monospecific antiserums. Electron microscopic examination of isolates for typical herpesvirus morphology is useful.

Following intravenous inoculation, researchers noted a slight drop in hemoglobin concentration and red blood cell counts. Leukopenia appeared 2 days after inoculation and lasted from 2 to 8 days followed by leukocytosis (Castrucci et al. 1978).

Histopathologic diagnosis involves biopsy of an early lesion with some normal appearing peripheral tissue. The histologic appearance includes intracellular edema, cellular infiltration, syncytia, and possibly intranuclear inclusion bodies. These signs are useful in differentiating the disease from poxvirus infections that are associated with intracytoplasmic inclusions.

Fresh and fixed tissues near the periphery of early lesions, vesicular fluid, and serum are the most productive specimens.

EPIDEMIOLOGY

Antibody surveys indicate that infection is far more common than clinical manifestations. Serologically positive cattle are potentially latent infected carriers subject to stress-induced recrudescence and viral shedding that may explain some outbreaks. Insect transmission is suspected.

Generally BHM is the principal syndrome in temperate climates, and PLSD is more common in tropical and subtropical regions. PLSD is most common in summer. BHM is most common in colder months, and lesions are larger and appear more rapidly when the skin is colder (Letchworth and Carmicheal 1984).

Questions exist regarding the mode of transmission and the usual means by which the virus enters new herds or new areas.

Incubation periods vary with the route of inoculation and the nature of the observations. Teat lesions can appear in 1 to 3 days after intradermal inoculation, and generalized skin lesions appear within 4 to 8 days of intravenous inoculation.

It appears that cattle are the natural host and usual source of infection, and open lesions excrete high quantities of virus.

Outbreaks have occurred, however, that cannot be explained by introduction of new cattle. This fact suggests that the source could be latent persistent infections, intermediate nonbovine hosts, or arthropod vectors.

The virus has been isolated from buffaloes, and antibody has been detected in wild herbivores in Africa.

Assumptions of exclusive transmission of BHM by milking fall into disrepute because maiden heifers sometimes develop lesions. Epidemiologic observations and seasonal distribution of BHV-2 in some parts of Britain and Australia and of PLSD in South Africa tend to implicate insect vectors. The successful transmission by intradermal inoculation and failure of transmission between cattle in direct contact support the vector hypothesis. The distribution of lesions may coincide with sites at which the virus enters the skin.

BHM appears to spread through dairy herds in 2 to 7 weeks.

IMMUNITY

Infected cattle develop neutralizing antibody, which can persist for years. Cattle with antibody titers can be infected and reinfected and antibody may be an indicator of latent infection.

Colostrally acquired maternal antibodies can be demonstrated in calves that have nursed.

VIRUS PERSISTENCE

Viral persistence and latent infections characterize most herpesviruses. It is assumed that the same is true of BHV-2.

PREVENTION AND CONTROL

Aside from insect control, good management practices, and sound basic hygiene, no specific control or preventive procedures are known. Infected cattle should not be introduced into susceptible herds.

Experimental vaccines using formalized cultures have not been greatly successful, nor have attenuation procedures.

Researchers injected unattenuated virus intramuscularly; it afforded protection (Letchworth and Ladue 1982) and was shown to be safe even for pregnant cattle (Gibbs and Rweyemamu 1977). To date, no commercial vaccines are available.

THERAPY AND MANAGEMENT OF OUTBREAKS

When BHM occurs, all precautions must be taken to limit its spread and minimize the number of cattle developing secondary mastitis. Milking affected cows last has been recommended. However, spread by milking machines has not been conclusively established, and insect control measures may actually make more sense. The udders of affected cows should be kept clean and dry if possible. Topical antibiotic ointments may control secondary infections and expedite healing, but antibiotic contaminated milk must be discarded.

Attempts to limit the spread of PLSD by insect control have had mixed success.

LIKELIHOOD OF ERADICATION

Until more information is available on the mode of transmission of BHV-2 and the presence of persistent latent infections (if any), eradication considerations are premature.

IMPACT ON INTERNATIONAL TRADE

Neither BHM nor PLSD is considered a List A or List B disease by the Office International Des Epzooties (OIE); both should have minimum trade impacts.

PLSD should not be confused with true lumpy skin disease (Chapter 33), which is an OIE List A disease and can be the object of international trade measures.

PUBLIC RESPONSIBILITY

When these diseases are suspected, owners should be advised to increase hygienic procedures and insect control activities and isolate cattle with open lesions. Animals with teat lesions should be examined carefully for lameness or mouth lesions that may indicate presence of FMD, VS, MCF, or other DABM.

When PLSD signs are presented, all possible effort is required to differentiate it from true lumpy skin disease.

AREAS IN NEED OF RESEARCH

Research should be continued on the pathogenesis and mode of transmission of BHV-2.

REFERENCES

Anderson RA, Plowright W, Haig, DA, 1953. Cytopathic agents associated with lumpy skin disease of cattle. *Bull Epizoot Dis Afr* 5:489–492.

Barnard, BJH, 1994. Pseudolumpyskin disease/bovine herpes mammillitis. In *Infectious Diseases of Livestock With Special Reference to Southern Africa,* edited by JAW Coetzer, GR Thomson, and RC Tustin. Capetown: Oxford University Press, pp. 942–945.

Castrucci G, Frigeri F, Cilli V, Rampichini L, Ranucci S, 1978. Distribution of bovid herpes virus 2 in calves inoculated intravenously. *Am J Vet Res* 39:943–947.

Dardiri AH, Stone SS, 1972. Serologic evidence of dermopathic bovine herpesvirus infection of cattle in United States of America. *Proc US Anim Health Assoc* 76:156–171.

Ehlers B, Goltz M, Ejercito M, Dasika GK, Letchworth GJ, 1999. Bovine herpesvirus type 2 is closely related to the primate alphaherpesviruses. *Virus Genes* 19:197–203.

Gibbs EPJ, Rweyemamu MM, 1977. Bovine herpesviruses. II. Bovine herpesviruses 2 and 3. *Vet Bull* 47:411–425.

Letchworth GJ, Ladue R, 1982. Bovine herpes mammillitis in two New York dairy herds. *J Am Vet Med Assoc* 180:901–902.

Letchworth GJ, Carmicheal LE, 1984. Local tissue temperature: a critical factor in the pathogenesis of bovine herpesvirus-2. *Infection and Immunity* 43:1072–1079.

Martin WB, 1973. Bovine mammillitis: Epizootiologic and immunologic features. *J Am Vet Med Assoc* 103:915–917.

Martin WB, 1990. Bovine mammillitis virus. In *Infectious Diseases of Ruminants,* edited by Z Dinter and B Morein. Amsterdam: Elsevier Scientific Publishers, pp. 109–118.

Woods JA, Herring JA, Nettleton PF, Kruger M, Scott FMM, Reid HW, 1996. Isolation of bovine herpesvirus-2 (BHV-2) from a case of pseudo lumpy skin disease in the United Kingdom. *Vet Rec* 138:114.

Yedloutschnig RJ, Breese SS, Hess HR, Dardiri AH, Taylor WD, Barnes DM, Page RW, Ruebke HJ, 1970. Bovine herpes mammillitis-like disease diagnosed in the United States. *Proc US Anim Health Assoc* 74:208–212.

18

INFECTIOUS BOVINE RHINOTRACHEITIS AND INFECTIOUS PUSTULAR VULVOVAGINITIS

INTRODUCTION

Infectious bovine rhinotracheitis (IBR), a respiratory disease characterized by rhinitis, tracheitis, and fever is caused by bovine herpesvirus-1 (BHV-1), which also causes infectious pustular vulvovaginitis (IPV), abortion, conjunctivitis, balanoposthitis, a fatal systemic condition in newborn calves, and mild inapparent and latent infections. So-called IBR encephalitis, actually caused by BHV-5, is included in this chapter.

BHV-1 is readily transmitted and has worldwide distribution. Its manifestations can be diagnosed clinically and confirmed by laboratory tests. Some countries have attempted eradication, but control is based largely on vaccination.

IPV was recognized in Europe for decades before IBR was described as a respiratory disease of feedlot cattle in western United States. Multiple syndromes caused by BHV-1 infection have been identified and clarified over the years.

IBR/IPV has been reviewed by Barnard and Collett (1994) Straub (1990), and Murphy et al. (1999).

ETIOLOGY

BHV-1, also called the IBR/IPV virus, is a DNA virus in the genus *Varicellavirus* in the family Herpetoviridae. It replicates in a variety of cell cultures, producing distinctive cytopathic changes that expedite diagnosis and studies on pathogenicity, epizootiology, and vaccine technology.

All IBR and IPV isolates are immunologically and genetically related, and it is difficult to distinguish between isolates obtained from reproductive and respiratory mucosa or to tell modified live virus (MLV) vaccine viruses from field isolates except by molecular methods.

BHV-1 is relatively stable at refrigerator temperature in cell culture media but readily inactivated by disinfectants and environmental conditions.

BHV-1 is immunologically and genetically distinct from the herpesviruses that cause African malignant catarrhal fever, bovine herpes mammillitis, pseudorabies, and other herpesviruses isolated from cattle.

CLINICAL SIGNS AND LESIONS

The variety of clinical manifestations associated with BHV-1 infections and the variations in their severity are determined by the strain of virus, the dose and route of exposure or inoculation, the immunologic status of exposed animals, and environmental influences such as stress and concomitant infections. Each clinical form will be discussed separately.

Respiratory IBR is manifested by fever, reduced appetite, rapid respiration, dyspnea, and a nasal discharge that is initially clear and later becomes mucopurulent, accumulating in the nasal passages and trachea and causing dilated nostrils and occasional openmouthed breathing. Hyperemia and reddening of the muzzle and nasal turbinates inspired the now-defunct synonym "red nose."

Careful examination of the anterior nasal mucosa, which requires restraint and a flashlight, may reveal adherent white necrotic debris caused by coalescence of initially discrete pustules. These lesions are almost pathognomonic for IBR but must be distinguished from nose lead injuries and mucopurulent material lodged in the nostrils.

Some cattle with respiratory IBR have conjunctivitis and excess ocular secretions that change from clear to mucopurulent over time.

Pulmonary auscultation reveals increased vesicular murmur (the resonant sound of normal breathing) or referred sounds caused by partial occlusion of the upper airways. Pulmonic pasteurellosis or other complications should be considered if rales are heard.

The case-fatality rate from respiratory IBR is low unless complicated with bacterial infections, as occurs in feedlots where deaths are more common than in dairy herds. Occasionally animals will suffocate from tracheal blockage by mucopurulent material.

When pregnant animals are present, abortions may occur in cattle with respiratory signs or subclinical infections and can continue for 90 to 100 days.

BHV-1 conjunctivitis, characterized by initially clear and later mucopurulent ocular discharge, can occur with or without respiratory signs and may be misdiagnosed as pinkeye. Its diagnosis is strengthened if pustules or plaques of white necrotic debris are found on the conjunctiva. The eyelids must be inverted to view these lesions and cattle object to this painful procedure.

Affected cattle occasionally have corneal opacities that appear to originate at the corneoscleral junction and expand inwardly. Cattle with pinkeye, caused by *Moraxella bovis,* have opacities that originate in the center of the cornea and spread outward. IBR conjunctivitis can occur simultaneously with pinkeye. It may be accompanied by abortions and may be incriminated retrospectively when BHV-1 abortion is diagnosed in a laboratory and the herd history includes an outbreak of a peculiar form of pinkeye.

IPV, a BHV-1 infection of vaginal and vulvar mucosa manifested by pustules and mucopurulent discharge, was known as blaschenausschlag in Europe for many years before the identification of respiratory IBR and isolation of the virus in the early 1950s (McKercher 1963).

When IPV is mild, it may not be noticed. If severe, there is edema and mucopurulent discharge that is usually first noticed when, because of pain, the animal's tail fails to return to the normal position after defecation or urination. Internal examination reveals pustules or plaques of white necrotic material on the vulva and vaginal mucosa and pools of odorless mucopurulent material on the vaginal floor.

IPV can be transmitted by natural breeding, by cattle sniffing one another, or by dogs licking the vulvas of recumbent cattle.

Although IPV is usually not observed in respiratory outbreaks (and vice versa), occasionally respiratory IBR and IPV occur simultaneously in herds where nose-to-vulva contact is common (Kahrs and Smith 1965). Thus the vulvar mucosa should be examined for pustules when respiratory IBR is suspected.

The differential diagnosis of IPV includes necrotic vaginitis from parturition injuries or sadism; irritation from caustic materials; and the brownish or off-orange colored elevated lesions of granular vaginitis found on the vulvar mucosa in many clinically normal cattle. Some granular vaginitis lesions may be hypoplastic lymphoid follicles. They are smaller than IPV lesions, do not increase in size, and usually don't cause mucopurulent discharge or discomfort.

IBR balanoposthitis, sometimes called infectious pustular balanoposthitis, can be transmitted to bulls breeding cows with IPV. This BHV-1 infection causes severe balanoposthitis with lesions similar to those of IPV. Such bulls can transmit BHV-1 during natural breeding. BHV-1 can be detected in the semen of bulls experiencing primary clinical balanoposthitis and bulls with reactivated latent infections. Contaminated semen and semen collection equipment can constitute a hazard in artificial insemination. The virus can survive in frozen semen. The artificial insemination industry has worked to prevent semen contamination by clinically infected bulls or healthy seropositive bulls with latent infections. Carefully collected semen from bulls in studs with rigorous herd-health programs is unlikely to distribute BHV-1.

Insemination of susceptible cattle with semen containing BHV-1 can cause endometritis, shortened estrous periods and reduction in conception rates (Parsonson and Snowdon 1975).

Systemic, frequently fatal, febrile BHV-1 infection can occur in neonatal calves infected in utero during late gestation or exposed shortly after birth.

Affected calves have respiratory distress and may have white necrotic lesions on the mucosa of the mouth, tongue, esophagus, and all 4 stomachs. They may develop diffuse peritonitis. They may have diarrhea and be diagnosed as having calf septicemia. At necropsy, the characteristic white necrotic abomasal lesions are easily overlooked or confused with curdled milk.

EFFECTS ON THE DEVELOPING FETUS

BHV-1-induced abortion requires the female to be both pregnant and susceptible when exposed. Pregnant cattle may abort following nonclinical BHV-1 infections or during and following IBR respiratory or conjunctivitis outbreaks. Fetuses exposed to BHV-1 at any stage of gestation can be aborted, but most are in the last third of gestation when expelled. The interval between exposure and abortion can range from 8 days to several months and abortions may occur while clinical IBR is evident in the herd and up to several months afterward. Fetuses exposed in late gestation may be dead at birth or carried to term and die within a few days with signs of fatal septicemic neonatal IBR.

Fetuses aborted because of BHV-1 can be dead in utero for several days before expulsion. Autolysis, brownish-stained friable tissues, a lack of gross lesions, and fluid in body cavities are characteristic findings. Gross lesions are difficult to find in autolyzed fetuses but microscopically, focal necrosis of liver, kidneys, and adrenal glands can sometimes be observed. Intranuclear inclusion bodies are easily seen in the rare fetus presented in fresh condition, and may be seen in autolyzed adrenal glands. The stomachs of aborted fetuses should be examined carefully for focal necrotic lesions.

BHV-1 abortions can be prevented by successful vaccination prior to pregnancy and by administration of nonabortifacient vaccines in early pregnancy (Cravens et al. 1996).

Diarrhea and epithelial ulcerations occasionally accompany fatal systemic neonatal IBR or respiratory IBR. It is difficult to unequivocally attribute these signs and lesions to BHV-1 because of the many causes of diarrhea in neonatal and adult cattle.

Encephalomyelitis occurs sporadically in young cattle infected with an IBR-like virus. It is a herpesvirus encephalitis and nonpurulent leptomeningitis characterized by incoordination, occasional circling or licking at the flanks, recumbency, and death. Once considered a variant IBR virus, this condition is now known to be caused by BHV-5, which is genetically distinct but indistinguishable from BHV-1 by serologic and immunofluorescent techniques. This condition appears to be controllable by IBR vaccines (Cascio et al. 1999).

Retrospective application of polymerase chain reactions to detect BHV-5 and BHV-1 DNA in collected fixed specimens of brains of calves with undiagnosed fatal nonsuppurative encephalitis indicates this condition, while sporadic, is more common than generally suspected (Ely et al. 1996).

BHV-5 encephalitis must be differentiated from polioencephalomalacia, lead poisoning, rabies, pseudorabies and other central nervous diseases.

Experimental inoculation of IBR virus into the bovine udder produces mastitis, and the virus has been isolated from clinical mastitis (Roberts and Carter 1974). BHV-1, however, is not a major cause of mastitis.

NECROPSY FINDINGS

Unless complicated, BHV-1 infections are rarely fatal for mature cattle. When cattle die with IBR the lesions are either unusually severe or the result of complications.

Initial exposure and primary BHV-1 infection may cause nonclinical infection or plaques of adherent whitish necrotic material raised above mucosal surfaces. These result from coalescence of discrete pustules and consist of leukocytes, fibrin, and necrotic epithelial cells. Intranuclear inclusion bodies are a histologic feature. Lesions appear at the site of inoculation or at target organs after systemic viral distribution by macrophages. If plaques are scraped off or slough off, underlying ulceration can be observed.

In respiratory IBR, these lesions are in the mucosa of the trachea and nasal passages, which may also be congested or contain petechial or ecchymotic hemorrhages and mucopurulent material. Fetuses and newborn calves are more likely to suffer serious systemic effects than mature animals. Focal necrosis is a common lesion in the parenchyma of organs of aborted fetuses or calves with systemic IBR.

Infections involving mucosal surfaces of the reproductive tract are not fatal.

DIAGNOSIS

The diagnostic profile and differential diagnosis for each clinical form of IBR was described above. Although not pathognomonic, pustules that coalesce to form adherent white necrotic lesions on respiratory, reproductive, or ocular mucosa are the best aid to clinical diagnosis. When clinical signs and history suggest IBR, these lesions support a field diagnosis, which can be confirmed by virus isolation and serology.

Differential Diagnosis

The differential diagnosis of each clinical manifestation of BHV-1 infection is discussed in the section on Clinical Signs and Lesions. The telltale clinical features of BHV-1 infections are the characteristic white necrotic plaques seen on the nasal, conjunctival, or vulval mucosa. They must be distinguished from free-flowing mucopurulent material by dislodging the material to make sure that it is attached to the mucosa.

Pulmonic pasteurellosis may be a sequel to IBR, and the two diseases may occur simultaneously. Care must be taken, however, to avoid incriminating IBR as a principal culprit in pasteurellosis, because it may also be a complication of other virus infections.

Laboratory Diagnosis

Laboratory confirmation of suspected BHV-1 infections can be obtained by serologic tests, virus isolation, fluorescent antibody (FA) staining of tissues, or identification of viral DNA by molecular technology.

While virus isolation is convincing, care is essential in laboratory identification of virus isolates because other herpesviruses have been found in cattle, and latent BHV-1 infections reactivated by stress or disease could be mistakenly declared the etiologic agent of observed conditions. Therefore, a specific etiologic diagnosis of BHV-1 requires virus isolation accompanied by appropriate signs, history, and seroconversion from negative to positive. All specimens submitted to laboratories should be accompanied by serum, and efforts should be made to collect a second serum 2 to 3 weeks later. Studies on enzyme-linked immunosorbent assay (ELISA) for detection of BHV-1-induced serum IgM, which is present only in early infections, offer hope for diagnostic tests based on a single serum specimen (Graham et al. 1999).

Laboratory specimens should be collected on the basis of the form of disease and collected carefully to minimize bacterial contamination. Specimens for virus isolation are inoculated into cell cultures, which are then observed for cytopathic changes. Isolates can then be identified by serologic, FA, or molecular procedures. Specimens collected for virus isolation should be accompanied by a serum sample.

For live animals with respiratory IBR, nasal swabs should be taken in the early febrile stages, when nasal discharges are serous rather than mucopurulent. They should be frozen or placed in the viral transport medium preferred by recipient laboratories. Diagnosis of BHV-1 conjunctivitis utilizes the aforementioned concepts, but the swabbing is from the conjunctival sac rather than from the nasal mucosa.

IPV or infectious balanoposthitis is diagnosed by swabbing vulvar, vaginal, or penile mucosa. BHV-1 can be identified in semen by cell culture techniques and nested polymerase chain reactions, which are more sensitive (Masri et al. 1996).

To identify BHV-5 as the cause of encephalitis, a brain specimen is necessary for standard isolation procedures or identification by FA techniques.

Laboratory diagnosis of the fatal systemic form can be accomplished by nasal or conjunctival swabs taken before the animal dies, and virus isolation from blood (preferably buffy coat) may establish viremia. When gross lesions are observed at necropsy, specimens of spleen, lymph node, liver, brain, or forestomachs can be inoculated into cell cultures. In fatal neonatal IBR, the necropsy materials are useful in FA assays, using smears or thin frozen sections of tissues with lesions for detecting virus. In addition, histologic examination of mucosal lesions, liver, or other organs with gross lesions can reveal intranuclear inclusion bodies, whose presence supports the diagnosis when other lesions and signs are consistent with BHV-1 infection.

The confirmation of BHV-1 as a cause of abortion requires identification of virus in fetal liver, brain, or spleen. Occasionally fetuses aborted because of

BHV-1 have focal necrosis on the mucosa of the forestomachs. The focal hepatic necrosis is usually not evident grossly, but it is recommended that liver and adrenal glands of fetuses be submitted in fixatives that permit visualization of inclusion bodies and focal necrosis.

Serum from aborting cows or heifers should be tested. It is usually difficult, however, to demonstrate a fourfold rise in titer (Cravens et al. 1996), and the major usefulness of serology on aborting females is to eliminate BHV-1 when specimens collected at the time of abortion and several weeks later are both free of antibody. IBR-aborted fetuses rarely have measurable BHV-1 antibody, because death usually occurs before a fetal immune response is mounted.

It is possible to identify BHV-1 in milk of cows with IBR infection of the udder.

Clinical pathology usually does not facilitate the diagnosis of BHV-1 infection. Affected animals are usually not anemic. Total white blood counts vary from leukopenia to leukocytosis.

EPIDEMIOLOGY

The epidemiology of IBR focuses on the multiple clinical manifestations and methods of viral shedding by sick and clinically normal cattle and the capacity of cattle to develop latent BHV-1 infections that can be reactivated.

Following exposure of susceptible cattle to BHV-1, the incubation period varies from 2 to 6 days, depending on dose, route of inoculation, and acuity in recognizing the onset of disease.

Cattle are the principal reservoir and usual source of infection of BHV-1, which is perpetuated in bovine populations by direct contact between infected cattle and by occasional virus shedding due to reactivated latent infections. Goats, swine, eastern cottontail rabbits, and water buffalo can be infected, but the epidemiologic significance of these species is unknown.

BHV-1 is globally distributed in cattle populations except for some European countries, which have undertaken eradication programs. BHV-1 is considered ubiquitous in the United States. Unless isolated, most cattle have a high probability of eventual exposure.

BHV-1 infection is easily transmitted because large quantities of virus are shed in respiratory, ocular, and reproductive secretions of infected cattle.

The case-fatality rate is higher in susceptible neonates (calves less than 2 weeks old) than in adults. The protective effect of maternally acquired antibody in calves that have suckled immune dams undoubtedly alters the age distribution of infected cattle.

The sex and breed distribution of clinical BHV-1 infections parallels the distribution of sexes and breeds in exposed populations. Feedlot cattle have higher attack rates, more severe disease, and higher fatality rates than do range or dairy cattle, a fact attributable to the stress of shipment, aggregation, social acclimatization, and exposure to multiple pathogens rather than from age, sex, or breed variations in susceptibility.

IMMUNITY

Immunity to IBR involves complex interactions of humoral antibody and cell-mediated immunity (CMI), which are both activated following natural BHV-1 infection or vaccination.

Locally deployed elements of the CMI system play a crucial role in resistance and recovery from early infection.

Presence of neutralizing antibody in serum is not an accurate indicator of resistance to infection and disease. It merely indicates either previous infection or vaccination and in calves less than six months old can result from ingestion of colostrum on the first day of life.

Cattle with humoral antibody induced by natural infection or successful vaccination are partially immune. This partial immunity may persist for life, but to be maintained at detectable levels, it may require occasional restimulation by exogenous exposure or endogenous virus release. Partially immune cattle can experience superficial infections of mucosal surfaces, but they are less likely to abort or experience clinical disease than susceptible cattle undergoing primary infection.

Colostrally acquired antibody has importance in vaccination and resistance to disease. Colostral antibody appears in the serum of calves that suckle immune dams on the first day of life and diminishes rapidly via metabolic degradation. The titers of colostrally acquired antibody vary from calf to calf depending on antibody levels in colostrum; the amount of colostrum ingested; and the efficiency of intestinal absorption. Some calves lose maternal antibody as early as one month of age, and a few may still have titers up to six months of age.

The protective value of waning, passively acquired antibody may be overridden by severe challenge and some vaccines. There is no certainty, however, that vaccination in the presence of maternal antibody will be successful. Calves vaccinated prior to 6 months of age should be revaccinated if long-term protection is desired.

VIRUS PERSISTENCE

Latent infections can occur following natural infection or vaccination with MLV vaccines. These latent infections, which amount to viral DNA sequestered in ganglia of nerves supplying sites of primary infection, are unidentifiable clinically but can be reactivated by stress or corticosteroids. Virus excretion during reactivation is usually not accompanied by clinical signs. Careful examination, however, may reveal localized discrete lesions, similar to cold sores caused by the human herpes simplex virus, at some sites. The fact that reactivation of latent BHV-1 infections can occur years after primary infection and may boost humoral antibody titers partially explains the lifelong seropositivity of some animals.

Reactivated latent BHV-1 infections may explain outbreaks when obvious sources of infection are not evident. In addition, potential reactivation of latent infections justifies saying that animals with humoral antibody should be considered potential sources of infection for susceptible cattle. This latency complicates control efforts and has implications for importing cattle and semen, especially in countries undertaking eradication programs.

PREVENTION AND CONTROL

The control of IBR can be attempted by hygiene, management, and isolation procedures. Because the success of these measures is limited by its ease of spread and by the wide distribution of active and latent BHV-1 infections, most control efforts are based on vaccination.

Vaccines come as inactivated products: MLV vaccines for intramuscular, subcutaneous, or intranasal use, temperature-sensitive mutants (Cravens et al. 1996), and gene-deleted marker vaccines (Kit et al. 1993). Vaccines approved by regulatory agencies are available in a bewildering number of types and combinations for inoculation by multiple routes under various circumstances. They should be used only within expiration dates and as directed in package inserts.

A general recommendation is that all female animals kept for breeding purposes, except those with export potential, should be vaccinated one or more times prior to their first breeding. Vaccination of beef breeds destined for early slaughter is most effective when accomplished with minimum stress at or before weaning and before assembly, transport, and arrival at feedlots (Wren 1994). Choice of vaccine, route of vaccination, and frequency of revaccination are factors that must be evaluated by veterinarians for each farm, ranch, or feedlot.

Early IBR vaccines developed were MLV products for intramuscular inoculation. Their principal advantages are ease of administration and availability in combination with other virus vaccines. Some are contraindicated for pregnant cattle, and inoculation-site blemishes have caused increased use of subcutaneous inoculations.

Intranasally administered MLV IBR vaccine was introduced in 1969. Some intranasal vaccines are safe for use on pregnant cattle, but package inserts should be studied carefully before pregnant cattle are vaccinated. Protection from these products is partly attributable to interferon production and rapid induction of secretory antibody at mucosal surfaces.

Inactivated IBR vaccine has been available in combination with other inactivated viruses and bacterins against *Pasteurella* species. As with many inactivated vaccines, levels of protection vary, the initial vaccination procedure should be repeated, and periodic boostering is recommended. If properly inactivated, so-called killed vaccines overcome concerns about postvaccination abortion, postvaccination shedding of vaccine virus, or establishment of latent vaccine virus infections capable of future reactivation. Disadvantages of inactivated vaccines include uncertain efficacy, need for frequent revaccination, injection site blemishes, and rare postvaccination reactions.

Gene-deleted marker vaccines that enable vaccinated seropositive animals to be distinguished from animals that are seropositive due to natural infections can contribute to eradication strategies (Kit et al. 1993).

Subunit vaccines consisting of viral proteins derived by detergent treatment of infected cell cultures showed brief promise of protecting cattle from IBR and solving many problems associated with MLV vaccines (Kit at al. 1993).

The issue of vaccinating breeding bulls against IBR is complicated. Some purchasers of purebred stock discriminate against seropositive bulls. If bulls on a farm have potential for sale as breeding animals, for export, or for commercial semen production, they should remain unvaccinated so purchasers can make the vaccination decision. A possible alternative is documented vaccination with gene-deleted marker vaccines. When considered on a population basis, the impact on herd immunity of leaving a few valuable bulls unvaccinated should be minimal, as would be the risk of serious disease from natural infection of the unvaccinated bull.

Vaccination decisions for artificial insemination units are complex. Managers of some units endeavor to keep the population free of IBR by quarantine measures and will not purchase seropositive bulls because of potential latent infections. Some workers argue that maintenance of seronegative artificial-insemination units is virtually impossible because of the ubiquitousness of BHV-1 and that exclusion of seropositive bulls causes loss of valuable genetic material, which cannot be justified by the minimal risk of transmission of the virus through semen.

Managers of some insemination units conduct periodic vaccination of all bulls in an effort to maintain high titers as protection against introduction of field strains of virus and subsequent development of latent infections. Thus, in artificial-insemination units, the vaccination decision must be based on the serologic status of the population, the available vaccine technology, the requirements of importers, and the disease-control philosophy of the management.

THERAPY AND MANAGEMENT OF OUTBREAKS

In respiratory IBR, treatment is directed at controlling complications. The welfare of affected cattle is maintained by good nursing care and supportive therapy. When clinical signs suggest bacterial complications, the value of antibiotic and other therapies must be evaluated regarding the hazard of residues in milk or meat. All withdrawal times must be observed.

In animals with hypoxia due to partial laryngeal or tracheal occlusion, tracheotomy may afford temporary relief but such cattle frequently die with necrotic tracheitis attributable to fungal and bacterial infections acquired through the incision.

Early administration of MLV intranasal vaccines to unaffected cattle in herds in which BHV-1 is diagnosed may provide early protection due to production of interferon and secretory antibody and may limit clinical signs in cattle incubating or not yet exposed to field virus. Vaccination decisions for exposed cattle must consider confidence in the clinical diagnosis and the tendency to blame vaccines for postvaccination diseases even if natural infection was present at the time of vaccination.

IPV can be treated locally with mild antiseptics or antibiotic ointments, but it is usually uncomplicated and self-limiting. In bulls with balanoposthitis, treatment with ointments may reduce the likelihood of preputial adhesions.

LIKELIHOOD OF ERADICATION

In most countries, the question of eradicating IBR is not considered a high priority because BHV-1 lacks pathogenicity for humans and because of resource priorities. If a nation or island continent with strong animal health infrastructure and strict border controls embarks on an eradication program, disease-control officials must understand the obstacles involved. They should first ascertain that the virus is not already present, then limit imports to seronegative cattle, quarantine imported cattle, carefully screen semen imports, and test, then slaughter all IBR-seropositive cattle. The potential for reactivation of latent infections and the potential of other animal reservoirs make it a relatively difficult and expensive disease to eradicate from infected regions. Austria, Denmark, parts of France and Germany, Finland, the Netherlands, Norway, and Sweden have undertaken eradication by test and slaughter. If successful, this program could open markets for purebred cattle and semen (de Wit et al. 1998).

IMPACT ON INTERNATIONAL TRADE

IBR/IPV is categorized as a List B disease by the Office International Des Epizooties. BHV-1-free countries may exclude seropositive animals, establish quarantine and testing requirements, and impose special requirements on semen and embryos. Countries or regions imposing such measures need documented surveillance systems to support claims of disease freedom.

PUBLIC RESPONSIBILITY

Human disease has not been associated with BHV-1. People passing between herds with known clinical cases should take precautions to avoid spreading the disease.

The clinically ill animal is unfit for slaughter because of systemic disease and fever. After its recovery, however, it can pass inspection and be fit for human consumption. If a sick animal has been treated, all drug and antibiotic withdrawal periods must be observed before shipment of milk or slaughter.

AREAS IN NEED OF RESEARCH

Ongoing research is needed to improve vaccine safety and efficacy. Studies are also needed to fine-tune diagnostic differentiation of the bovine herpesviruses and to further clarify their epidemiology and clinical impact.

REFERENCES

Barnard BJH, Collett MG, 1994. Infectious bovine rhinotracheitis/infectious pustular vulvovaginitis. In *Infectious Diseases of Livestock With Special Reference to Southern Africa,* edited by JAW Coetzer, GR Thomson and RC Tustin. Capetown: Oxford University Press, pp. 932–941.

Cascio KE, Belknap EB, Schultheiss PC, Ames AD, Collins JC, 1999. Encephalitis induced by bovine herpesvirus 5 and protection by prior vaccination or infection with bovine herpesvirus 1. *Vet Diagn Invest* 11:134–139.

Cravens RL, Ellsworth DA, Sorenson CD, White KA, 1996. Efficacy of a temperature-sensitive modified-live bovine herpesvirus-1 vaccine against abortion and stillbirth in pregnant heifers. *J Am Vet Med Assoc* 208: 2031–2034.

de Wit JJ, Hage JJ, Brinkoff J, Westenbrink F, 1998. A comparative study of serological tests for use in bovine herpes 1 eradication in The Netherlands. *Vet Microbiol* 61:153–163.

Ely RW, d'Offay JM, Ruefer AH, and Cash CY, 1996. Bovine herpesviral encephalitis: a retrospective study on archived formalin-fixed, paraffin-embedded brain tissue. *J Vet Diagn Invest* 8:487–492.

Graham DA, Foster JC, German A, McLaren IE, Adair BM, Merza M, 1999. Evaluation of an immunofluorescent antibody test to detect bovine herpesvirus 1-specific IgM. *J Vet Diagn Invest* 11:324–329.

Kahrs RF, Smith RS, 1965. Infectious bovine rhinotracheitis, infectious pustular vulvovaginitis, and abortion in a New York dairy herd. *J Am Vet Med Assoc* 146:217–220.

Kit S, Otsukwa H, Kit M, 1993. Blocking ELISA for distinguishing infectious bovine rhinotracheitis virus (IBRV)-infected animals from those vaccinated with a gene-deleted marker vaccine. *J Virol Meth* 40:45–56.

Masri SA, Olson W, Nguyen PT, Prins S, Deregt, D, 1996. Rapid detection of bovine herpesvirus-1 in the semen of infected bulls by a nested polymerase chain reaction assay. *Can J Vet Res* 60:100–107.

McKercher DG, 1963. Studies of the etiologic agents of infectious bovine rhinotracheitis and blaschenausschlag (coital vesicular exanthema). *Am J Vet Res* 24:501–509.

Murphy FA, Gibbs EPJ, Horzinek, MC, Studdert MC, 1999. Infectious bovine rhinotracheitis (caused by bovine herpes virus-1) In *Veterinary Virology,* 3rd ed., edited by FA Murphy, EPJ Gibbs, MC Horzinek, MJ Studdert. San Diego: Academic Press pp. 309–311.

Parsonson IM, Snowdon WA, 1975. The effect of natural and artificial breeding using bulls infected with, or semen contaminated with IBR virus. *Aust Vet J* 51:365–369.

Roberts AW, and Carter GR, 1974. Infectious bovine rhinotracheitis virus recovered from the milk of a cow with mastitis. *J Am Vet Med Assoc* 164:413.

Straub OC, 1990. Infectious bovine rhinotracheitis virus. In *Infectious Diseases of Ruminants.* Edited by Z Dinter, B Morein. Amsterdam: Elsevier Scientific Publishers. pp. 71–108.

Wren G, 1994. Don't become complacent about IBR. *Bovine Veterinarian* July: 18–20.

19

MALIGNANT CATARRHAL FEVER

INTRODUCTION

Malignant catarrhal fever (MCF), also called malignant head catarrh, bovine malignant catarrh, and snotsiekte, is a highly fatal pansystemic syndrome characterized by mucosal lesions, severe rhinitis, panophthalmia, lymphadenopathy, encephalitis, and frequently diarrhea. These signs are similar to those of other diseases affecting the bovine mucosa (DABM), but MCF has more severe upper-respiratory, ocular, and neurologic involvement. It affects deer and bison as well as cattle.

MCF, transmitted across species by persistently infected carriers, occurs in two epidemiologic forms. They are sheep associated (SA) MCF and wildebeest associated (WA) MCF, caused by two host adopted herpesviruses. It occurs throughout the world, sometimes as individual sporadic cases and sometimes in epizootics.

WA MCF, largely seen in Africa and in zoos and wildlife preserves elsewhere, has reservoirs in wild ruminants, particularly the blue and black wildebeest and the hartebeest.

SA MCF, which occurs both in Africa and elsewhere in the world, has ovine reservoirs and is sometimes called American MCF. American and African MCF have slight differences but enough similarities to be discussed as a single disease.

Classic MCF is easy to diagnose on clinical signs and gross and histopathologic lesions. Control involves separating cattle from sheep or other ruminants that serve as healthy carriers.

MCF has been reviewed by Heuschele (1998), Barnard et al. (1994), and Plowright (1990).

ETIOLOGY

Two epidemiologically distinct but closely related DNA viruses of the family Herpesviridae cause MCF. These are alcelaphine herpesvirus-1 (AHV-1), which causes WA MCF and is well characterized, and ovine herpesvirus-2 (OHV-2), which causes SA MCF and has never been isolated and is largely uncharacterized.

AHV-1 virus, the cause of African MCF, is highly cell associated and can be adapted to grow with cytopathic effects (CPE) in bovine thyroid cells in which it produces syncytia, vacuolization, clumping of nuclei, and type A intranuclear inclusion bodies. Thyroid-adapted strains produce a more rapidly progressing CPE than do primary isolates. It has also been propagated in bovine, swine, and Vero monkey kidney cells.

OHV-2 has not been successfully propagated in cell cultures but has been quantitated by competitive polymerase chain reaction (PCR) (Hua et al. 1999) and identified by PCR in clinically affected bison (Schultheiss et al. 1998) and swine with clinical MCF (Loken et al. 1998).

Like other members of the family Herpesviridae, these viruses are sensitive to environmental influences and perpetuated by persistent latent infections.

CLINICAL SIGNS AND LESIONS

Although prolonged and variable incubation periods (usually exceeding 3 weeks) are usual, the appearance of clinical signs is almost always sudden, and MCF can be peracute, with death ensuing within 1 to 2 days of onset (Pierson et al. 1973). More often, however, affected cattle live 4 to 12 days before succumbing. A few cases may survive (O'Toole et al. 1995).

The first signs include fever, nasal discharge, and severe depression. Blinking of the eyes, photophobia, and conjunctivitis with excess lacrimation may occur early in the course of the disease. The eye involvement develops into a severe panophthalmitis, which is usually bilateral. In cattle it is almost always accompanied by a corneal opacity that progresses centrally from the limbus. Before the cornea is completely opaque, cattle frequently keep their eyes closed and strongly resist efforts to open them. There may be a bilateral miosis (pupillary constriction), hypopyon (pus in the anterior chamber), and terminal nystagmus.

The muzzle may become crusted and assume a burnt appearance. Occasionally the mucosa between the nasal openings becomes necrotic, and cracking and sloughing ensue. There is usually a copious mucopurulent nasal discharge, which is frequently fetid. The mucosa of the nasal septa become fiery red and assume a purple coloration due to hyperemic engorgement. Necrotic debris may be seen clinging to the mucosa of the nasal septa. The animal may snore as a result of partial occlusion of the upper airways.

There is frequently hyperemia of the oral mucosa and the mucosa on tips of buccal papillae may become necrotic and slough. The hard palate and tongue may have discrete punched-out ulcers like those seen in bovine viral diarrhea (BVD). The lymph nodes of the head are frequently visibly swollen, and palpation frequently reveals swelling of the prescapular and other lymph nodes.

Hematuria may be present and some animals will have diarrhea. Anorexia and fever frequently persist throughout the course of the disease, and the pulse rate is generally elevated.

Sometimes, the hoof separates from the skin at the coronary band. Most patients exhibit some degree of dehydration prior to death.

The skin lesions of MCF start as small areas of exanthema that may be mistaken for papules or small vesicles. These are purple blotches from which the superficial skin layer may slough or remain, leaving scabs on hairless areas like the teats. On skin areas covered by hair these eruptions are manifested as small elevations giving the hair a characteristic tufted appearance over the back, inside the hind legs, and on the escutcheon. These eruptions may be evident only to careful observers and may not be recognized unless the entire skin coat is palpated.

In most cases animals have neurologic signs such as severe depression or stupor. Affected cattle may stand with the head and neck extended, suggesting head and eye pain. Often, the head will appear to droop lower and lower as if the animal is dozing. At some point, the animal suddenly catches its head and returns it to a higher position. The process then resumes.

This head jerking is also seen in some early cases of acute infectious keratoconjunctivitis and in encephalitides of other origins. Periods of apparent stupor may be interrupted by sessions of extreme irritability and mania in which the animal may knock the shells off of its horns or otherwise injure itself, its caretakers, or veterinarians. Since their behavior is unpredictable, cattle and bison (particularly bulls) with MCF should be regarded as dangerous, and extreme caution should be used in examination and treatment.

MCF has emerged as a major disease of captive and feedlot bison in which high population densities induce a clinical and pathological picture somewhat different from the classic bovine model.

OHV-2-infected bison herds experience higher attack rates and a shorter clinical course and often resemble respiratory disease outbreaks. Usually bison have less profound corneal opacities and nasal encrustation and more pronounced hemorrhagic cystitis and bloody diarrhea than is seen in cattle. Bison outbreaks often lack direct contact with sheep and may result from stress-induced reactivation of previously acquired latent OHV-2 infections or bison-to-bison transmission.

EFFECTS ON THE DEVELOPING FETUS

In utero transmission of AHV-1, without abortion, may occur, and wildebeest calves so infected may contribute to transmission of the virus in Africa (Barnard et al. 1994). Most affected cattle die within a week. Bovine abortion is not commonly associated with MCF.

NECROPSY FINDINGS

MCF cases submitted for necropsy frequently have a dehydrated and sometimes feces-splattered carcass. The shells of the horns may be missing. In addition to the mucosal and ocular lesions visible upon careful examination of the live animal, necropsy may reveal severe inflammation, congestion, and necrosis of the nasal turbinates. Necrotic materials, often described as diphtheritic membranes, adhering to the turbinates and the trachea may resemble lesions of infectious bovine rhinotracheitis (IBR).

There is frequently esophageal necrosis or ulceration similar to that seen in BVD. The abomasal mucosa may be hyperemic and contain petechial hemorrhages and ulcers, which frequently have jagged areas of hemorrhage on the periphery. There may be petechial hemorrhages throughout the intestinal tract, as with BVD. Necrosis and hemorrhages in Peyer's patches as seen in BVD are rare in SA MCF.

There may be severe hyperemia and petechial hemorrhage in the trachea. The lungs may be normal, have some emphysema, or have areas of secondary bronchopneumonia and consolidation.

A characteristic gross lesion of MCF is white foci in the kidney cortex due to focal infiltration with lymphocytes and mononuclear cells.

The retropharyngeal, cervical, and prescapular lymph nodes are frequently swollen and edematous. The brain and meninges may appear grossly swollen or edematous, pericarditis is sometimes present, the liver may be enlarged, there may be hemorrhages in the bladder and the gallbladder, and the kidney may contain grayish white foci and petechial hemorrhages.

The most significant histopathologic lesion is a necrotizing vasculitis in vessels particularly where gross lesions are present (O'Toole et al. 1995), and lymphoid infiltration about small vessels in the brain, liver, kidney, heart, and adrenals. These vascular lesions are the basis for a pathologic diagnosis.

DIAGNOSIS

Except for atypical cases (Pierson et al. 1978), MCF can usually be diagnosed on the basis of the clinical and epidemiological picture.

Textbook cases of MCF occur in cattle sharing an environment with sheep or wild ruminants. They develop a fatal febrile disease characterized by inflammation, necrosis, and erosions of gastrointestinal and respiratory mucosa, panophthalmitis, and neurologic signs.

The clinical diagnosis of bovine MCF is relatively easy when signs, visible lesions, and history are integrated. Clinical diagnosis is supported by necropsy findings. The focal kidney lesions and lack of Peyer's patch involvement help to distinguish MCF from the other DABM.

Histopathologic confirmation is based on characteristic necrotizing vasculitis and lymphocytic infiltrations, particularly around blood vessels in brain, kidney, and liver.

Differential Diagnosis

Bovine MCF must be distinguished from IBR and other forms of upper respiratory distress; from BVD, rinderpest, bluetongue, and other DABM; from salmonellosis, various toxicoses, and other causes of diarrhea; and from infectious keratoconjunctivitis and other eye disorders. It must also be differentiated from a wide variety of encephalitides of cattle including rabies, thromboembolic meningoencephalitis, Buss disease, thiamine-responsive polioencephalomalacia, and a variety of toxicoses. Although atypical cases may present difficulty in clinical diagnosis, none of the above-mentioned diseases presents the mucosal, lymphadenopathic, ophthalmic, neurologic syndrome that is unique to MCF in cattle.

Laboratory Diagnosis

Isolation of AHV-1 from cattle contracting MCF from contact with wild species can be accomplished from lymph nodes or buffy coat cells taken from acute clinical cases soon after death. Some success has been achieved by explanting cultures of the thyroids of acute clinical cases. In these instances, cytopathic changes can be seen in 3 to 5 days. Efforts to isolate the OHV-2 have met with limited success.

Serologic tests for the AHV-1 are done at some national laboratories and a few research facilities, but such tests require special arrangements. Except in unusual circumstances, clinical and pathologic diagnosis is adequate in cattle. Cases of illness, being less distinctive, may require laboratory tests.

Laboratory procedures for SA MCF are being worked out using assays that detect genomic OHV-2 DNA (Crawford et al. 1999).

Many animals with MCF have leukopenia. This finding is not consistent, however, and the blood picture may be equivocal and of minimal diagnostic value. The packed cell volume is usually normal but may increase when dehydration occurs. Hematuria and albuminuria may be present.

EPIDEMIOLOGY

The reservoirs of AHV-1 are the blue and black wildebeest, the hartebeest, and probably other wild ruminants. Sheep are the natural host and reservoir of OHV-2. In these natural hosts, persistent infections are usually inapparent. As with other herpesviruses, after nasal and lacrimal shedding associated with primary infection early in life, intermittent shedding occurs at times of stress. Clinical signs have been reported in buffaloes, deer (Wyand et al. 1971), antelopes, and other ruminants (Boever and Kurka 1974) and in swine (Loken et al. 1998). The agent probably escapes from the reservoir host in secretions and excretions, particularly nasal fluids. The placenta may be one immediate source of infection, suggesting that wildebeest calves and possibly lambs infected in utero can be persistently infected and serve as carriers for prolonged periods. This hypothesis is unsubstantiated.

Most evidence suggests that MCF is not naturally transmitted from cow to cow. Infections occurring in Africa without direct contact with reservoir species have caused speculation that occasional wind-borne or vector-borne transmission may occur. It is presumed that entry of the agent into the new susceptible host occurs via the mouth or through inhalation but this hypothesis requires further elaboration.

Under natural conditions the incubation period may range from 2 to 8 weeks or longer. When experimental transmission is accomplished using parenteral injections of blood or lymph node material from affected animals, the incubation period may be shorter, ranging from 7 to 50 days.

MCF occurs in cattle of all ages and breeds and in both sexes. In epizootics, the onsets of new cases may all occur within several weeks (suggesting simultaneous exposure to a common source), or the appearance of new cases may spread over 4 to 5 months, leading to conclusions that cow-to-cow spread is occurring.

IMMUNITY

Studies of the few documented survivors of WA MCF indicate presence of low levels of neutralizing antibodies.

VIRUS PERSISTENCE

MCF viruses establish persistent infections in inapparent host reservoirs, and trans-species infection by persistently infected carriers appears to occur regularly. Most bovine infections are fatal, and it is not known if latent persistent infections occur in the rare bovine survivors.

PREVENTION AND CONTROL

Control is accomplished by preventing cattle from contacting sheep or wild ruminants. Progress with the OHV-2 has not yet developed to the point where vaccine development is feasible. An experimental inactivated vaccine against the AHV-1 has met only limited success, and further studies are needed to bring it to practical usage.

THERAPY AND MANAGEMENT OF OUTBREAKS

Treatment is usually to no avail. Clinicians sometimes administer aspirin in an effort to combat the fever. Corticosteroids and antibiotics may be helpful (O'Toole et al. 1995). Efforts to restore electrolyte balance with fluid therapy usually have no effect on the eventual fatal outcome.

The most positive method of control is to immediately eliminate contact with sheep or other ruminant sources of infection. This step has no effect on the fate of cattle already infected, and the variable incubation periods indicate that owners should be warned that new cases may continue to occur for several months after the presumed reservoir hosts have been removed or the herd has been isolated.

LIKELIHOOD OF ERADICATION

Eradication of AHV-1 is unlikely because of the numerous wild species that are persistently infected. The question of eradication of SA MCF can be addressed only if molecular technology provides definitive information on the distribution and extent of persistent OHV-2 infections in sheep.

IMPACT ON INTERNATIONAL TRADE

The major trade impact of MCF lies in movement of wild ruminants for zoos or game preserves. Persons so involved must separate potential carriers including sheep, wildebeest, and other exotic ruminants from susceptible bovine and cervid species or anticipate MCF outbreaks. Because of the long incubation period, in apparently healthy exported cattle that have contacted sheep or wild ruminants, MCF may break out after the animals have arrived at their destination.

PUBLIC RESPONSIBILITY

The clinician encountering MCF should recommend isolation of the cattle from the inapparently infected host species (sheep or wild ruminants). Healthy exposed cattle should not be sold without the warning that they could be incubating the disease. Clinically ill animals are unsuitable for human consumption because of the fulminating septicemia-like nature of the disease. This admonition is reasonable even though human infection has not been reported.

AREAS IN NEED OF RESEARCH

Research is needed to elaborate the etiology and pathogenesis of SA MCF. The feasibility of vaccines should be explored further.

REFERENCES

Barnard BHJ, van der Lugt JJ, Mushi EZ, 1994. Malignant catarrhal fever. In *Infectious Diseases of Livestock With Special Reference to Southern Africa,* edited by JAW Coetzer, GR Thomson, RC Tustin. Capetown: Oxford University Press, pp. 946–957.

Boever WJ, Kurka B, 1974. Malignant catarrhal fever in Greater Kudus. *J. Am. Vet. Med. Assoc.* 165:817–819.

Crawford TB, Li H, O'Toole D, 1999. Diagnosis of malignant catarrhal fever by PCR using formalin-fixed, paraffin-embedded tissues. *J. Vet. Diagn. Invest.* 11:111–116.

Heuschele WP, 1998. Malignant catarrhal fever. In *Foreign Animal Diseases,* edited by WW Buisch, JL Hyde, CL Mebus. Richmond: U.S. Animal Health Assoc., pp. 311–321.

Hua Y, Li H, Crawford TB, 1999. Quantitation of malignant catarrhal fever viral DNA by competitive polymerase chain reaction. *J. Vet. Diagn. Invest.* 11:117–121.

Loken T, Aleksanderson M, Reid H, Pow I, 1998. Malignant catarrhal fever caused by ovine herpesvirus-2 in pigs in Norway. *Vet. Rec.* 143:464–467.

O'Toole D, Li H, Roberts S, Rovnak J, Demartini J, Cavender J, Williams B, Crawford T, 1995. Chronic generalized obliterative arteriopathy in cattle: a sequel to sheep-associated malignant catarrhal fever. *J. Vet. Diagn. Invest.*:108–121.

Pierson, RE, Thake D, McChesney AE, Storz J, 1973. An epizootic of malignant catarrhal fever in feedlot cattle. *J. Am. Vet. Med. Assoc.* 163:349–350.

Pierson RE, Liggitt HD, DeMartini JC, McChesney AE, Storz J, 1978. Clinical and clinicopathologic observations in induced malignant catarrhal fever of cattle. *J. Am. Vet. Med. Assoc.* 173:833–837.

Plowright W, 1990. Malignant catarrhal fever. In *Infectious Diseases of Ruminants,* edited by Z Dinter, B Morein. Amsterdam: Elsevier Scientific Publishers. pp. 123–150.

Schultheiss PC, Collins JK, Austgen LE, DeMartini JC, 1998. Malignant catarrhal fever in bison, acute and chronic cases. *J. Vet. Diagn. Invest.* 10:255–262.

Wyand DS, Helmboldt CF, Nielsen, SW, 1971. Malignant catarrhal fever in white-tailed deer. *J. Am. Vet. Med. Assoc.* 159:605–610.

PAPULAR STOMATITIS

INTRODUCTION

Bovine papular stomatitis (BPS) is a widely distributed poxvirus infection that produces diagnostically confusing papular (and occasionally erosive) lesions on the muzzle and buccal mucous membranes of young cattle. Although occasionally invasive, these lesions, which may be mistaken for erosions of mucosal disease or healing vesicles, usually do not cause overt clinical signs. Diagnosticians who examine the bovine oral mucosa will eventually encounter BPS.

BPS has been associated with skin lesions in humans, teat lesions in milking cattle, esophageal ulcers and hyperkeratosis in calves, and a "rat-tail syndrome" in feedlot cattle. Diagnosis is based on visual examination of the lesion, histopathology or virus isolation, or electron microscopic visualization of the virus in lesions.

Occasionally, under certain conditions, the infection may cause clinical signs, particularly if it occurs in newborn calves or concomitantly with deficiencies or toxicoses. The major importance of BPS lies in its role in the differential diagnosis of diseases affecting the bovine mucosa (DABM).

BPS has been reviewed by Mayr and Buttner (1990), Munz and Dumbell (1994), and Yeruham et al. (1994).

ETIOLOGY

Bovine papular stomatitis virus (BPSV) is a DNA virus of the genus *Parapoxvirus* in the family Poxviridae. It has been cultivated (with some difficulty) on the chorioallantoic membranes of embryonating hens' eggs. Primary isolation and cultivation has also been accomplished on calf kidney, calf testicle, and bovine turbinate cell cultures in which it causes cytopathogenic effects characterized by cytolysis, cytoplasmic stranding, cellular necrosis, and development of horseshoe-shaped intracytoplasmic inclusions (Crandell and Conroy 1974).

The BPSV is large, and when viewed by electron microscopy it resembles orf virus, the type species of the genus *Parapoxvirus* and the cause of contagious pustular dermatitis in sheep. The virus is even more similar to paravaccinia virus, the cause of pseudocowpox, but the three viruses can be distinguished serologically and by DNA hybridization studies.

CLINICAL SIGNS AND LESIONS

Usually, BPSV produces no evident disease aside from the lesions in the mouth and on the muzzle. These lesions may be sequelae to an unnoticed viremia (Mayr and Buttner 1990). They begin as raised hyperemic areas and quickly become roughened plaque-like lesions with irregular edges. Mature lesions are usually red but may have a brownish or yellow color. Occasionally, some degenerate into erosions and can be confused with the lesions of the DABM.

These lesions may persist for several months in an individual calf, although most heal without scar formation in 3 to 5 weeks. Lesions on the muzzle and lips are raised (papular). On the gums and hard palate they frequently are flat and at a glance resemble irregular red-bottomed erosions. Close examination and gentle palpation of lesions is necessary to determine that the mucosa is intact and possesses cornified discolored epithelium that is level with the surrounding mucosa or slightly elevated above it. This differentiating examination is frequently difficult in living cattle because they resent manipulation of the head and mouth.

Occasionally, lesions on the muzzle and lips develop a white necrotic center that eventually sloughs, leaving an ulcerated area that is confusing if one feels that papules are the only landmark of BPS.

BPS usually occurs in calves or young cattle and appears to spread rapidly. When one case is found, other cases are usually present in herdmates. The lesions are usually found when a complete physical examination, including examination of the oral mucosa of calves, is undertaken prior to sale or when other diseases are suspected. Occasionally, calves have severe involvement, possibly stress-induced reactivation of latent infections, with lesions extending to the posterior oral cavity, the esophagus (Crandell and Gosser 1974), and the stomach mucosa, where they may be confused with the focal necrotic lesions of infectious bovine rhinotracheitis (IBR) or mycotic infections.

When fever or extensive distribution of lesions is observed, the possibility that BPS is a complication of another disease or that the calf is immunologically compromised should be considered. As is true of most mild infections, occasionally an animal may develop severe systemic disease.

The disease is occasionally seen concomitantly with pseudocowpox lesions on the teats of milk cows and the hands of milkers (Nagington et al. 1967). In this case, the nomenclature becomes confusing because pseudocowpox is considered a distinct entity.

A necrotic dermatitis of the tail of feedlot cattle, designated rat-tail syndrome, has been associated with papular stomatitis virus. Cattle with this condition lose the switch of the tail, leaving a raw, denuded area. They become chronically unthrifty and are usually culled from feedlots. Affected cattle sometimes have hyperkeratotic lesions in the mouth, esophagus, and omasum (Brown et al. 1976).

EFFECTS ON THE DEVELOPING FETUS

The effects (if any) of BPSV on the developing fetus are not known.

NECROPSY FINDINGS

Most infected animals survive without serious harm and thus are not subjected to necropsy. When BPS lesions are found at necropsy, they are usually incidental findings, and unless widely distributed throughout the body, they are probably not etiologically involved in the animal's demise. Sometimes, however, BPS causes extensive proliferative lesions and ulceration of mucosa throughout the upper alimentary tract.

Histologic examination of specimens taken for biopsy reveals the typical features of poxvirus infections. If a series of early and late proliferative lesions are examined, the pathogenesis of the lesion can be appreciated. The lesion is focal and characterized by vacuolization, hydroptic degeneration, and hyperplasia of epithelial cells. There is capillary distention, moderate infiltration of involved areas with inflammatory cells, and accumulation of necrotic material in the center of the lesion. Eosinophilic inclusions are frequently found in cytoplasm of degenerating cells. Most experienced pathologists recognize the lesion, which is similar to pseudocowpox on the teats of milk cows.

Aside from collection of specimens for histopathologic or electron microscopic examination, diagnostic tests are usually not conducted for BPS.

DIAGNOSIS

Diagnosis is based on finding lesions in the mouths of calves and can be verified histologically.

The diagnostic profile involves dairy calves between 1 and 20 months of age (but usually less than 6 months old) or older beef cattle on poor pasture. Affected animals usually show no systemic disturbance but have raised papular or flat, irregular-edged, brown lesions on the oral mucous membranes and muzzle. Affected animals may have clinical signs of other diseases, warranting examination of the buccal mucosa, but BPS lesions themselves do not usually produce serious illness. The rare widely distributed extensive lesions and the rat-tail syndrome are exceptions to this classic description.

Clinical diagnosis is based on finding the lesions.

Differential Diagnosis

The differential diagnosis includes ingestion of caustic substances, and DABM that cause ulceration, erosion, vesiculation, necrosis, or hemorrhage in the mouth of cattle. These include BVD, malignant catarrhal fever, rinderpest, bluetongue, vesicular stomatitis, and foot-and-mouth disease. Usually, the distinctive lesions and lack of other clinical signs are adequate for a diagnosis, which may be confirmed histopathologically.

Laboratory Diagnosis

The experienced clinician can diagnose BPS by the nature and location of the lesions. To familiarize themselves with BPS, those who have never seen the disease should carefully examine the mouths of calves until suspicious lesions are seen. The suspicion can be confirmed by sending a lesion and some adjacent normal tissue in fixative to a histopathologist, who will confirm the diagnosis by reporting a pox-like lesion with intracytoplasmic inclusions. The virus can be visualized by direct electron microscopy and can be isolated in some cell culture systems.

EPIDEMIOLOGY

The reservoir and usual source of infection is probably latently infected cattle (Mayr and Buttner 1990). While nursing infected cattle may be a major mode of transmission, BPS is seen in bucket-fed as well as nursing calves and probably also spreads on feeding utensils. Because it is seen commonly in calves under 20 months of age, many modes of transmission may exist. The virus probably enters through abrasions in the oral mucosa.

IMMUNITY

Recovered animals are probably resistant to serious subsequent infections. It has been difficult to demonstrate humoral antibody against BPSV and colostrally acquired passive immunity is probably not protective.

VIRUS PERSISTENCE

One school of thought holds that BPSV can become a chronic persistent infection capable of producing lesions periodically upon stress-induced reactivation (Mayr and Buttner 1990).

PREVENTION AND CONTROL

Because of the benign nature of the disease, no specific control or eradication procedures other than good hygiene and management practices are usually undertaken. An experimental orf virus vaccine has been developed in Europe but is not widely used.

THERAPY AND MANAGEMENT OF OUTBREAKS

BPS is generally self-limiting, benign, and untreated. If seen in time, transmission to other calves may possibly be limited by isolation, hygiene, and use of separate feeding equipment.

Because transmission to humans occasionally occurs, workers should be advised to avoid contacting calves if they have abrasions or lesions on the skin (Schurrenberger et al. 1980), or are immunologically compromised.

Where disseminated lesions occur, a search should be made to determine what (if any) complicating factor such as stress, dietary deficiency, or low-level toxicosis may be contributing to the pathogenesis of the infection, which is usually benign.

LIKELIHOOD OF ERADICATION

It is unlikely countries will attempt eradication of BPS because of its limited economic impact.

IMPACT ON INTERNATIONAL TRADE

BPS is not categorized as a List A or List B disease by the Office International Des Epizooties and it is unlikely that BPSV-based import measures would be imposed. However, individuals preparing health certificates should always examine the mouths of cattle before certifying that the animals are free of contagious diseases.

PUBLIC RESPONSIBILITY

Knowledge of the diagnosis of BPS is necessary to avoid misdiagnosis and to alert workers of the zoonotic potential.

Because BPS occasionally causes a benign, self-limiting lesion in humans, caretakers with skin abrasions, severe dermatitis, acne, or other skin problems or those with known immunologic deficiencies or on immunosuppressive therapy should stay away from infected calves and use extreme care on infected premises.

AREAS IN NEED OF RESEARCH

Research is needed on the serologic response to infection and on other diagnostic features of BPS, with emphasis on differentiation from other pox-like and ulcerative lesions. Further work is needed on the conditions required for manifestation of the pathogenic potential of BPSV.

REFERENCES

Brown LN, Irwin LR, Bucerra VM, 1976. "Rat-tail syndrome" of feedlot cattle and bovine papular stomatitis virus infection. *Proc. Am. Assoc. Vet. Lab. Diagn.* 19:405–410.

Crandell RA, Conroy JD, 1974. The isolation and characterization of a strain of papular stomatitis virus. *Proc. Am. Assoc. Vet. Lab. Diagn.* 17:223–234.

Crandell RA, Gosser HA, 1974. Ulcerative esophagitis associated with a poxvirus infection in a calf. *J. Am. Vet. Med. Assoc.* 165:282–283.

Mayr A, Buttner M, 1990. Bovine Papular Stomatitis Virus. In *Infectious Diseases of Ruminants,* edited by Z Dinter, B Morein. Amsterdam: Elsevier Scientific Publishers, pp. 23–28.

Munz E, Dumbell K, 1994. Bovine papular stomatitis. In *Infectious Disases of Livestock With Special Reference to Southern Africa,* edited by JAW Coetzer, GR Thomson, RC Tustin. Capetown: Oxford University Press, pp. 623–624.

Nagington JE, Lauder M, Smith JS, 1967. Bovine papular stomatitis, pseudocowpox, and milkers nodules. *Vet. Rec.* 81:306–313.

Schurrenberger PG, Swango LJ, Bowmwan GM, Lutgen PO, 1980. Bovine papular stomatitis in veterinary students. *Can. J. Comp. Med.* 44:239–243.

Yeruham I, Abraham A, Nyska A, 1994. Clinical and pathological description of a chronic form of bovine papular stomatitis. *J. Comp. Pathol.* 111: 279–286.

21

PARAINFLUENZA TYPE-3

INTRODUCTION

Bovine parainfluenza type-3 virus (PI-3) was once called "the shipping fever virus" because of its frequent association with pulmonic pasteurellosis. It is now known to be one participant in the multifactorial etiology of shipping fever (SF) and other bovine respiratory disease (BRD), including enzootic calf pneumonia.

PI-3 was isolated in the late 1950s from cattle with SF (Reisinger et al. 1959). Since then, it has been recovered repeatedly throughout the world from normal cattle, calves with enzootic calf pneumonia, cattle with SF and a variety of BRD, and occasionally from aborted fetuses. Its role as a singular primary pathogen is probably minimal, but it is involved in several multiple-etiology syndromes.

In the decades since the PI-3 virus was first isolated, information has emerged on its epizootiology, pathogenicity, and immunology. Vaccines have been produced, improved, and widely used in combination with various other viral and bacterial products.

Despite these advances, the problems of enzootic calf pneumonia, BRD, and SF remain without totally effective preventive measures. Management factors, stress of movement and assembly, bacteria, and numerous other viruses including infectious bovine rhinotracheitis virus (IBRV), bovine respiratory syncytial virus (BRSV), adenoviruses, respiratory coronaviruses, and bovine viral diarrhea virus (BVDV) have been implicated as contributing factors in BRD, and concern over PI-3 has diminished.

PI-3 has been reviewed by Bryson (1990), Frank (1992), and van Vuuren (1994).

ETIOLOGY

The family Paramyxoviridae contains three genera, including the genus *Paramyxovirus,* which includes the parainfluenza viruses. The Paramyxoviridae are enveloped RNA viruses, varying in size from 120 to 300 microns, that infect the respiratory tract and contain surface receptors that agglutinate red blood cells. Even though "parainfluenza" means "influenza-like," the paramyxoviruses are antigenically and biologically distinct from the true influenza viruses, which are classified in the family Orthomyxoviridae.

PI-3, one of four parainfluenza virus types in the genus *Paramyxovirus,* has worldwide distribution. All the parainfluenza viruses are antigenically related and have similar biological, biophysical, and cultural characteristics but are distinguished serologically and by species of origin. Human parainfluenza type-3 viruses are one cause of respiratory disease in children.

Unlike the true influenza viruses, which undergo frequent minor antigenic drift through mutation and occasional major antigenic shifts through viral recombination producing antigenically distinct viral populations in nature, PI-3 has been remarkably stable.

In cell cultures, PI-3 virus induces cytopathic effects (CPE), characterized by cytoplasmic stranding, formation of holes in monolayers, intranuclear and intracytoplasmic inclusion bodies, and syncytium formation. These CPE can be inhibited by addition of antibody, and a virus neutralization test based on this phenomenon can be used for serologic tests. When the virus is cultivated in monolayers under agar overlays, distinct plaques are formed and serum antibody can also be assayed using plaque-reduction neutralization tests.

Red blood cells of many species adhere to cell cultures actively infected with PI-3 virus (hemadsorption), and PI-3 virus suspensions will cause clumping (hemagglutination) of erythrocyte suspensions. Hemagglutination is a commonly employed laboratory marker, and the hemagglutination inhibition (HI) test is generally preferred over the neutralization test for diagnosis, strain identification, vaccine evaluation, and selection of susceptible experimental cattle.

CLINICAL SIGNS AND LESIONS

The widespread prevalence of HI antibody among cattle that have never been reported ill suggests that PI-3 virus is ubiquitous, and most singular uncomplicated infections are asymptomatic or mild or go unrecognized. Nonetheless, evidence for a pathogenic potential for PI-3 abounds. The consistent isolation of the virus from cattle with fever, cough, excess nasal and ocular discharge, and increased respiratory rates and pulmonary rales (Marshall and Frank 1975) and the numerous reports of respiratory disease following experimental infection of susceptible calves (Bryson 1990) all indicate that given the proper circumstances, cattle can sicken when infected with PI-3 virus.

The impact of these findings diminishes because, despite damage to respiratory epithelium, clinical signs are frequently mild and asymptomatic unless complicated by other infections.

After the evidence is evaluated, it must be concluded that PI-3 generally expresses its pathogenic potential as a predisposing infection working in concert with other agents and that certain environment-host-agent interactions are required for its participation in the multifactorial etiology of BRD. These interactions occur when cattle are shipped, assembled in feedlots, and commingled in intensive calf-raising operations, but they can also occur in other production-management situations if appropriate exacerbating cofactors are present (Li and Castleman 1990).

EFFECTS ON THE DEVELOPING FETUS

The PI-3 virus has been isolated from naturally and experimentally aborted fetuses (Sattar et al. 1967; Swift and Kennedy 1972).

HI antibody against PI-3 has been found in aborted fetuses, sometimes along with antibody to multiple viruses (Dunne et al. 1973). Fetuses at midgestation can respond immunologically to PI-3 virus, and fetal serology is sometimes used as a diagnostic procedure (Swift 1973).

Fetal infection is unlikely if the pregnant female possesses serum HI antibody at the time of exposure (Swift and Trueblood 1973) and the widespread seroprevalence of PI-3 antibody may preclude it as a major cause of bovine abortions (Swift and Trueblood 1974). This lack of major abortifacient significance is supported by a survey (Anderson et al. 1990). Nevertheless, PI-3 infection of the fetus occurs, and occasional abortions result.

NECROPSY FINDINGS

The majority of deaths from respiratory diseases in North America occur in feedlots. Many are attributed to SF pneumonia caused by pulmonic pasteurellosis or other bacterial infections that are secondary to viral infections. Thus, lesions of naturally occurring respiratory disease are not usually attributed to PI-3, even if it played a role in their development.

The gross respiratory lesions of experimental PI-3 infection are congestion of respiratory mucosa, consolidation of ventral portions of the lungs, and enlargement of the bronchial and retropharyngeal lymph nodes (Marshall and Frank 1975).

Histopathologic findings include bronchiolitis and peribronchiolitis. Variable degrees of cellular and exudative infiltration and intranuclear and intracytoplasmic inclusions may be found in cells that line the alveoli (Frank and Marshall 1973).

Calves examined from 5 to 12 days after aerosol exposure had more extensive microscopic lesions in the lungs than in the trachea (Tsai and Thomson 1975). There may be degenerative and proliferative changes in the epithelial cells of the alveoli and bronchioles, infiltration by mononuclear and polymorphonuclear cells, formation of multinucleated giant cells, and intranuclear and intracytoplasmic inclusion bodies. Electron microscopy may reveal viral particles associated with epithelial degeneration in the trachea and bronchioles. These findings support the hypothesis that PI-3 infection causes epithelial damage by permitting colonization of *Pasteurella* and other bacteria.

Slight depression in total leukocyte counts has been associated with experimental infection with PI-3 (Marshall and Frank 1975). Leukocytosis has also been reported and because multiple infections are frequently encountered, total white blood cell counts are probably a poor diagnostic tool for PI-3 infection.

DIAGNOSIS

Clinical signs and lesions are not distinctive enough for diagnosis of PI-3 infection. Outbreaks of acute pneumonia in calves, chronic enzootic calf pneumonia, or SF warrant consideration of PI-3 infection as a contributing or predisposing factor. This suspicion can be confirmed by virus isolation or immunofluorescent identification of viral antigen in tissues. Confirmation by seroconversion is less convincing.

Differential Diagnosis

The differential diagnosis includes IBRV, BRSV, BVDV, respiratory coronaviruses, as well as *Pasteurella* and a multitude of bacteria, all of which contribute, along with management factors, to the multifactorial etiology of BRD.

Laboratory Diagnosis

Because of the nondescript nature of clinical signs and lesions, PI-3 infection is definitively diagnosed only by laboratory procedures.

The antibody prevalence is high in most bovine populations and single serum specimens are relatively useless for diagnostic purposes. Seroconversion from negative to positive or significant (fourfold) rises in HI titers are indicative of infection but do not necessarily establish that PI-3 caused the observed clinical signs.

The presence of PI-3 antibody in serum of aborted fetuses or stillborn calves indicates prenatal infection.

The PI-3 virus can be isolated by inoculating cell cultures with nasal and ocular secretions or blood of live animals during the early stages of the infection. If characteristic CPE appear, the virus can be identified by hemagglutination inhibition or neutralization tests using specific antiserums.

At necropsy within a few days of exposure, PI-3 can be recovered from lung tissue, which is the specimen of choice (Frank 1992), and from trachea, larynx, turbinates, and lymph nodes draining the respiratory tract. Frequently, by the time necropsy is conducted on naturally occurring cases of BRD, virus is no longer present.

PI-3 can also be isolated from homogenates of fetal tissues (Swift and Trueblood 1974) and the thoracic fluid and lungs of aborted fetuses (Sattar et al. 1967). People seeking virus isolations should first contact the laboratory for instructions on sample collection and shipment.

EPIDEMIOLOGY

Virus shed in nasal discharges is acquired via the respiratory tract of susceptible cattle, especially those in close contact in cold weather. It replicates in respiratory epithelium where it depresses phagocytosis by alveolar macrophages and causes cell damage that permits secondary invasion by bacteria.

The high antibody prevalence among adults suggests frequent reinfection or prolonged persistence of serologic titers or both. Fetal infection probably requires primary infection of susceptible pregnant cattle, a rare event in populations with high antibody prevalences.

The incubation period is short but hard to estimate in the field because many infections are inapparent and asymptomatic. Nonetheless, careful monitoring indicates that fever appears within 2 days of aerosol exposure and lasts for 6 to 10 days.

Cattle are probably the principal reservoir, and their nasal and ocular discharges are the immediate source of infection. Virus probably enters susceptible cattle via the nasal passages and mouth.

Antibody surveys indicate that water buffalo, deer, horses, and monkeys can also be infected. Sheep infected with certain BPI-3 may develop severe respiratory disease, but the role of nonbovine animals in virus transmission and maintenance is probably minimal.

As with most endemic viruses, antibody prevalence increases with increasing age, and younger cattle manifest most severe clinical signs. The seriousness of clinical disease may be more related to immune status, complicating infections, and environmental conditions than to age per se. There appears to be no significant difference in susceptibility among the sexes and breeds.

IMMUNITY

The immunity following vaccination or natural exposure is partial rather than complete. Cattle with serum or nasal antibody can be infected but then illnesses are likely to be less severe than those of immunologically naive animals.

Cattle with measurable serum antibody are unlikely to support transplacental transmission to their fetuses (Swift and Trueblood 1974), so previous exposure or successful vaccination may afford protection from PI-3 abortion.

Following aerosol exposure, neutralizing antibody appears in both the serum and nasal secretions (Frank and Marshall 1971). Nasal antibody produced locally or spilled over from the circulation may help resist infection but probably requires frequent restimulation for maintenance of protective levels.

Because of the high prevalence of serum antibody among adults, many newborn calves have passive antibody acquired by colostrum ingestion. This antibody may persist from 10 weeks to 8 months. Depending on the titer of the calf, the vaccine dose, and the route of inoculation, colostrally acquired maternal antibody may interfere with vaccination. Calves with colostrally acquired maternal antibody have less severe infections than colostrum-deprived calves (Marshall and Frank 1975).

Cattle with actively induced antibody frequently experience a secondary immune response and rising titer upon subsequent exposure. This response and the fact that calves with actively acquired antibody can become infected and sicken (Frank and Marshall 1971) support the thesis of partial rather than absolute immunity and reaffirm recommendations for repeated vaccinations.

VIRUS PERSISTENCE

Most experimentally infected cattle stop shedding virus in nasal secretions after 8 to 10 days of exposure (Marshall and Frank 1975). Evidence of active shedding cessation, however, does not necessarily ensure total virus clearance. Naturally infected calves have been detected shedding PI-3 for several months (Stott et al. 1980). The frequency of infections with PI-3 suggests that persistent infections occur, that immunity is extremely short-lived and that reinfection is common, or that nonbovine reservoirs frequently reseed cattle populations. Tsai (1977) found noncytolytic PI-3 infections of alveolar macrophages of infected calves and indications that these cells can produce and liberate mature virus when exposed to lowered temperatures. This phenomenon could explain the ubiquity of PI-3 virus in cattle populations and the association of outbreaks with cold weather.

PREVENTION AND CONTROL

The production-management systems under which PI-3 expresses its maximum pathogenic potential are characterized by close contact among cattle, stress, and commingling of cattle harboring different microbiologic flora. The management style of feedlots, calf-rearing areas, and veal production units is changing as the relationship between comfortable, noncompetitive environments and production efficiency becomes apparent. Thus, control efforts may gradually de-emphasize vaccines in favor of less crowding, improved ventilation, and stress-reduction measures. The safety and efficacy considerations concerning PI-3 immunization reviewed by Gale (1968) are still applicable.

Inactivated and modified live virus PI-3 vaccines for intramuscular, subcutaneous, or intranasal installation are widely used despite gaps in information regarding their mechanism of action and duration of effectiveness. The uncertainty about the pathogenesis of simple singular PI-3 infection has caused these vaccines to be used largely in combination with IBRV, BRSV, BVDV vaccines or *Pasteurella* bacterins. This pattern of use implies that the diseases they are designed to prevent have multifactorial etiology and that PI-3 (by itself) does not justify the expense of vaccination.

Inactivated adjuvanted PI-3 vaccine was released for marketing in the United States combined with bacterins for *Pasteurella multocida* and *P. hemolyticum* in the late 1960s. In the early 1970s, it was combined with inactivated IBR vaccine, and this combination has been available intermittently since then. Inconsistency of PI-3 challenge studies and questions about the protective role of serum antibody, a major indicator of vaccine response, has complicated evaluations of the efficacy of inactivated PI-3 vaccines. Nevertheless, the consistent production of PI-3 antibody following vaccination, the clamor for a product against BRD, and marketing programs have resulted in continued use of vaccines.

The safety of the inactivated vaccines gives them appeal for use on pregnant cattle and in stressful situations where clinical judgment weighs against use of MLV vaccines. Fatal or nonfatal anaphylactic reaction has followed their use, but this is an extremely rare occurrence.

The inactivated vaccines can be used on cattle of all ages. Revaccination is recommended for any calves vaccinated before 6 months of age because of uncertainty about possible blocking effects of colostrally acquired maternal antibody.

When compared with MLV vaccines, the inactivated products are probably less effective, and their use requires more frequent revaccination. However, what they sacrifice in efficacy they gain in safety.

Like the inactivated vaccines, the MLV products are hard to evaluate because of the insidious nature of the infection. Also, by being available only in combination vaccines, the PI-3 components tend to lose their identity to IBRV, BRSV, and BVDV, which produce more distinctive clinical syndromes.

The early MLV vaccines were tissue-culture-propagated viruses attenuated by a small number of serial passages and inoculated intramuscularly (IM). They were contraindicated for pregnant cattle. With emerging knowledge of local immunity, the use of serum antibody as an indicator of immunity to PI-3 was questioned, and in the late 1960s intranasal (IN) application of MLV PI-3 vaccines was proposed. IN MLV vaccines are still used today and appear to be moderately effective (Bryson et al 1999).

Today, PI-3 MLV vaccines are available for both IN and IM administrations. The major differences are ease of administration of IM vaccines and utility of IN vaccines for pregnant cattle. Both IN and IM vaccines can be used on calves of all ages. Because of possible interference by colostrally acquired maternal antibody, calves vaccinated under 6 months of age probably should be revaccinated (Marshall and Frank 1975). Because of the frequency of neonatal problems, extreme caution is advised in using MLV vaccines on neonates unless these vaccines are specifically labeled for such use.

Both IM and IN vaccines can contribute to calfhood vaccination programs when administered to healthy, unstressed dairy calves as a means of reducing the probability of catastrophic outbreaks from new introductions into totally susceptible herds. In other production-management systems and stressful situations, they should be used with caution.

When combined with MLV vaccines that are abortifacient, they are contraindicated for pregnant cattle.

THERAPY AND MANAGEMENT OF OUTBREAKS

Primary infections are rarely recognized until secondary events lead to enzootic calf pneumonia, SF, or other BRD. These diseases are treated with good nursing care, supportive therapy, and stress management measures. Bacterial pneumonia is treated with recommended doses of approved antibiotics in strict observance of appropriate withdrawal times.

The question of use of MLV PI-3 vaccines upon suspicion of PI-3 infection is controversial and confused by the inability to obtain an etiologic diagnosis based solely on clinical signs. Also, the incorporation of IBRV, BRSV, and BVDV into PI-3 virus-containing products complicates the decision by forcing consideration of the contraindications and hazards associated with each virus in vaccine combinations. The vaccination question must be evaluated individually for each situation using the guidelines presented in the section on Vaccination of Infected, Exposed, or Stressed Cattle in Chapter 5.

LIKELIHOOD OF ERADICATION

Because of its apparent ubiquitousness and the lack of a clear-cut clinical syndrome for PI-3, eradication seems unlikely.

IMPACT ON INTERNATIONAL TRADE

PI-3 has not been categorized as a List A or List B disease by the Office International Des Epizooties. It is unlikely to impact international trade unless identified in association with sick cattle moving internationally.

PUBLIC RESPONSIBILITY

The retrospective nature of laboratory diagnosis means specific action regarding infected herds cannot be recommended. Cattle with respiratory disease should not be transported.

AREAS IN NEED OF RESEARCH

The immunologic approaches to PI-3 control need further elaboration, and the mechanisms of persistent infection (if any) need exploration.

REFERENCES

Anderson MJ, Blanchard PC, Barr BC, Hoffman RL, 1990. A survey of causes of bovine abortion in the San Joaquin Valley of California. *J. Vet. Diag. Invest.* 2:283-287.

Bryson DG, 1990. Parainfluenza-3 virus in cattle. In *Infectious Diseases of Ruminants,* edited by Z Dinter, B Morein. Amsterdam: Elsevier Scientific Publishers, pp. 319-333.

Bryson DG, Adair BM, McNulty MS, Mcaliskey H, Bradford H, Allan G, Evans RT, Forster F, 1999. Studies on the efficacy of intranasal vaccination for the protection of experimentally induced parainfluenza type-3 virus pneumonia in calves. *Vet. Rec.* 145:33-39.

Dunne HW, Ajinka FM, Bubash GR, Griel LC, 1973. Parainfluenza-3 and bovine enteroviruses as possible important causative factors in bovine abortion. *Am. J. Vet. Res.* 34:1121-1126.

Frank GH, 1992. Parainfluenza type-3. In *Veterinary Diagnostic Virology: A Practitioners Guide,* edited by AE Castro, WP Heuschele. St. Louis: Mosby Yearbook, pp. 114-116.

Frank GH, Marshall RG, 1971. Relationship of serum and nasal secretion-neutralizing antibodies in protection of calves against parainfluenza-3 virus. *Am. J. Vet. Res.* 32:1707-1713.

Frank GH, Marshall RG, 1973. Parainfluenza-3 virus infection of cattle. *J. Am. Vet. Med. Assoc.* 163:858-860.

Gale C, 1968. Bovine parainfluenza-3 immunization procedures. *J. Am. Vet. Med. Assoc.* 152:871-877.

Li X, Castleman WL, 1990. Effects of 4-Epomeanol on bovine parainfluenza type-3 virus induced pneumonia in calves. *Vet. Pathol.* 28:428-437.

Marshall RG, Frank GH, 1975. Clinical and immunological response of calves with colostrally acquired maternal antibody against parainfluenza-3 virus to homologous viral infection. *Am. J. Vet. Res.* 36: 1085-1089.

Reisinger RC, Heddleston KI, Manthei CA, 1959. A myxovirus (SF-4) associated with shipping fever of cattle. *J. Am. Vet. Med. Assoc.* 135:147-152.

Sattar SA, Bohl E, Trapp HC, Hamdy AH, 1967. Infection of bovine fetuses with myxovirus parainfluenza-3 virus. *Am. J. Vet. Res.* 28:45-49.

Stott EJ, Thomas LH, Collins, AP, Crouch S, Jebbett, J, Smith GS, Luther PD, Caswell R, 1980. A survey of virus infections in the respiratory tract of cattle and their association with disease. *J. Hyg. (Camb.)* 85:257-270.

Swift BL, 1973. Bovine parainfluenza-3 virus experimental fetal disease. *J. Am. Vet. Med. Assoc.* 163:861-862.

Swift BL, Kennedy PC, 1972. Experimentally induced infection of in utero fetuses with bovine parainfluenza-3 virus. *Am. J. Vet. Res.* 33: 57-63.

Swift BL, Trueblood MS, 1973. Failure to induce fetal infection by inoculation of pregnant immune heifers with bovine parainfluenza-3 virus. *J. Infect. Dis.* 127:713-717.

Swift BL, Trueblood, MS, 1974. The present status of the parainfluenza-3 (PI-3) virus and fetal disease of cattle and sheep. *Theriogenology* 2:101-107.

Tsai KS, 1977. Replication of parainfluenza type-3 virus in aveloar macrophages: Evidence of in vivo infection and of in vitro temperature sensitivity in virus maturation. *Infect. Immunol.* 18:780-791.

van Vuuren M, 1994. Parainfluenza infection. In *Infectious Diseases of Livestock With Special Reference to Southern Africa,* edited by JAW Coetzer, GR Thomson, RC Tustin. Capetown: Oxford University Press, pp. 766-768.

22

PARVOVIRUSES

INTRODUCTION

Bovine parvoviruses (BPoV) are found in aborted fetuses and in the feces of normal calves and of calves with diarrhea. Antibody prevalence studies indicate BPoV are globally distributed in cattle, and most infections are inapparent. Under certain conditions, however, BPoV can be significant pathogens deserving consideration in the diagnosis of abortion and calf diarrhea.

BPoV have been reviewed by Storz (1990), Sandals et al. (1995), and Thomson (1994).

ETIOLOGY

Parvovirus is a genus of small, nonenveloped DNA viruses in the family Parvoviridae. The name comes from the Latin word *parvus,* which means very small. Most parvoviruses require rapidly dividing cells for optimal replication and thus favor fetal and gastrointestinal tissues.

The first BPoV, isolated from the feces of healthy calves before the term parvovirus evolved, was called HADEN virus, an acronym for hemadsorbing enteric virus (Abinanti and Warfield 1961). Over the years, additional isolations from sick and healthy cattle have occurred, and it is now known that BPoV are widely distributed among cattle populations.

BPoV induce cytopathic effects (CPE) in some cell cultures, but these changes are not always evident because they require rapidly dividing cells and cultures free of inhibiting substances. They are more easily recovered from feces than from tissues.

Like other parvoviruses, the BPoV hemagglutinate red blood cells of guinea pigs and human type O erythrocytes. Even though serum from infected animals neutralizes viral activity, hemagglutination inhibition (HI) tests are usually used for serodiagnosis, typing isolates, and determining the susceptibility of experimental cattle. Using HI, most isolates appear to be parvovirus type 1 (related to the prototype HADEN virus), but a few differ and are designated parvovirus type 2.

BPoV are antigenically distinct from parvoviruses that infect humans, swine, cats, dogs, and rabbits. Occasional BPoV serotiters in human and porcine serums may result from ingestion of bovine milk or milk products containing BPoV or BPoV antibodies (Mengling and Mathews 1990).

Although sensitive to some disinfectants, BPoV are generally resistant to chemicals and physical influences.

CLINICAL SIGNS AND LESIONS

BPoV have been isolated from clinically normal cattle, aborted fetuses, and animals with respiratory disease, conjunctivitis, and diarrhea. Their role in field outbreaks is obscured by the difficulty of obtaining isolates from clinical specimens and the fact that they commonly occur in multiple infections with other viruses (Storz 1990).

The experimental production of diarrhea in neonatal calves (Storz 1990) leaves little doubt that BPoV have considerable pathogenic potential, but their importance as a cause of neonatal diarrhea and the conditions required for expression of this potential need further clarification.

EFFECTS ON THE DEVELOPING FETUS

BPoV can cause fetal death and abortion when virus gains access to fetuses in the first and second trimesters of pregnancy. Fetuses exposed in the last trimester may respond immunologically and survive (Storz 1990). Fetal viremia may persist in the presence of fetal antibody and can hinder virus isolation from fetuses (Liggitt et al. 1982).

NECROPSY FINDINGS

Following natural or experimental infection of fetuses and calves, virus can be demonstrated throughout the body by fluorescent antibody (FA) techniques and isolated from erythrocytes and leukocytes. Specific gross lesions of diagnostic value do not occur. Aborted fetuses have nonspecific lesions such as generalized edema and fluids in body cavities.

Histologically, unique intranuclear inclusion bodies are found in infected cell cultures and in the adrenal glands of experimentally infected calves and cells of liver, intestinal mucosa, and lymph nodes of aborted fetuses.

DIAGNOSIS

Clinical diagnosis can only be presumptive; laboratory tests are necessary to confirm the diagnosis. Although BPoV may contribute to neonatal diarrhea and abortion, the associated clinical signs and lesions are nonspecific, and a characteristic diagnostic profile cannot be described.

Differential Diagnosis

BPoV deserve consideration in the diagnosis of bovine abortion and calf diarrhea and must be differentiated from the multiple other causes of these problems.

Laboratory Diagnosis

Virus isolation and identification are prerequisites for diagnosis. Virus isolation can be achieved in rapidly replicating cultures of bovine fetal testicle, spleen and adrenal cells. Most field isolates have come from feces. These findings must be interpreted cautiously because BPoV is shed in feces for some time after primary infection and development of serum antibody.

Isolation from tissues is expedited by direct culture of infected tissues or by inoculation of parasynchronous cell cultures (Stolz 1990). These cultures have been synchronized to achieve optimal cell division and subsequently stimulated for continued cell division by periodic partial cell harvests and addition of serum free from parvovirus antibody.

BPoV isolation techniques are not routinely conducted in all diagnostic laboratories. The actual importance of BPoV will not be appreciated until this technology is more widely applied.

FA assay can be useful for locating viral antigen in tissues from infected cattle and in cell cultures inoculated with diagnostic specimens. For serologic testing, HI tests are commonly used, but other tests such as indirect FA and virus neutralization test are adaptable to BPoV studies and offer potential for detecting seroconversion or rising titers. Because of widespread antibody prevalence and the nondescript nature of the clinical signs and lesions, all precautions applicable to viral serology are necessary. Fetal serology holds promise for diagnosing parvovirus-induced abortion.

Those seeking BPoV diagnostic procedure should contact the laboratory to inquire if serology, virus isolation procedures, or FA assay is available and for instructions on specimen collection.

EPIDEMIOLOGY

Current information indicates that cattle are the reservoir and usual source of infection. Transmission occurs by the oral–fecal route, and healthy carriers shed virus in their feces, making the infection virtually ubiquitous and accounting for the high antibody prevalence.

IMMUNITY

Colostrally acquired immunity may afford some protection against infection. Actively induced humoral antibody is widespread and may protect or merely indicate that local immune functions have been stimulated. Prior exposure may be adequate to prevent BpoV-induced abortion upon exposure during pregnancy.

VIRUS PERSISTENCE

The virus continues to multiply in the gut of infected cattle even after development of serum antibody, thus establishing a healthy infected carrier state of unknown duration.

PREVENTION AND CONTROL

The management and hygiene procedures appropriate to all viral infections are applicable to BPoV infections. Care should be taken to restrict movement between groups of cattle if one group is experiencing abortions or neonatal diarrhea. To date, BPoV vaccines have not been developed.

THERAPY AND MANAGEMENT OF OUTBREAKS

Symptomatic treatment and good nursing care, coupled with antibiotics, antidiarrheals, and replacement of fluids to maintain body hydration, are indicated for calves with neonatal diarrhea, whatever the cause. Management practices should be adjusted to minimize transmission and ensure colostrum acquisition.

LIKELIHOOD OF ERADICATION

Current information indicates BPoV lack the economic importance to justify eradication attempts.

IMPACT ON INTERNATIONAL TRADE

BPoV infection is not included as a List A or List B disease by the Office International Des Epizooties and international trade measures have not been adopted.

PUBLIC RESPONSIBILITY

There is no evidence of pathogenicity for humans. Aside from hygienic considerations, biosecurity, and good management, no special public responsibilities are currently advised.

AREAS IN NEED OF RESEARCH

Further studies are needed in the diagnosis, epidemiology, immunology, and pathogenicity of BPoV.

REFERENCES

Abinanti FR, Warfield MS, 1961. Recovery of a hemadsorbing virus (HADEN) from the gastrointestinal tract of calves. *Virology* 14:288–289.

Liggitt HD, DeMartini JC, Pearson LD, 1982. Immunologic responses of the bovine fetus to parvovirus infection. *Am. J. Vet. Res.* 43:1355–1359.

Mengling WI, Mathews PJ, 1990. Antibodies to bovine parvovirus acquired by neonatal pigs through ingestion of virus and antibody in the dict. *Am. J. Vet. Res.* 51:632–635.

Sandals WC, Povey RC, Meek AH, 1995. Prevalence of bovine parvovirus infection in Ontario dairy cattle. *Can. J. Vet. Res.* 59:81–86.

Storz J, 1990. Bovine parvoviruses. In *Infectious Diseases of Ruminants,* edited by Z Dinter, B Morein. Amsterdam: Elsevier Scientific Publishers. pp. 203–214.

Thomson GR, 1994. Bovine parvovirus infection. In *Infectious Diseases of Livestock With Special Reference to Southern Africa* edited by JAW Coetzer, GR Thomson, RC Tustin. Capetown: Oxford University Press, pp. 895–987.

POXVIRUS INFECTIONS OF THE TEATS

INTRODUCTION

Vaccinia virus, cowpox virus, and pseudocowpox virus are among the many causes of bovine teat lesions. Poxvirus lesions are frequently sporadic but can occur in epizootic proportions, causing economic loss associated with mastitis and lowered milk production.

Pseudocowpox virus causes pseudocowpox, the most common poxvirus lesion of the teats, and milker's nodules, the most common lesion on the hands of milkers.

Cowpox and vaccinia (the laboratory strain used as human smallpox vaccine) viruses occasionally infect the teats of cattle. This discussion will include vaccinia virus and make historic reference to smallpox vaccination.

All these viruses can be transmitted from cattle to the hands of milkers, causing painful but usually self-limiting lesions.

Worldwide smallpox eradication, discontinuance of smallpox vaccination, and emergence of a totally susceptible human population may usher in a new era in poxvirus lesions on the hands of people and the teats of cows.

ETIOLOGY

Vaccinia virus, cowpox virus, and pseudocowpox virus are large DNA viruses in the family Poxviridae. Vaccinia and cowpox are of the genus *Orthopoxvirus*. Pseudocowpox virus is of the genus *Parapoxvirus*.

In the past, human poxvirus infections were modified by immunity to vaccinia from smallpox vaccination, which has now ceased.

These poxviruses are highly resistant to disinfectants, heat, and drying and are capable of maintaining their infectivity in scabs or other tissue fragments. They can be preserved for prolonged periods by freezing.

They produce cytopathic changes in cell cultures and intracytoplasmic inclusions in cell cultures and animal tissues. They are readily transmittable by intradermal inoculations, which induce lesions in cattle.

Vaccinia and cowpox are similar, but pseudocowpox has many differentiating characteristics. All three can be distinguished by monoclonal antibody and DNA restriction analyses.

Vaccinia virus, the most studied poxvirus and type species of the genus *Orthopoxvirus,* is the virus to which most poxviruses are compared. Its exact origin is unclear. It is probably a cowpox isolate dating back to the late 1700s, when it was first used to vaccinate people against smallpox.

It has been perpetuated and possibly modified by serial passage on the shaved, scarified skin of calves and laboratory animals sacrificed at peak inflammatory reaction to harvest the "lymph," which constituted smallpox vaccine. Later, chick embryo and tissue-culture technology provided superior production methods.

When used intradermally as a human vaccine, it produced a discrete, transient lesion and immunity to serious infection with variola (true smallpox) virus. Before cessation of human smallpox vaccination in the late 1980s, postvaccination encephalitis occasionally occurred, and stillbirths resulting from fetal vaccinia infection sometimes followed vaccination of pregnant women.

On rare occasions, vaccination of people with immunologic deficiencies resulted in sometimes fatal vaccinia necrosum (progressive vaccinia). With the global eradication of smallpox, the risk of these sequelae exceeded the risk of contracting smallpox, and smallpox vaccination was discontinued.

Vaccinia virus from newly vaccinated milkers occasionally caused outbreaks of pox-like lesions on the teats of cattle. In such cases, a history of recent smallpox vaccination was more useful diagnostically than the nature or distribution of the lesions, which are hard to distinguish clinically from cowpox and may be confused with pseudocowpox.

Cowpox virus, a member of the genus *Orthopoxvirus* and of uncertain origin, has been associated occasionally with pox-like teat lesions in cattle in Europe, where it may have a reservoir in field mice and voles (Bennett et al. 1997). It is rarely reported elsewhere. Early observers surmised that "true cowpox" differed from pseudocowpox and correctly speculated that the two conditions had distinct viral etiologies. They also realized that cowpox spread to the hands of milkmaids, rendering them immune to smallpox. The first vaccination (*vacca* means *cow* in Latin) evolved by scarification of people with material from cowpox lesions.

Cowpox virus can also infect buffalo, camels, goats, sheep, and cats. In domestic cats, it occasionally causes generalized illness, which can be fatal. Occasionally cowpox virus causes outbreaks in large felidae in European zoos.

The cowpox virus grows on the CAM of chick embryos, in various cell cultures, and on the skin of laboratory animals (Mayr and Czerny 1990).

Today, diagnosis of bovine cowpox is rare even in Europe, where it was once considered endemic (Munz and Dumbell 1994). The cowpox virus is closely related to vaccinia virus. The two can be distinguished immunologically by the nature of lesions produced on the chorioallantoic membranes of embryonating hens' eggs, by the nature of intracytoplasmic inclusion bodies induced in cell cultures, and by growth preferentials in cell cultures. Transmission of true cowpox to humans by cattle or cats rarely occurs in individuals who have been vaccinated against smallpox.

Pseudocowpox virus is the cause of pseudocowpox (or spurious cowpox), the most common lesion on the teats of cattle and milker's nodules, the most common lesion on the hands of people working with cattle. It appears to have worldwide distribution. Pseudocowpox virus belongs in the genus *Parapoxvirus,* whose members are smaller and morphologically distinct from those of the genus *Orthopoxvirus.*

Pseudocowpox virus has little if any cross-immunity with vaccinia or cowpox viruses. It grows in cell cultures, producing cytopathic effects (CPE), but some strains resist isolation and adaptation to cell cultures (Gibbs et al. 1970).

Pseudocowpox virus closely resembles bovine papular stomatitis virus (Munz and Dumbell 1994) and orf virus, which is the cause of contagious pustular dermatitis in sheep and the type species of the genus *Parapoxvirus.*

Distinctive clinical features permit field differentiation of pseudocowpox from other bovine teat lesions, but detecting these differences requires careful examination of unaltered lesions.

CLINICAL SIGNS AND LESIONS

A wide variety of proliferative, ulcerative, and scab-forming lesions occur on the teats of cattle. The poxvirus infections involved include cowpox, pseudocowpox, and before smallpox vaccination was discontinued, teat infections with vaccinia virus from the hands of recently vaccinated milkers.

In herds with sound hygienic practices, these infections are frequently benign and may not cause major problems. Individual discrete, sometimes painful, pox-like lesions are considered a fact of life by dairy farmers and are usually not distinguished from teat and teat-end lesions of other origins (Timms et al. 1998). When they reach epizootic proportions in a herd, the owner requests veterinary assistance and expects a diagnosis.

In the field, these infections, particularly pseudocowpox, sometimes present a relatively characteristic clinical picture. More often however, observers are presented with advanced lesions that are traumatized by milking procedures, altered by medications, and complicated by secondary infections. Sometimes serious herd outbreaks of teat lesions have multifactorial etiology.

The teat lesions caused by cowpox and vaccinia viruses are virtually identical and cannot be distinguished clinically (Gibbs et al. 1970). The various stages of the lesions are redness and edema, vesicle formation, pustule development and rupture, followed by ulceration and scab formation. When cows are milked or nursed, scab formation is impeded, or scabs are dislodged, leaving ulcerative areas of varying size, some scabbed areas, and minimal extension to areas beyond the teat. With cessation of smallpox vaccination, vaccinia should cease to appear on bovine teats.

Pseudocowpox (spurious cowpox) is the most common poxvirus infection of the teats. The lesions produced by pseudocowpox virus involve early pain, edema, erythema, a small intradermal vesicle (which may be evident only histologically), or an exudative film over the edematous area. A papule emerges, scab formation ensues, the lesion expands centrifugally, and the center becomes depressed (umbilicated).

After about 10 days the central scab scales off, leaving a slightly raised series of tiny scabs described as "horseshoe," "ring," or "circinate" lesions that are virtually pathognomonic of pseudocowpox (Gibbs et al. (1970). The individual lesions caused by pseudocowpox are usually smaller and shallower than lesions of cowpox and vaccinia.

In 1961, the author investigated an outbreak of pseudocowpox complicated by warts that lasted 18 months in a 40-cow herd in New York state. During this period, every milch cow had one or more papules, pustules, or scabbed sores on the teats, and a few discrete lesions appeared on some udders. Some cattle had recurrences after the initial lesions had healed.

Papules, pustules, scabs, and warts were frequently present on the same teat. Horny, narrow-based, filamentous warts appeared near some papules, and broad-based nodular warts were present on many teats. Many cases of mastitis developed, presumably in association with failure of milk letdown, which may have been exacerbated by malfunctioning milking machines and inefficient milking practices.

The owner and his wife had nodules and scabs on their hands and arms. These lesions itched, were indifferent to medical treatment, and yielded cultures of *Staphylococcus aureus*. Specimens for biopsy taken from the cows' teats yielded a histopathologic diagnosis of pseudocowpox based on presence of ballooning epidermal cells and intracytoplasmic inclusions of varying size. Other, more proliferative lesions were identified as fibropapillomas. Lesions were ground and inoculated into cell cultures, but cytopathic changes were not observed. The herd was eventually sold, and the owner sought another occupation.

EFFECTS ON THE DEVELOPING FETUS

True cowpox virus sometimes causes a generalized infection that can result in abortion in pregnant cows (Mayr and Czerny 1990). Abortion is usually not associated with vaccinia or pseudocowpox infection.

NECROPSY FINDINGS

These infections are rarely fatal; pathologic examinations are based on histopathologic examination of lesions. Pathologists have difficulty distinguishing cowpox lesions from vaccinia virus lesions in specimens from field cases.

The histopathologic appearance of pseudocowpox is more distinctive and closely resembles that of papular stomatitis. Depending on the age of the lesion, there will be a papulovesicular reaction, with ballooning, degeneration, and enlargement of epithelial cells and intracytoplasmic inclusion bodies and neutrophilic infiltration of the papillae of the lamina propria.

DIAGNOSIS

When observed clinically, the lesions caused by these infections are frequently in an advanced stage and recognizable as little more than scabs or ulcerations (Gibbs et al. 1970). It is difficult to determine the precise etiology.

If warranted, an epidemiologic investigation can be undertaken and the hands of people who milk the cows should be examined for lesions. A thorough examination of the teats and udders of affected and unaffected cattle is necessary to view lesions in various stages of development and observe thereby some of the distinctive features. In addition, cattle should be examined for lameness, systemic disease, and lesions of the oral mucosa. These efforts will be particularly revealing if typical papular stomatitis lesions are found in calves that have suckled affected cows.

Differential Diagnosis

Unless thorough investigation is done or laboratory diagnosis is attempted, individual cases may be indistinguishable from injuries, frostbite, sunburn, insect bites, bacterial infections, traumatized warts, bovine herpes mammillitis, or the teat lesions accompanying the diseases affecting the bovine mucosa (DABM).

In the case of mild and ordinary occurrences of pox-like lesions on the teats, a casual diagnosis of pseudocowpox may be sufficient and will have a high probability of being correct. In severe or unusual outbreaks or when exotic diseases are suspected, an etiologic determination becomes important, and laboratory tests and regulatory intervention are warranted.

Laboratory Diagnosis

Any laboratory diagnostic procedure should be prearranged, and laboratory personnel should provide specific instructions regarding required specimens.

Virus isolation in cell culture and serologic characterization of isolates can be conducted by laboratories that are adequately equipped and that have trained personnel and appropriate diagnostic reagents. Electron microscopy (EM) is useful for identifying cytopathic agents grown in cell cultures, and on the basis of size, distinction can be made between the orthopoxviruses (vaccinia and cowpox) and pseudocowpox, which is a member of the genus *Parapoxvirus*. Histopathologic examination by light microscopy can usually distinguish poxvirus lesions from herpes mammillitis or non-poxvirus lesions, but distinctions within the family Poxviridae are difficult.

Specimens for biopsy should include some normal-appearing tissue on the periphery of the lesions. Restraint is required for collecting suitable specimens from bovine teat lesions, and scissors are less apt to damage the teat in the event of sudden movement than razor-sharp scalpels.

Neutralization and agar gel diffusion tests for serum antibody may be done, but few laboratories routinely conduct them. Also, the retrospective nature of investigations makes demonstration of seroconversion unlikely.

EPIDEMIOLOGY

The epidemiology and natural history of poxvirus infections of the teats has evolved over the years and contains considerable speculation. The reservoir of vaccinia virus used to be vaccine-production establishments, and recently vaccinated milkers served as the source of infection.

Rodents and cattle may be the reservoir and source of infection for cowpox virus. Cattle are probably the reservoir and usual source of infection of pseudocowpox.

Transmission is usually by milking machines or the hands of milkers. Entry of the virus into new hosts through the skin probably requires abrasions or open lesions that are universally present on the teats of milch cows. True cowpox virus may also be acquired by ingestion or inhalation of infected dust particles (Mayr and Czerny 1990).

IMMUNITY

Cattle probably develop effective protection following infection with vaccinia and cowpox viruses.

Pseudocowpox, on the other hand, seems less immunogenic, and reinfection can occur within several months of the healing of lesions. Also, previous vaccinia or cowpox infections appear not to protect cattle from pseudocowpox infection. The role (if any) of colostrally acquired maternal antibody is unknown.

VIRUS PERSISTENCE

Chronic pseudocowpox infections occur (Gibbs et al. 1970), but the mechanism of actual persistent infections, if they actually occur, is not known. Likewise, it is conceivable that latent cowpox infections occur (Mayr and Czerny 1990).

PREVENTION AND CONTROL

A certain amount of pseudocowpox is inevitable among dairy cattle. Major problems are avoided by minimizing conditions for its spread and by reducing udder and teat trauma and limiting exposure to irritating influences like frostbite, sunburn, sharp objects, and malfunctioning or improperly operated milking machines. Good milking hygiene is essential, as is milking healthy cows first, and those with teat lesions later.

Prepurchase udder and teat examination may help limit introduction of pseudocowpox virus into herds. To date, no workable vaccination procedures have been developed.

THERAPY AND MANAGEMENT OF OUTBREAKS

Cows with lesions should be milked last to limit spread and after milking may be treated with a variety of ointments, lotions, and salves. The udder must be cleansed of medications prior to the next milking to avoid contaminating milk.

Contaminated milk must be discarded. Handlers should be warned of the zoonotic potential and encouraged to wear rubber gloves or wash meticulously after handling lesions, particularly if they have skin abrasions, eczema, or other skin diseases or are immunodeficient or undergoing immunosuppressive therapy.

Milking machines should be checked for malfunctions, and milking procedures evaluated to make certain they are not contributing to teat irritation and exacerbating the condition or expediting its spread. Use of common udder towels should be discontinued, and post-milking teat-dipping procedures should be examined.

Investigators must question owners about introduction of new cattle to determine possible sources of infection. Prior to discontinuance of human smallpox vaccination, emergency vaccination of cattle with vaccinia virus was occasionally practiced in Europe.

LIKELIHOOD OF ERADICATION

Bovine vaccinia mammillitis will probably eventually disappear as long as smallpox vaccination is not practiced.

Cowpox infection has apparently diminished in concert with the reduction of smallpox. Although this apparent association may be coincidental and the role of rodent or feline reservoirs needs clarification, this trend could continue.

Pseudocowpox virus is firmly established and eradication seems unfeasible.

IMPACT ON INTERNATIONAL TRADE

Poxvirus infections of the teats are not categorized as List A or List B diseases by the Office International Des Epizooties. They are usually not subject to international sanitary measures. Individuals signing health certificates for live animals, however, cannot certify that the animals are free from infectious diseases if lesions are present.

PUBLIC RESPONSIBILITY

The zoonotic potential of these infections requires a public-minded approach, including the recommendations outlined above.

In addition, dairy farmers with affected herds deserve advice on procedures for minimizing disease spread and should be advised not to sell cattle with lesions, except for immediate slaughter.

AREAS IN NEED OF RESEARCH

Further studies are needed on the nature of persistence of cowpox and pseudocowpox viruses and on conditions supporting their transmission within and between herds. The role of rodents and felidae in transmission of cowpox needs elucidation.

REFERENCES

Bennett M, Crouch AJ, Begon M, Duffy B, Feore S, Gaskell RM, Kelly DF, McCracken CM, Vicary L, Baxby D, 1997. Cowpox in British voles and mice. *J. Comp. Pathol.* 116:35–44.

Gibbs EPJ, Johnson RH, Osborne AD, 1970. Differential diagnosis of viral skin infections of the bovine teat. *Vet. Rec.* 87:602–609.

Mayr A, Czerny CP, 1990. Cowpox virus. In *Infectious Diseases of Ruminants,* edited by Z Dinter, B Morein. Amsterdam: Elsevier Scientific Publishers, pp. 9–15.

Munz E, Dumbell K, 1994. Pseudocowpox. In *Infectious Diseases of Livestock With Special Reference to Southern Africa,* edited by JAW Coetzer, GR Thomson, RC Tustin. Capetown: Oxford University Press, pp. 625–626.

Timms LI, Van der Maaten MJ, Kehrli ME Jr, Ackerman MR, 1998. Histologic features and results of virus isolation tests of tissues obtained from teat lesions that developed in dairy cattle during winter. *J. Am. Vet. Med. Assoc.* 213:862–865.

24

PSEUDORABIES

INTRODUCTION

Pseudorabies (PR), infectious bulbar paralysis, or mad itch is also called Aujeszky's disease in honor of the Hungarian microbiologist who first described it (Aujeszky 1902). PR is a sometimes serious infection of swine that is the object of eradication efforts in many countries.

In cattle and other nonporcine animals, PR is a sporadic nonsuppurative encephalomyelitis. Bovine PR is unique because it is characterized by self-mutilation, is usually fatal, and is preventable by separation of cattle from swine.

Pseudorabies has been reviewed by Mullaney (1986), Mohanty (1990), Mare (1994), and Murphy et al. (1999).

ETIOLOGY

Pseudorabies virus (PRV), also called porcine herpesvirus-1, belongs in the Alphaherpesvirinae subfamily of the family Herpesviridae. It possesses all the biochemical and biophysical properties of the Herpesviridae, including double-stranded DNA and 162 capsomeres arranged in icosahedral symmetry.

The natural host of PRV is swine, in which latent persistent infections occur. PRV is globally present except in countries without swine, some island regions, areas without supportive ecosystems, and countries that have successfully eradicated it. PRV also infects dogs, cats, horses, sheep, goats, rats, and feral animals. In nonporcine animals, it is usually fatal. Thus, they are terminal or dead-end hosts.

PRV grows readily in a variety of cell cultures, in which it causes a rapidly appearing cytopathic effect (CPE) characterized by foci of rounded cells arranged in grape-like clusters. This appearance is typical of herpesviruses, and agents thus isolated must be specifically identified by immunofluorescent techniques or neutralization of CPE with monospecific antiserum.

PRV is relatively stable and can survive 10 to 30 days at room temperature if dried. It will survive on feed or bedding if appropriate conditions are present, and for years if frozen. It is, however, readily destroyed by detergents, fat solvents, and many common disinfectants.

CLINICAL SIGNS AND LESIONS

Knowledge of porcine PR and PRV infections of other species is essential to understanding the bovine disease.

Swine are the natural host species for PRV. Until the mid-1900s, it was assumed most North American porcine infections were inapparent and followed by latent persistent infections whose reactivation kept many swine populations immunized, permitting only sporadic clinically perceptible economic losses.

With advancing diagnostic technology, the ever-increasing worldwide movement toward large concentrations of confinement-reared swine, and the eradication of hog cholera, porcine PR has emerged as a swine disease of major economic and regulatory importance in the United States and elsewhere.

Porcine PR control utilizes gene-deleted vaccines and biosecurity measures. Eradication programs are based on serologic testing followed by isolation or herd depopulation by slaughter to establish disease-free herds, zones, regions, or countries. These efforts are increasingly successful but have not addressed the challenge of populations of PRV-infected feral swine.

In swine, infection with PRV is frequently nonclinical but upon introduction into groups of susceptible pregnant gilts or sows, can cause fetal infections with embryonic death and resorption, abortion storms, and mummified or stillborn fetuses. In baby pigs, the same scenario produces acute death and a febrile respiratory disease, which terminates fatally with neurologic signs. In adult swine, the infection is usually mild or nonclinical, but sometimes, fully susceptible adult swine develop fever and neurologic signs and succumb.

Other species including cattle usually develop a fatal encephalomyelitis and are dead-end hosts.

In cattle the most prominent clinical signs are associated with pruritus. Affected animals bite, lick, scratch, and rub against objects. This activity causes abrasions and eventual destruction of skin and underlying tissues by a process best described as self-mutilation. The areas most commonly involved are the flanks, hindquarters, anus, and vulva. In some outbreaks, however, the face and neck are most involved.

These signs are often accompanied by fever, rapid respiration, excess salivation, twitching of facial muscles, licking at the nostrils, bellowing, convulsions, and rarely by aggressive behavior. Cattle may lick at themselves or kick out aimlessly. Affected animals refuse feed and water, become recumbent, and die. There are suggestions that the site of the lesions may correlate with the site of inoculation.

Occasionally, cattle, perhaps those infected by the oral or nasal routes, die of PR without exhibiting the pruritus and self-mutilation syndrome. Such animals demonstrate fever and depression and sometimes convulsions or circling prior to paralysis and death. Occasional cattle survive (Hagermoser and Moss 1978).

Trauma-induced lesions visible in the intact animal are the result of self-mutilation. They consist of hyperemia, hemorrhage, abrasion, and laceration of

skin or vulva mucosa. Frequently edema, hemorrhage, and mutilation of subcutaneous tissues and underlying muscles are evident.

In addition to cattle, cats, dogs, horses, goats, sheep, rats, and other wild animals sporadically develop fatal encephalomyelitis after direct contact with
PRV-infected swine, by eating infected carcasses, or by aerosol transmission. A
flock of newly shorn sheep in Northern Ireland acquired air-borne virus through
abrasions resulting from sheep shears, and many died of encephalomyelitis
after exhibiting severe pruritus at wound sites (Henderson et al. 1995).

EFFECTS ON THE DEVELOPING FETUS

Although fetal wastage is a sequel to infection of pregnant sows and gilts,
there are no reports of PRV-induced bovine abortions, possibly because most
diagnosed cases succumb rapidly.

NECROPSY FINDINGS

The gross necropsy findings are usually associated with the mutilation and
are described under Clinical Signs and Lesions. In addition, there may be agonal pulmonary edema, atelectasis, and petechial hemorrhages on lung and tracheal mucosa. Meningeal congestion may be evident.

Histologically, the traumatic nature of the lesions on the body surface is verified by presence of edema, laceration, and hemorrhage. There may be lymphocytic infiltration of the peripheral nerves supplying the affected area. This
finding tends to support the neurologic origin of the irritation stimulating the
self-mutilation.

The most significant histologic lesions are found in the central nervous system
and consist of nonsuppurative encephalomyelitis, meningitis, and ganglioneuritis.
These lesions may contain sparsely distributed intranuclear inclusion bodies and
have varying degrees of lymphocytic infiltration and indications of moderate
degrees of neuronal degeneration or necrosis.

DIAGNOSIS

The clinical diagnosis of PR in cattle is usually relatively easy because of the
distinctive clinical signs and short clinical course. Occasionally, atypical cases
occur. When cattle in contact with swine show signs of itching that progresses
to frenzied self-mutilation, recumbency, and death, PR is the logical diagnosis.

Differential Diagnosis

Typical bovine cases are rarely confused with other diseases. Atypical cases
must be differentiated from the major causes of encephalitis in cattle. These
include rabies, thromboembolic meningoencephalitis, polioencephalomalacia,

listeriosis, and other encephalitides, as well as nervous acetonemia, lead poisoning, and other toxicoses.

Laboratory Diagnosis

Because most affected cattle die within 3 days of the onset of clinical signs, serologic testing is rarely employed in the diagnosis of bovine PR.

In regulatory programs, serologic tests on swine serums are commonly employed.

Isolation of PRV from brain tissue by means of cell culture inoculation is the diagnostic procedure most used in cattle. The virus can frequently be identified in brain tissue using specific immunofluorescent microscopy. Subcutaneous inoculation of rabbits with brain, spinal cord, or fluid from local lesions usually causes an intense pruritus, frenzied scratching and biting, and death. Rabbit inoculation has been replaced largely by tissue culture techniques.

Leukopenia is occasionally observed in acutely ill cattle.

The brain is the specimen of choice for laboratory diagnosis. If brain cannot be obtained, nasal swabs or swabs of tissues from areas where cattle have self-inflicted wounds may be used as specimens for virus isolation.

EPIDEMIOLOGY

The epidemiology of bovine PR relates to contact with swine.

The incubation period can be as short as 48 hours when experimental cattle are inoculated parenterally with large doses of virus. Under natural conditions, cattle have been observed to begin rubbing themselves against fences and other objects within 7 days of being put in direct contact with swine. Likewise, when cattle are excluded from contact with swine, new cases can continue to be observed for about 7 days or more.

Swine are generally regarded as the natural host and usual reservoir of PRV. They secrete virus in saliva, nasal secretions, and semen (Mare 1994). In swine, infection may be inapparent, and latent persistent infection capable of reactivation is common. Evidence suggests PRV acquired orally or by inhalation infects the superficial mucosa prior to generalization and when virus enters through the skin, it spreads via peripheral nerves to the central nervous system.

The immediate source of infection for cattle is probably the nasal discharge of infected swine, and PRV is sometimes acquired by bite inoculation when swine nip at the noses of cattle. In rare cases, air-borne porcine-to-bovine transmission may occur (Power et al. 1990) and some speculation suggests that cow-to-cow transmission is possible.

For some time it was believed rats played a major role in perpetuation of PRV in nature. Current thought, however, supports the idea that rats are likely to be dead-end hosts unless eaten by susceptible swine or other animals (McFerran and Dow 1970). Rats probably play a very minor role in the transmission of PRV to cattle.

Cattle, sheep, dogs, and cats are all terminal hosts and rarely transmit the disease unless their tissues are eaten by susceptible animals.

Cattle of all ages and breeds and both sexes appear to be equally susceptible. The major factor in the distribution of clinical cases is contact with swine.

IMMUNITY

In swine, immunity develops concurrently with latent infection. Since most infected cattle succumb, immunity and serologic procedures have not been elaborated for cattle.

VIRUS PERSISTENCE

Persistent latent infections are common in swine but are not reported in cattle that are terminal hosts.

PREVENTION AND CONTROL

Bovine PR is prevented by keeping swine from contact with cattle. Dogs and cats can develop fatal PR and should not be permitted to eat tissues of infected animals. While vaccination of swine is effective, vaccination of cattle is problematic and should be approached with caution.

THERAPY AND MANAGEMENT OF OUTBREAKS

Once clinical signs appear, the disease is usually fatal. If the diagnosis is evident, tranquilizers or sedatives can be used to reduce the discomfort of affected cattle. Separation of swine and cattle is imperative in handling outbreaks.

LIKELIHOOD OF ERADICATION

Eradication of PR in swine is underway in Europe and the United States. Its widespread distribution, however, the presence of latent persistent infection, and the established infection in feral swine populations suggest that eradication is a formidable challenge.

IMPACT ON INTERNATIONAL TRADE

PR is categorized as a List B disease by the Office International Des Epizooties (OIE). Most focus is on international reporting and import standards for pigs and porcine products rather than cattle.

PUBLIC RESPONSIBILITY

The diagnostician suspecting pseudorabies should advise immediate separation of swine from cattle or sheep and inform the owners that carcasses of affected animals should be burned or buried where cats, dogs, people, or wildlife cannot eat them.

There have been a few unconfirmed reports of asymptomatic human infections; for this reason precautions are advised in the handling of infected animals or materials or the performing of necropsies particularly by immunologically compromised individuals.

Bovine veterinarians must remain aware of PR. It presents characteristic clinical signs but may become rare enough to be ignored in veterinary curricula and continuing education programs as its occurrence declines. This decrease in bovine PR could possibly result from protective effects of IBR vaccination (Zuffa et al. 1986), reduction of contacts between swine and cattle, and declining PR incidence in domestic (but not feral) swine due to eradication efforts.

AREAS IN NEED OF RESEARCH

Research and regulatory emphasis on PR should probably focus on the infection in swine, because cattle are dead-end hosts and the disease is preventable by keeping them from contact with swine.

REFERENCES

Aujeszky A, 1902. Uber eine neue infecktions-krankheit bei haustieren. *Centralbl. Bakteriol. Parasitol. Infekt.* 32:353–373.

Hagermoser WA, Moss EW, 1978. Nonfatal pseudorabies in cattle. *J. Am. Vet. Med. Assoc.* 173:205–206.

Henderson JP, Graham DA, Stewart D, 1995. An outbreak of Aujeszky's disease in sheep in Northern Ireland. *Vet. Rec.* 36:555–557.

Mare CJ, 1994. Aujeszky's disease. In *Infectious Diseases of Livestock With Special Reference to Southern Africa,* edited by JAW Coetzer, GR Thomson, RC Tustin. Capetown: Oxford University Press, pp. 958–962.

McFerran JB, Dow C, 1970. Experimental Aujeszky's disease (pseudorabies in rats). *Br. Vet. J.* 126:173–179.

Mohanty SB, 1990. Pseudorabies virus. In *Infectious Diseases of Ruminants,* edited by Z Dinter, B Morein. Amsterdam: Elsevier Scientific Publishers, pp. 117–121.

Mullaney TP, 1986. Pseudorabies in cattle. *Proc. Am. Assoc. Vet. Lab. Diag.* 29:497–503.

Murphy FA, Gibbs EPJ, Horzinek MC, Studdert MC, 1999. Pseudorabies (caused by porcine Herpesvirus-1). In *Veterinary Virology,* 3rd ed. San Diego: Academic Press.

Power EP, O'Connor M, Donnelly WJC, Dolan CE, 1990. Aujeszky's disease in a cow. *Vet. Rec.* 126:13–15.

Zuffa A, Zuffa T, Zajac J, 1986. A proof of protection of cattle with differing degrees of immunity against infectious bovine rhinotracheitis against experimental infection by Aujeszky's disease. *J. Med. Vet.* 33:425–433.

25

RABIES

INTRODUCTION

Rabies, also called *hydrophobia* or *the rage,* is an acute, bite-transmitted, inevitably fatal, nonsuppurative encephalomyelitis that occurs sporadically in cattle and other mammals. It occurs throughout the world except in rabies-free areas (usually islands) such as Great Britain, New Zealand, Hawaii, Japan, Antarctica, and other areas that have imposed quarantines on carnivores.

In humans, rabies is dreaded and almost always fatal. In Asia and Africa, dogs are a source of most human infection, and bovine rabies receives less attention. Where dog rabies is controlled by vaccination, as in the United States, wildlife, including bats, are sources of human exposure.

Bovine rabies is frequently acquired by bites from skunks, foxes, mongooses, and bats. Affected cattle manifest a variety of neurologic and behavioral signs prior to death and rabies is often not considered until human exposure has occurred. Thus, although cattle are generally dead-end hosts, considerable anxiety and apprehension accompanies bovine rabies. Confirmative laboratory tests are essential for a definite diagnosis.

Rabies has been reviewed by Baer (1990), Swanepoel (1994) and Murphy et al. (1999).

ETIOLOGY

The rabies virus is a highly neurotropic, bullet-shaped, RNA-containing member of the genus *Lyssavirus* in the family Rhabdoviridae. It is commonly isolated and cultivated by intracerebral inoculation of mice and will replicate in brains of most mammals. It can also be grown in chick embryos, duck embryos, and a variety of cell cultures but rarely produces cytopathology.

Strains of rabies virus from different geographic areas and various species are antigenically similar to the extent that cross-neutralization occurs and polyvalent vaccines are usually not required. Antigenic distinctions between isolates can be detected, however, by agar gel and neutralization tests. These tests use monoclonal antibodies and detect host-adapted genotype variants that are maintained in specific hosts and prevail in differing ecosystems.

Rabies virus has been studied experimentally since the time of Pasteur and a unique vocabulary has evolved. The term "street virus" was coined by Pasteur to describe virus isolated from naturally occurring canine cases. The term "fixed virus" originally designated *canine-origin virus* attenuated by serial passage in rabbit brains until experimental animals survived subcutaneous inoculation. Today "fixed virus" connotes any strain attenuated by serial passage in experimental animals.

The Flury strain, a classic rabies virus, was isolated from a human brain and passed repeatedly in numerous host systems and is the basis from which many vaccines have evolved. Other strains, named for the animal from which they were originally isolated, include skunk, fox, bobcat, and vampire bat strains. They may vary in virulence for different experimental animals and can be distinguished using monoclonal antibodies or by analysis of their genomes.

Rabies virus is relatively fragile and is temperature and pH sensitive. It is inactivated by most disinfectants and many detergents but is partially resistant to phenol.

CLINICAL SIGNS AND LESIONS

Aside from fatal termination with central nervous system (CNS) involvement, the clinical signs of bovine rabies, when acquired from terrestrial animals, are variable, inconsistent, and can be confused with those of many other bovine afflictions.

Vampire bat-transmitted rabies, also called bovine paralytic rabies (BPR), has a unique clinical course and geographic distribution and will be described separately.

Bovine rabies transmitted by terrestrial mammals does not follow a standard clinical course. It can resemble most bovine diseases. No two cases look exactly alike and it is frequently misdiagnosed (Stoltenow et al. 1999).

Following a variable and usually prolonged incubation period, rabies-infected cattle pass through a prodromal period, an excitatory stage, and a paralytic stage that terminates fatally.

During the prodromal stage there may be vague uneasiness, a temperature rise of 1 or 2 degrees, partial anorexia, and other nonspecific signs.

As the disease progresses, almost anything can happen. Some cattle move rapidly into the excitement stage. Others show nonspecific signs of rumen atony and anorexia that can be diagnosed as traumatic gastritis or indigestion. Veterinarians may be exposed while passing stomach tubes or administering medication. Because rabies presents signs suggesting need to examine the mouth and throat and is transmitted by saliva, veterinarians should consider preexposure rabies vaccination.

During the subsequent excitatory stage, a variety of neurologic and behavioral signs appear. These may be subtle or very obvious. The temperature is usually normal or in the high-normal range and occasionally reaches 104° F or higher. There may be slight shivering or trembling or subtle twitching of contiguous muscle groups, particularly around the face.

Experienced observers suspect rabies when they see a characteristic facial expression that features a staring, alert look in the eyes and a listening attitude with an erect, forward-turned ear position. Such cattle are unusually attentive and stare intently at moving objects. They may appear otherwise normal, but frequently exhibit excitability and exaggerated movements (particularly over flexion of joints) in their gait. Some continuously emit a characteristic high-pitched bellow and some exhibit tenesmus.

The principal complaint varies. It may be anorexia, cessation of milk production, mania, recumbency, paralysis, tenesmus, or sexual excitement.

Occasionally, rabid cattle go berserk and smash their stanchions, run into walls or fences, or chase dogs, people, or equipment. Such aggressive behavior is rare.

The characteristic tenesmus, when present, is a forceful, unproductive straining as if to defecate and is frequently accompanied by violent contractions of abdominal muscles. After straining, there is a sudden relaxation and a noisy inrush of air into the flaccid anus producing a sucking sound. This sign has been confused with calving by owners suspecting dystocia. Sometimes there is frequent urination, usually minimally productive, with straining efforts producing mere dribbles. Bulls may have a persistent erection or prolapse of the penis, and females may appear to be in estrus.

During the excitatory stage, anorexia progresses until it is complete. Some cattle will hold uneaten food in their mouths, and some will drool as a result of paralysis of facial muscles and muscles of deglutition. Occasionally the tongue will protrude, and the inability to swallow suggests that the animal is choking. Many people have been exposed while searching for nonexistent objects stuck in the throat.

The excitatory period usually ends in recumbency and paralysis. Death soon follows. Paralysis may be the first sign observed in pastured cattle that are not observed frequently. The clinical signs in 91 bovine rabies cases were reported by Schnurrenberger et al. (1970).

In South and Central America, cattle develop a unique disease transmitted by vampire bats with characteristic clinical signs. It is called BPR, but it rarely elicits the variety of clinical signs and progressive stages seen in bovine rabies as transmitted by terrestrial mammals.

BPR, also known as vampire bat rabies, derriengue, or mal de caderas, is one of Latin America's most important cattle diseases and causes thousands of bovine deaths annually. In BPR the excitatory stage is brief and usually absent. It is frequently first noticed when cattle on pasture are found down and unable to rise with the head thrown back as in milk fever. Sometimes, prior to recumbency, affected animals are weak or ataxic in the hind legs and have slight to marked tail paralysis. Knuckling of the fetlock joint may be apparent during walking, or the affected animal may merely appear stiff.

Cattle frequently become recumbent with paralysis of the hind legs and a flaccid tail and anus. Before the ascending paralysis reaches the head, affected animals may appear bright and alert and may eat. Within a few days, however, they refuse feed, and death rapidly ensues.

BPR cases increase during the wet season with an influx of a new generation of susceptibles into bat populations (Lord et al. 1992). Few cattle have obvious bite wounds, but during the dry season a trail of dried blood on the skin may indicate that bites occurred earlier.

EFFECTS ON THE DEVELOPING FETUS

Transplacental infection from a rabid cow to its fetus has been reported (Swanepoel 1994). Rabies is not, however, an important cause of bovine abortion or congenital defects.

NECROPSY FINDINGS

Cattle dying of rabies may dig up the ground during agonal seizures or thrashing. Aside from lacerations, bruises, and evidence of weight loss and dehydration, there are usually no gross lesions except for meningeal congestion and agonal pulmonary congestion and atelectasis.

Histological features of bovine rabies include a nonsuppurative encephalomyelitis characterized by sparse perivascular lymphocytic infiltration and neuronal degeneration. Prior to introduction of fluorescent antibody techniques in the late 1950s, the finding of Negri bodies in stained impression smears or histologic sections was the key to early rabies diagnosis.

These distinctive histopathologic rabies lesions are round, acidophilic intracytoplasmic inclusions in neurons in the cerebellum, hippocampus, and brainstem. Their characteristic matrix of inner granules and intracytoplasmic location between the nucleus and the corner of neurons permits their rapid identification. They may, however, be absent or overlooked in 10% to 15% of cattle ultimately shown to be rabid.

DIAGNOSIS

Early clinical suspicions of bovine rabies is crucial to avoid unnecessary human exposure and the anxiety and apprehension associated with the long, variable incubation period and usually fatal outcome. Except for BPR in Latin America, most cases are treated for something else before rabies is considered.

Because rabies occurs sporadically and is uncommon in cattle in most regions, livestock owners and veterinarians tend to forget about it unless an epidemic is in progress (Haag 1996). Frequently rabies comes to mind only when all examinations, including bare-handed examination of the mouth, prove negative. Early misdiagnosis is frequent because the initial signs are vague and extremely variable.

In North America bovine rabies occurs in individual cattle on pasture, during seasons of wildlife activity in summer or autumn. Affected individuals develop a vague malaise that is first regarded as indigestion, injury, a nondescript metabolic disorder, or an infection. As the prodromal stage passes, neurologic involvement is evident, and some of the previously described signs can be observed. Within 2 to 4 days, recumbency results and death follows.

Differential Diagnosis

Any disease causing neurologic signs in cattle can be confused with rabies. The protean nature of bovine rabies makes its differential diagnosis resemble a treatise on cattle diseases. Rabies must be considered when clinical signs suggest listeriosis, lead poisoning, botulism, pseudorabies, polioencephalomalacia, thromboembolic meningoencephalitis, and organophosphate poisoning or other toxicoses. It must also be distinguished from abscesses, tumors, or trauma to the central nervous system, and from nervous acetonemia, dystocia, choke, indigestion, and milk fever.

In some cases where such conditions are initially suspected, rabies comes to mind as the disease progresses and the animal fails to respond to treatment. Bellowing, tenesmus or characteristic facial expressions are other suggestive signs.

Frequently, rabies is not considered until necropsy reveals negative gross pathologic findings, and Negri bodies are observed histologically. Retrospective histologic diagnosis is common when rabies is absent from the area or when the initial clinical diagnosis is listeriosis, lead poisoning, or botulism.

BPR must be differentiated from malnutrition and parasitism, which also causes weakness and recumbency. Laboratory studies are needed to differentiate it from botulism and from poisoning by the seeds of *Melochia pyramadatum* (the purple bush), a plant native to Central America.

Rabies must always be kept in mind when excessive salivation or neurologic signs are observed. The veterinarian must consider it before examining the mouth of cattle or prescribing oral medication.

Laboratory Diagnosis

In cattle, laboratory diagnosis of rabies is essential because clinical diagnosis is hampered by the extremely variable clinical signs. When human exposure has occurred, it is crucial to obtain a rapid diagnosis so a physician can initiate postexposure prophylaxis (PEP). Uncertainty during the long and variable incubation and the high fatality rate imposes a tremendous psychological impact on potentially exposed people.

Until introduction of fluorescent antibody (FA) tests in the late 1950s, rabies diagnosis involved a search for Negri bodies in sections or impression smears of the cerebellum and the mouse inoculation test. Currently, the rabies FA test is the most commonly used diagnostic test if fresh brain tissue is available and (along with virus isolation) is the standard to which other procedures are compared (Hanlon et al. 1999).

Some laboratories employ reverse transcriptase polymerase chain reactions to detect rabies virus RNA in specimens that are too deteriorated for other procedures (Murphy et al. 1999). Where human exposure has occurred or other uncertainty exists, confirmatory virus isolation by mouse inoculation may be undertaken.

The mouse inoculation test consists of intracerebral inoculation of suckling mice with a suspension of the brain of the suspect animal. The mice are observed for 4 weeks and periodically sacrificed for examinations of brain for Negri bodies and FA tests. If the suspect materials contain rabies virus, some mice usually succumb with signs of rabies.

Serum neutralization (SN) tests for rabies can be used to determine the antibody response of vaccinated individuals. The antibody titer of antiserums used for postexposure treatment can be similarly tested. The immune status of carnivores imported from rabies-infected regions is also measurable by SN tests. SN tests using mouse inoculations are being replaced by indirect FA techniques, or the rapid fluorescent focus inhibition test, which can be completed within 24 hours (Peharpre et al. 1999).

Serology is rarely employed as a diagnostic tool, because virus identification is urgent. Because the disease is usually fatal, paired samples cannot be obtained.

The brain is the specimen of choice in all species. If there has been human exposure to the saliva, cattle salivary glands may be submitted. If it is certain that they will arrive while still refrigerated, entire bovine heads can be packed in double watertight plastic bags and placed in trash barrels packed with ice. The whole head makes it possible for diagnosticians to dissect out the brain specimen.

In cattle, the cerebellum with attached brainstem is the most productive and readily accessible specimen. It can be obtained by entering the foramen magnum of cattle decapitated at the atlantooccipital joint, severing nerve trunks with a scalpel, and removing the cerebellum and brainstem with a teaspoon. Gloves should be worn for this procedure.

When Negri body detection was the major rapid diagnostic tool, it was recommended that suspect cattle be allowed to die to provide time for inclusion bodies to develop. This procedure also eliminated arguments over possible recovery and ensured the fatality portion of the definition of rabies. Where indemnities are paid for cattle dying of rabies, premature killing may preclude death certification.

The FA test can detect virus before Negri bodies are present. If all other considerations are satisfied, it is not required to await death before submitting the specimen for FA assay. Although the virus survives freezing, the specimen should be refrigerated or packed in ice rather than frozen so that histologic integrity is maintained and delay for thawing is avoided. Because such specimens are hazardous material, some postal services will not handle specimens for rabies diagnosis.

Rabies specimens should be packed in at least two containers. The innermost should be watertight and the outermost of unbreakable material. For protection of laboratory workers and parcel handlers and to ensure timely delivery and prompt attention, the package should be clearly marked "rabies specimen," and its submission should be announced to laboratory personnel by telephone or e-mail.

If refrigeration or ice is unavailable or the laboratory is distant, the specimen can be shipped unrefrigerated in a mixture consisting of equal parts glycerol and isotonic saline solution. This medium preserves viral infectivity and tissue integrity and minimizes growth of bacterial contaminants. Its disadvantage is that specimens so preserved provide poor impression smears. Another disadvantage of this transport medium is that it hinders the culturing of *Listeria monocytogenes* or other bacteria.

Rabies specimens must be accompanied by forms required by the testing laboratory and regulatory authorities. These should be firmly attached to the outer container and indicate the history of the case, the nature of the human exposures (if known), and the rabies vaccination status of the cow. They must also indicate the name, address, and telephone number of the owner. The same data and the name and telephone number of the physician of any person believed exposed to the saliva, unpasteurized milk, or nervous tissues of the animal should also be provided. In some regions, health department laboratories perform all rabies testing.

EPIDEMIOLOGY

Cattle are usually dead-end hosts of rabies virus. The epidemiology of bovine rabies is dependent largely on the distribution of rabies infection in wildlife and contact with wildlife is usually required for exposure.

Rabies virus is not an "efficient parasite." Rather than coexisting with hosts, it requires bite-induced inoculation of saliva for transmission and causes an inevitably fatal disease in most species. This deficiency is overcome by the fact that many infected carnivores are driven to sprees of biting prior to death.

Rabies is largely a disease of wild animals and bats. It appears to cycle in wildlife, and times of epidemic spread are interspersed with periods with little rabies activity perceptible to humans.

Bovine rabies usually results from unobserved bites, and incubation periods are not obvious. Most observations suggest that incubation periods vary from 10 days to several months.

In humans, a mean incubation period of 34 days follows bites on the face, while bites on the upper extremities require a median of 78 days before onset of signs.

Vampire bats are the reservoir and usual source of infection for BPR in Latin America.

In other parts of the world, sylvatic rabies cycles in rabid foxes, skunks, mongooses, and sometimes felidae that serve as natural reservoirs and sources of infection for cattle.

Species compartmentalization occurs; dominant host animals prevail in defined ecosystems with occasional spillover to other species. Foxes are the principal reservoirs in Canada, raccoons are the principal host species in eastern United States, and skunks are the major sylvatic reservoir in the midwestern United States.

Until the 1960s, when it was learned that aerosol transmission to humans and other animals can occur in bat caves, bite-inoculation of saliva was considered the only natural means of rabies transmission. Laboratory-generated aerosols have resulted in transmission to technologists in vaccine preparation areas and human-to-human transmission has resulted from corneal transplants (Swanepoel 1994).

Bovine rabies, however, is almost always acquired from biting animals. Cattle owners often report seeing strange-acting skunks or foxes with cattle 10 to 30 days prior to signs. Cattle are naturally curious and are probably bitten on the face when they investigate rabid wildlife of species that normally do not mingle with cattle.

The virus probably reaches the CNS by traversing nerve trunks from peripheral nerves at inoculation sites. It may reach the salivary glands by migration along nerves from the brain.

Cattle of all ages, sexes, and breeds can develop rabies. Apparent differences in incidence among ages, sexes, and breeds are probably related to likelihood of exposure.

Time distribution of cases depends on time of exposure and varying individual incubation periods. BPR results from exposure of many cattle to different bats and can continue irregularly during seasons of bat feeding activity.

IMMUNITY

Natural immunity is believed to be rare because most infected animals eventually succumb. Studies on immunity induced by vaccination of animals indicates that serum antibody develops readily and indicates an animal's ability to resist challenge. Cattle vaccinated with live or inactivated rabies vaccine develop neutralizing antibody titers that gradually decline.

VIRUS PERSISTENCE

Virus persists for prolonged periods in the brown fat of certain bats. Following bite inoculation, virus may persist at the wound site for a "lag time" before beginning migration via nerves to the CNS. In skunks there is a prolonged incubation period during which the saliva is infective. These phenomena do not, however, qualify as persistent infections as usually defined.

PREVENTION AND CONTROL

Efforts to control wildlife rabies through bait-distributed vaccines have been successful in some European countries but have had mixed success elsewhere.

Because of the sporadic nature of the disease, control of terrestrial wildlife transmitted bovine rabies in North America is of limited concern. Unless wildlife-borne epidemics are in progress, little thought is given to bovine rabies control.

When epidemics occur in wildlife, some livestock owners restrict their cattle from pastures. Occasionally, valuable cattle in epidemic areas are vaccinated. Purebreds prepared for export to areas where BPR is endemic may be vaccinated against rabies.

Programs to reduce losses from BPR rabies in Latin America include vaccination of cattle and reduction of vampire bat populations by inoculating cattle with warfarin (an anticoagulant) in dosages harmless to cattle but lethal to blood-sucking bats (Crespo et al. 1979). Vampire bat control efforts have also involved smearing the backs of captured bats with petroleum jelly impregnated with another anticoagulant (diphacinone) and permitting them to return to their roosts, where the chemical is spread as the bats groom one another. Sometimes the material is applied directly to the roosts, smeared on cattle, or injected intramuscularly into cattle with the objective of delivering lethal doses to the bats.

The history of rabies vaccines goes back to Pasteur. Unlike most vaccines, human rabies vaccines are used largely for PEP. However, high-risk professionals like veterinarians should consider a preexposure vaccination regimen after evaluating their personal risks of exposure to rabid animals and the potential for postvaccination reactions that may consist of irritation at inoculation sites. They must also consider potential allergic reactions from booster vaccinations and rare systemic sequelae (Murray and Arguin 2000).

Many varieties of rabies vaccines have been developed over the years. Their history has been reviewed by Bunn (1988). Current rabies vaccinations and control recommendations, compiled by the National Association of Public Health Veterinarians are published each January in the *Journal of the American Veterinary Medical Association* as a compendium on rabies prevention and control. Research under way to develop viral subunit vaccines for humans will undoubtedly have future spin-offs for cattle.

THERAPY AND MANAGEMENT OF OUTBREAKS

Because of the inevitably fatal outcome of rabies, therapy, other than measures to provide comfort to dying animals, is of little avail. Wildlife rabies is usually beyond the control of individuals and must be addressed by public health and regulatory officials. When outbreaks are first suspected, cattle owners should be advised to remove cattle from pastures and consider all the issues, including vaccination, discussed in the preceding section on Prevention and Control.

LIKELIHOOD OF ERADICATION

It is unlikely that rabies eradication will succeed in endemic areas until methods are developed to eliminate it from wildlife reservoirs.

IMPACT ON INTERNATIONAL TRADE

Rabies is categorized as a List B disease by the Office International Des Epizooties (OIE). Control of international spread focuses on movement of carnivores. The OIE International Animal Health Code recommends that rabies-free countries require carnivores entering from infected countries to carry a certificate of vaccination or be held in quarantine for six months.

PUBLIC RESPONSIBILITY

Although uncommon, there are reports of humans acquiring rabies from cattle. These dangers are real and cannot be minimized.

Veterinarians suspecting bovine rabies should take all precautions to prevent human exposure. They should immediately refer people suspected of being exposed to saliva or unpasteurized milk to physicians and report the incident to local health officials. They must take all actions necessary to achieve a prompt, accurate diagnosis.

Veterinarians seem to understand rabies better than most health professionals. During epidemics, they sometimes emerge as community rabies authorities. They are obligated to be sure that the information they disseminate is current and accurate. They should limit their professional opinions and activities to animal species, leaving diagnosis and treatment of humans to physicians.

Information on prevention of human exposure to rabid animals is, however, clearly the responsibility of veterinarians, as is encouragement of dog and cat vaccinations as a means of reducing the likelihood of human exposure.

AREAS IN NEED OF RESEARCH

Research is needed to improve vaccines for humans, domestic animals and wildlife. Research on control of BPR is indicated.

REFERENCES

Baer GM, 1990. Rabies virus. In *Infectious Diseases of Ruminants*, edited by Z Dinter, B Morein. Amsterdam: Elsevier Scientific Publishers, pp. 393–404.

Bunn TO, 1988. Vaccines and vaccination of domestic animals. In *Rabies*, edited by JB Campbell, KM Charlton. Boston: Kluwer Academic Publishers, pp. 323–333.

Crespo RP, Fernandez SS, Lopez DDE, Verlarde FI, Anaya RM, 1979. Intramuscular inoculation of cattle with warfarin: A new technique for control of vampire bats. *Bull Pan Am Health Organ* 13:147–161.

Haag KL, 1996. Bovine rabies—more common than you think. *Bovine Vet* May 18–22.

Hanlon CA, Smith JA, Anderson GR, 1999. Article II. Laboratory diagnosis of rabies. Recommendations of a national working group on prevention and control of rabies in the United States. *J Am Vet Med Assoc* 215:1444–1446.

Lord RD, 1992. Seasonal reproduction of vampire bats and its relation to bovine rabies. *J Wildlife Dis* 28: 292–294.

Murphy FA, Gibbs EPJ, Horzinek MC, Studdert MJ, 1999. Rabies. In *Veterinary Virology,* 3rd ed. San Diego: Academic Press, pp. 432–439.

Murray KO, Arguin PM, 2000. Decision-based evaluation of recommendations for pre-exposure rabies vaccination. *J Am Vet Med Assoc* 216:186–191.

Peharpre D, Cliquet F, Sange E, Renders C, Costy F, Aubert M, 1999. Comparison of visual microscopic and computer-automated fluorescence detection of rabies neutralizing antibodies. *J Vet Diagn Invest* 11:330–333.

Schnurrenberger PR, Martin RJ, Meerdink GL, 1970. Rabies in Illinois farm animals. *J Am Vet Med Assoc* 156: 1455–1459.

Smith JS, and Baer GM, 1988. Epizootiology of rabies in the Americas. In *Rabies,* edited by JB Campbell, KM Charlton. Boston: Kluwer Academic Publishers pp. 267–299.

Stoltenow CL, Shively LA, Jones T, Rupprecht CE, 1999. Clinical report—atypical rabies in a cow. *Bov Pract* 33:4–5.

Swanepoel R, 1994. Rabies. In *Infectious Diseases of Livestock With Special Reference to Southern Africa,* edited by JAW Coetzer, GR Thomson, RC Tustin. Capetown: Oxford University Press, pp. 493–552.

26

RESPIRATORY SYNCYTIAL VIRUS

INTRODUCTION

Bovine respiratory syncytial virus (BRSV) causes a globally distributed, frequently inapparent infection. It is also a primary respiratory pathogen and principal player in bovine respiratory disease (BRD). In cattle of all ages, it causes an acute, rapidly spreading respiratory infection.

Clinical signs and lesions are generally inadequate for a specific etiologic diagnosis, which must be based on serology, virus isolation, or identification of viral antigens in tissues. Inactivated and modified live virus BRSV vaccines are widely used.

BRSV has been reviewed by Belknap et al. (1995), van Vuuren (1994), Wellemans (1990), and Murphy et al. (1999).

ETIOLOGY

Respiratory syncytial viruses (RSV), so named for their capacity to induce formation of syncytia (multinucleate protoplasmic masses) in cell cultures and tissues, are enveloped DNA viruses that infect most vertebrates. They are classified in the genus *Pneumovirus* of the family Paramyxoviridae.

Human RSV cause respiratory infection characterized by cough and rhinitis and sometimes bronchiopneumonia in infants and young children. While distinct, they share biochemical, biophysical, epidemiologic, immunologic, and pathologic characteristics with BRSV. Some bovine isolates cross-react serologically with human RSV.

BRSV is a relatively labile, pleomorphic RNA virus of variable size, first isolated in the late 1960s (Paccaud and Jacquier 1970). It can be visualized by electron microscopy in pulmonary alveolar cells of infected animals and in eosinophilic cytoplasmic inclusions formed in cell cultures in which it also induces slowly developing cytopathic changes. These changes include syncytia, giant cells, and focal necrosis.

It has been isolated from nasal or ocular secretions following outbreaks of respiratory disease in adult cattle (Inaba et al. 1972) and calves (Lehmkuhl et al. 1979). In early reports of a massive outbreak of respiratory disease in Japan it was called Nomi virus (Inaba et al. 1972). BRSV replicates in tracheal and pulmonary epithelium.

Since its discovery there have been conflicting opinions about the extent and patterns of pathogenicity of BSRV and its role in BRD. These differences have been based on clinical observations, experimental infections, and apparent inconsistencies in immunologic responses to infection.

Differences in field manifestations have been attributed to potentiation by simultaneous infection with bovine viral diarrhea (BVD) (Kelling et al. 1995), parainfluenza-3 (Inaba et al. 1972), bovine adenoviruses (Lehmkuhl et al. 1979), and bacteria of the genus *Pasteurella, Hemophilus,* or *Actinomyces* (Larsen et al. 1999). They have also been attributed to exacerbation by three-methylindole generated by rumen microflora after sudden exposure to tryptophan-rich lush green pastures or feedlot diets (Bingham et. al 1999). Clinical and experimental observations indicate that BRSV is a primary pathogen, but its effects can be modified by concurrent conditions.

In the case of experimental infections this variability has been attributed to virus strain differences, varying doses of inoculum, and loss of viral infectivity through continued tissue culture passage. Other reasons cited for variability include partial inactivation of inocula while in transit to calf units, differing immunopathologic responses by nasal and pulmonary epithelium, and variability among experimental animals.

Some cattle manifest an early febrile reaction followed by apparent recovery only to experience relapse manifested by pulmonary emphysema, labored breathing, and anorexia. This phenomenon, believed to occur also in human RSV infections, has been hypothesized to be an immune-mediated reaction, (possibly but not necessarily due to reexposure or a secondary immune response). Pulmonary production of immunoglobulin E (IgE) may exacerbate the effects of infection (Gershwin et al. 2000) and explain some intricacies of its pathogenesis.

CLINICAL SIGNS AND LESIONS

BRSV outbreaks are usually characterized by rapid onset, fever, cough, increased respiratory rates with occasional openmouthed breathing, conjunctivitis, and watery nasal and ocular discharge. The course varies from 3 to 10 days. Some cases have excess salivation, depression, decreased milk production, and pneumonia. Fatalities are rare unless multiple infectious agents are involved.

Experimental BRSV exposures, reviewed by Belknap et al. (1995), have produced a continuum of results including unsuccessful efforts to infect, nonclinical infections, and mild respiratory disease characterized by early leukopenia, fever, anorexia depression, rhinitis, excess nasal and ocular discharge, and cough. In some reports the experimental disease has been severe (Woolums et al. 1999). In others, it has been so mild that workers suggest BRSV may play its major role as a triggering agent for secondary or concomitant infections.

Lesions of diagnostic value are usually absent in intact live animals infected with BRSV.

EFFECTS ON THE DEVELOPING FETUS

The occurrence of abortions was reported in Japan (Inaba et al. 1972). This aspect of the disease was not studied in detail, however, and subsequent observations suggest BRSV is not a major cause of abortion.

NECROPSY FINDINGS

The case fatality rate is low in uncomplicated BRSV infections. The lungs of animals dying in naturally occurring BSRV outbreaks may have atelectasis, interstitial emphysema, and pneumonia (which may be secondary).

Histopathologically, multinucleated cells may be seen in cells lining the alveolar lumen.

DIAGNOSIS

Because of the complexity and overlapping clinical characteristics of the many agents causing BRD, a diagnosis of BRSV infection requires laboratory confirmation.

Uncomplicated classic BRSV outbreaks in susceptible herds involve an acute, rapidly spreading respiratory disease characterized by fever, rapid respiration, clear nasal and ocular discharge, and cough. In individual cattle, the disease runs its course in 2 to 10 days. A few cattle may develop pneumonia and a small percentage may succumb. In herds in which the infection has become endemic, individual cases and inapparent infections may occur.

Differential Diagnosis

The differential diagnosis includes all infections associated with BRD. The presence of multiple infections in some cases raises the question of which agent has the primary etiologic role.

It is essential to carefully examine the nasal passages and vulvar mucosa for white plaque-like lesions of infectious bovine rhinotracheitis. The oral mucosa must be examined for erosions or ulcers characteristic of the diseases affecting bovine mucosa (DABM) including BVD, malignant catarrhal fever, and rinderpest.

BRSV outbreaks may resemble ephemeral fever, although BRSV lacks the unique partial paralysis and one-legged lameness of ephemeral fever. BRSV is common in winter months in temperate climates, while insect-borne ephemeral fever is more common in summer and in tropical regions where competent vectors abound.

Since there are no distinctive clinical signs or lesions, laboratory studies are needed to establish a diagnosis of BRSV.

Laboratory Diagnosis

Isolation of BRSV is tricky because inapparent infections are common and virus is present for very brief periods after infection. Because BRSV is heat labile, specimens require constant refrigeration. For virus isolation attempts, swabbings of nasal secretions or tracheal lavage washings from incubating or acutely infected cattle are specimens of choice. The ability to isolate virus disappears early in the course of the disease. Therefore, swabbings from unaffected cattle in close contact with clinical cases may result in selection of incubating cases and increased probability of successful virus isolation.

Virus isolation is surpassed as a diagnostic procedure by detecting nucleoprotein BSRV antigen using antigen capture enzyme-linked immunosorbent assay (ELISA) or by detecting BRSV fusion protein after polymerase chain reaction (West et al. 1998).

Blood for serology should be taken from acute cases and from any animal from which specimens are taken for virus isolation. The same cattle should be bled 3 weeks later in order that paired serums can be tested. Because of the likelihood of previous nonclinical infections, single positive serum specimens should not be regarded as diagnostic without additional laboratory findings.

Serologic tests for BRSV include serum neutralization, indirect immunofluorescence, plaque-reduction, or complement fixation tests.

Seroconversion or significant rises in titer are demonstrated readily in large outbreaks involving highly susceptible populations (Inaba et al. 1972). Some evidence (Lehmkuhl et al. 1979) suggests, however, that some cattle manifesting serious clinical signs may not seroconvert. They may possess serum antibody of maternal origin at the time of infection and secretory immunoglobulins in nasal mucus may be more suitable than serum for testing in calves.

Another consideration, raised by studies of human respiratory syncytial virus, suggests that humoral antibody does not prevent subsequent clinical infection and that sensitivity reactions involving humoral antibody may contribute to the pathogenesis of the disease.

Leukopenia has been observed in the early stages of naturally occurring and experimental infections.

EPIDEMIOLOGY

The epidemiology reflects a pattern of a highly infectious rapidly spreading virus that causes frequent inapparent infections.

Outbreaks of rapidly spreading, usually mild respiratory disease have been associated with BRSV in Japan (Inaba et al. 1972), the United Kingdom (Jacobs and Eddington 1971), Switzerland (Paccaud and Jacquier 1970), and the United States (Lehmkuhl et al. 1979). Further, antibody is prevalent in South Africa (van Vuuren, 1994). Most evidence suggests worldwide distribution of BRSV. It appears that most regions with the diagnostic capacity and willingness to look for evidence of BRSV have found it.

In the field the disease has sudden onset and the incubation period, which usually lasts from 2 to 4 days, can vary from 2 to 10 days.

Cattle are probably the principal reservoir and usual source of infection. Introduction into susceptible populations is accompanied by rapid spread and many clinical infections. Although sheep and goats have been infected experimentally, their role in the epidemiology of BRSV infection is unclear. The serologic cross-reactions with human respiratory syncytial virus suggests a common ancestry, but human infection has not occurred concurrently with major BRSV outbreaks.

Typical antibody prevalences vary from 25% to 80%. Thus, it appears that inapparent infections are common, and the virus is endemic in many areas.

Virus is present in nasal secretions and it appears that aerosol transmission can occur. The route of entry into susceptible cattle is probably via the respiratory tract.

While some reports indicate calves between 3 and 9 months of age are most susceptible, attack and fatality rates do not appear to be affected by age, sex, or breed of cattle.

IMMUNITY

The ability to isolate virus declines with appearance of humoral antibody. It remains to be established, however, that humoral antibody is protective since infection and reinfection may occur in the presence of serum antibody. Nasal antibody protects against some infections. Calves with colostrally acquired antibody can be clinically infected (Lehmkuhl et al. 1979; West and Ellis 1997). Finer details of the immune response to BRSV remain to be elucidated (Gershwin et al. 2000).

VIRUS PERSISTENCE

Virus persistence has been suggested but not confirmed (Wellemans 1990); this area of study probably deserves exploration.

PREVENTION AND CONTROL

Inactivated and modified live vaccines against BRSV infection are in use throughout the world (Ellis et al. 1995; Ferguson et al. 1997). They are frequently used in combination with other viral vaccines and bacterins directed against bovine respiratory disease. Care and thoughtful deliberation are needed to ensure that products chosen achieve maximum efficacy and safety possible for each production-management system.

Inactivated vaccines have been unsuccessful for controlling human respiratory syncytial virus infection, and clinical impressions suggest that they actually exacerbate lung lesions by immunologically mediated sensitivity reactions.

THERAPY AND MANAGEMENT OF OUTBREAKS

Therapy probably has no effect on BRSV infection per se. Antibiotic treatment is probably indicated, however, for cattle developing bacterial pneumonia.

The apparent rapid spread suggests that uninfected herds should not be visited by people contacting diseased cattle. Infected cattle should not be introduced into uninfected herds.

LIKELIHOOD OF ERADICATION

At present, not enough is known about BRSV infection to appraise the feasibility of eradication programs. However, its communicability and widespread distribution suggest successful eradication would be unlikely except in unique small isolated regions.

IMPACT ON INTERNATIONAL TRADE

Because BRSV appears to be globally ubiquitous, and because it is not listed by the Office International Des Epizooties, BRSV is currently not a factor in international trade.

PUBLIC RESPONSIBILITY

The lack of human infections in major outbreaks makes it appear that BRSV infection is not transmissible to humans (Paccaud and Jacquier 1970; Inaba et al. 1972). People working with infected cattle should avoid contact with other cattle, and sick cattle should not be sold, traded, or otherwise allowed to contact other cattle.

Cattle undergoing infections should not be slaughtered until recovery is complete and drug withdrawal times have been observed.

AREAS IN NEED OF RESEARCH

Further studies are needed to elaborate the pathogenicity and immunity of BRSV, explore the role of immune complexes in BRSV pathogenesis, and improve vaccines.

REFERENCES

Belknap EB, Ciszewski DK, Baker JC, 1995. Review article. Experimental respiratory syncytial virus infection in calves and lambs. *J. Vet. Diag. Invest.* 7:285–298.

Bingham HR, Morely PS, Wittum TE, Bray TM, West KH, Selmons RD, Haines DM, Levy MA, Sarver CF, Saville WJA, Cortese VS, 1999. Synergistic effects of concurrent challenge with bovine respiratory syncytial virus and three-methylindole in calves. *Am. J. Vet. Res.* 60:563–570.

Ellis JA, Hassard LE, Morely PS, 1995. Bovine respiratory syncytial virus-specific immune responses in calves after inoculation with commercially available vaccines. *J. Am. Vet. Med. Assoc.* 206:354–361.

Ferguson JD, Galligan GT, Cortese V, 1997. Milk production and reproductive performance in dairy cows given bovine respiratory syncytial virus vaccine prior to parturition. *J. Am. Vet. Med. Assoc.* 210:1779–1784.

Gershwin LJ, Gunther RA, Anderson ML, Woolums AR, McArthur-Vaughn K, Randel K, Boyle GA, Friebertshauser KE, McIntruff PS, 2000. Bovine respiratory syncytial virus-specific interleukin-2 and 4, and interferon-y expression in pulmonary lymph of experimentally infected calves. *Am. J. Vet. Res.* 61:291–297.

Inaba Y, Tanaka Y, Sato K, Omori T, Matumoto M, 1972. Bovine respiratory syncytial virus, studies on an outbreak in Japan 1968–1969. *Jpn. J. Microbiol.* 16:373–383.

Jacobs JW, Eddington N, 1971. Isolation of respiratory syncytial virus from cattle in Britain. *Vet. Rec.* 88:694.

Kelling CL, Brodersen BW, Perino LJ, Cooper, VI, Doster AR, Pollreisz JH, 1995. Potentiation of bovine respiratory syncytial virus infection in calves by bovine viral diarrhea virus. *Proc. U.S. Anim. Health Assoc.* 98:273–278.

Larsen LE, Tjornehoj B, Viuff NE, Jensen NE, Uttenthal A, 1999. Diagnosis of enzootic pneumonia in Danish cattle: reverse transcription-polymerase chain reaction assay for detection of bovine respiratory syncytial virus in naturally and experimentally infected cattle. *J. Vet. Diag. Invest.* 11:416–422.

Lehmkuhl HD, Gough PM, Reed DE, 1979. Characterization and identification of a bovine respiratory syncytial virus isolated from young calves. *Am. J. Vet. Res.* 40:124–126.

Murphy FA, Gibbs EPJ, Horzinek MC, Studdert MJ, 1999. Bovine respiratory syncytial virus. In *Veterinary Virology,* 3rd ed. San Diego: Academic Press, pp. 426–427.

Paccaud MF, Jacquier C, 1970. A respiratory syncytial virus of bovine origin. *Arch. Gesamte Virusforsch.* 30:327–342.

van Vuuren M, 1994. Bovine respiratory syncytial virus infection. In Infectious Diseases of Livestock With Special Reference to Southern Africa, edited by JAW Coetzer, GR Thomson, RC Tustin. Capetown: Oxford University Press, pp. 769–772.

Wellemans G, 1990. Bovine respiratory syncytial virus. In *Infectious Diseases of Ruminants,* edited by Z Dinter, B Morein. Amsterdam: Elsevier Scientific Publishers, pp. 363–375.

West K, Ellis J, 1997. Functional analysis of antibody responses of feedlot cattle to bovine respiratory syncytial virus following vaccination with mixed vaccines. *Can. J. Vet. Res.* 61:28–33.

West K, Bogdan J, Hamel A, Nayar G, Morley PS, Haines D, Ellis J, 1998. A comparison of diagnostic methods for the detection of bovine respiratory syncytial virus in experimental clinical infections. *Can. J. Vet. Res.* 62:245–250.

Woolums AR, Anderson ML, Gunther RA, Schelegle ES, LaRochelle DR, Singer RS, Boyle GA, Friebertshauser KE, Gershwin LJ, 1999. Evaluation of severe disease induced by aerosol inoculation of calves with bovine respiratory syncytial virus. *Am. J. Vet. Res* 60:473–480.

27

RHINOVIRUSES

INTRODUCTION

Bovine rhinoviruses (BRV) have been isolated from nasal and tracheal washings of normal cattle and from cattle with respiratory disease. They are often found in combination with other disease-producing agents. They have not been much studied, but they are widely distributed and are probably ubiquitous in cattle populations throughout the world. Their pathogenic potential needs to be further elaborated.

BRV have been reviewed by Thomson (1994) and Sellers (1990).

ETIOLOGY

Rhinoviruses are small icosahedrally symmetrical RNA viruses, usually measuring less than 30 nm in diameter. They are classified in the genus *Rhinovirus* in the family Picornaviridae. Rhinoviruses were so named because human isolates have been associated with the common cold. In humans, multiple rhinovirus serotypes are distinguished by neutralization tests and genetic analyses (Rodrigo and Dopaso 1995). Members of the genus *Rhinovirus* are sensitive to many disinfectants and are acid liable.

BRV have been known since 1962 (Bogel 1968). BRV of uncertain pathogenicity are isolated from nasal or tracheal swabs and cultivated in cell cultures, where they are recognized by their often slowly developing cytopathogenic effects (CPE). The CPE may be meager on primary isolation (Rosenquist 1971) but improve after adaptation to susceptible cell cultures (Bogel 1968).

Unlike bovine enteroviruses, which are also in the family Picornaviridae, BRV are sensitive to mild acids and probably do not survive passage through the acid pH of the digestive tract; thus they are not usually found in feces. They do survive and replicate in the respiratory mucosa. Some BRV are thermosensitive and grow better at 30° to 34° C than they do at conventional incubator temperatures of 36° C. This phenomenon may reflect adaptation to the lower temperatures of their natural habitat in the nasal passages (Bogel 1968). At least three serotypes of BRV have been identified (Yamashita et al. 1985).

CLINICAL SIGNS AND LESIONS

BRV have been isolated from cattle with classic bovine respiratory disease signs including fever, depression, anorexia, excess nasal discharge, rapid respiration, pneumonic rales, coughing, conjunctivitis, and ocular discharge (Lupton et al. 1980). These signs, however, are characteristic of most bovine respiratory diseases and are not specific to BRV or any other infectious agent.

BRV have been found during epizootics of shipping fever (Rosenquist 1971). In Japan numerous rhinoviruses were isolated from nasal swabs taken from a group of assembled 8-to-9-month-old calves in an outbreak of nonfatal but rapidly spreading respiratory disease characterized by fever, depression, decreased appetite, lacrimation, conjunctivitis, salivation, nasal discharge, cough, and respiratory distress (Kurogi et al. 1974).

A number of experimental infections have been mild and asymptomatic, although a transient temperature elevation and pneumonia may occur (Bogel 1968). Part of a group of calves inoculated intranasally or intratracheally developed increased temperatures, pulmonic rales, and other signs of pneumonia (Mohanty et al. 1969).

EFFECTS ON THE DEVELOPING FETUS

BRV appear to infect superficial respiratory mucosa with minimal systemic dissemination and probably rarely cause abortion.

NECROPSY FINDINGS

Reports of necropsy observations are sparse because few BRV-infected cattle die. Calves inoculated intranasally and intratracheally had mild signs. When calves were killed, areas of pulmonary consolidation and emphysema were observed (Mohanty 1973). Histologically, these lungs had interstitial pneumonia.

DIAGNOSIS

Clinical diagnosis is next to impossible because the signs are generally mild and nonspecific. If severe disease exists and BRV are isolated it is likely that other agents are also present. BRV infection should be considered in any respiratory disease, but no clear-cut diagnostic profile can be presented.

Differential Diagnosis

The differential diagnosis should include bovine respiratory syncytial virus, bovine parainfluenza-3, infectious bovine rhinotracheitis, respiratory coronavirus infection, bovine viral diarrhea, pasteurellosis, and other bacterial respiratory infections.

Laboratory Diagnosis

The virus is best isolated in cell cultures from nasal swabs taken in the early stages of infection (Kurogi et al. 1974). Seroconversion can be demonstrated using carefully selected paired blood specimens.

Leukopenia has been observed in the acute stages of infection (Kurogi et al. 1974).

EPIDEMIOLOGY

The vagueness of clinical signs makes calculation of a meaningful incubation period difficult. Mohanty (1973) reported excess nasal discharge 2 to 4 days after experimental exposure.

The reservoir is probably cattle, but nonbovine reservoirs may exist. Nasal secretions of acutely infected calves are the usual immediate source of infection and spread is usually by direct animal-to-animal contact. To date, mostly calves and young cattle have been identified as naturally infected, but cattle of all ages are likely to be susceptible. No particular breed or sex appears unusually susceptible. The infection spreads between animals in close contact.

IMMUNITY

Neutralizing antibody develops after infection (Bogel 1968), and rising titers can be demonstrated in field cases (Kurogi et al. 1974). An area that requires further study is the degree of protection conferred by actively induced antibody. Colostrally acquired passive immunity may not be adequate to prevent infection (Bogel 1968).

VIRUS PERSISTENCE

The possible role (if any) of persistent viral infections is unknown.

PREVENTION AND CONTROL

Management, hygiene, and stress reduction are the major preventive or control procedures.

THERAPY AND MANAGEMENT OF OUTBREAKS

When infection is associated with clinical signs, symptomatic treatment and hygienic measures aimed at limiting spread should be undertaken along with stress-reducing management practices.

LIKELIHOOD OF ERADICATION

The lack of definite knowledge about the pathogenicity and epidemiology of BRV precludes consideration of eradication at this time.

IMPACT ON INTERNATIONAL TRADE

BRV are not considered important enough to be placed on List A or List B by the Office International Des Epizooties and probably will not have a major effect on trade unless significant changes in pathogenicity occur or new knowledge is presented.

PUBLIC RESPONSIBILITY

Currently, human infection with BRV has not been reported. Veterinarians should make all efforts to determine an accurate diagnosis and prevent further spread.

AREAS IN NEED OF RESEARCH

There is need for research on the pathogenesis, immunology, and epidemiology of BRV infections.

REFERENCES

Bogel K, 1968. Bovine rhinoviruses. *J. Am. Vet. Med.* 152:780–784.

Kurogi H, Inaba Y, Goto Y, Takahashi A, Sato K, Omori T, Matumoto M, 1974. Isolation of rhinovirus from cattle in outbreaks of acute respiratory disease. *Arch. Gesamte. Virusforsch.* 44:215–226.

Lupton HW, Smith MH, Frey ML, 1980. Identification and characterization of a bovine rhinovirus from Iowa cattle with acute respiratory disease. *Am. J. Vet. Res.* 41:1029–1034.

Mohanty SB, 1973. New herpesviral and rhinoviral respiratory infections. *J. Am. Vet. Med. Assoc.* 163:855–857.

Mohanty SB, Lille, MG, Albert TF, Sass V, 1969. Experimental exposure of calves to a bovine rhinovirus. *Am. J. Vet. Res.* 30:1105–1111.

Rodrigo MJ, Dopaso J, 1995. Evolutionary analysis of the picornavirus family. *J. Mol. Evol.* 40:362–371.

Rosenquist BD, 1971. Rhinoviruses: Isolation from cattle with acute respiratory disease. *Am. J. Vet. Res.* 32:685–688.

Sellers RF 1990. Bovine rhinoviruses. In *Infectious Diseases of Ruminants,* edited by Z Dinter, B Morein. Amsterdam: Elsevier Scientific Publishers, pp. 517–518.

Thomson GR, 1994. Bovine rhinovirus infection. In *Infectious Diseases of Livestock With Special Reference to Southern Africa,* edited by JAW Coetzer, GR Thomson, RC Tustin. Capetown: Oxford University Press, pp 823–824.

Yamashita H, Atashi H, Inaba Y, 1985. Isolation of a new serotype of bovine rhinovirus from cattle. *Arch. Virol.* 83: 113–116.

28

ROTAVIRUS ASSOCIATED WITH NEONATAL DIARRHEA

INTRODUCTION

Neonatal calf diarrhea (NCD) causes deaths on dairy farms and in intensive veal-growing operations, where mortality may approach 90%. Mortality among range calves is usually less.

Many factors are involved in NCD etiology including diet, colostrum deprivation, management, sanitation, crowding, environmental temperature and humidity, stress, bacteria, and viruses.

The isolation of a virus from calves with NCD in 1968 (Mebus 1969) was a breakthrough. The agent was later named bovine rotavirus (BRoV) and classified in the genus *Rotavirus* of the family Reoviridae. BRoV is one of many causes of NCD.

Simple singular BRoV infections are frequently mild and nonfatal. However, in totally susceptible stressed calves, the outcome can be disastrous if initial infective doses are massive, as occurs in highly contaminated environments, and the BRoV infection is accompanied by other viruses or enteropathogenic bacteria.

Reviews have been prepared by (Gerdes 1994), (Mebus 1975), and (Mebus 1990).

ETIOLOGY

Rotaviruses are named for their wheel-like appearance. They are found in the feces of many species including cattle, sheep, swine, and horses, but minimal cross-species transmission appears to occur. They are frequently associated with neonatal diarrhea.

Rotaviruses are resistant to environmental influences and many disinfectants (Gerdes 1994) but are inactivated by appropriate concentrations of formaldehyde, hexachlorophene, Lysol, and chloramine T. Rotaviruses are classified immunologically into groups, subgroups, and serotypes (Parwnai et al. 1995).

BRoV is difficult to isolate in cell cultures because of the cytotoxic nature of feces and fecal filtrates and because BRoV is inconsistent in production of cytopathic effects (CPE) unless adapted to specialized cell lines. Thus, molecular technology including polymerase chain reactions (PCR) (Chinsangarum et al. 1994) and numerous immunologic procedures such as immunofluorescent and immunoelectron microscopy, enzyme-linked immunosorbent assay (ELISA) tests, and electrophoretic procedures (Parwani et al. 1995) are employed for identification and comparison of BRoVs and their antigens.

CLINICAL SIGNS AND LESIONS

The clinical signs associated with BRoV infections vary from inapparent infections and mild diarrhea to profuse watery feces the color of which is determined by the age of the animal and its diet. The diarrhea is usually yellow or tan in neonates on milk or milk replacement and darker in calves on solid diets. Severe dehydration is common, and some calves die before diarrhea is observed (Mebus 1969).

The temperature may be elevated, normal, or subnormal. The nose may be reddened and crusted and there may be excess salivation. There is commonly severe depression and reluctance to eat. Varying degrees of dehydration and electrolyte imbalances are evident prior to death, which occurs in up to 50% of cases in some outbreaks (Mebus et al. 1971).

The age at onset of diarrhea varies from herd to herd but is usually within 10 days of birth. There are generally no distinctive gross lesions visible in the intact calf.

EFFECTS ON THE DEVELOPING FETUS

To date, adverse effects on the developing fetus have not been demonstrated.

NECROPSY FINDINGS

Calves dying with BRoV diarrhea and its complications are usually dehydrated and have sunken eyes, roughened hair coat, and hind parts soiled with fetid fecal material. The principal gross lesion is an intestine distended with fluid consisting of unabsorbed milk and water, proteins, and electrolytes derived from the serum and destined for loss through diarrhea.

Except for intestinal distention, congestion of intestinal mucosa, and occasional petechial hemorrhages throughout the gut, calves are free of gross lesions distinctive enough to provide an etiologic diagnosis. Unless death is peracute, there is usually serous atrophy of fat, indicating malabsorption or malnutrition. The lungs may be congested or show signs of secondary pneumonia.

Histopathologically, the principal lesion is sloughing of the villous epithelial cells in the small intestine and their replacement by immature squamous epithelial cells.

DIAGNOSIS

A diagnosis of undifferentiated NCD or calf septicemia is warranted when a calf develops diarrhea, weakness, dehydration, prostration, and death. However, a diagnostic profile unique to BRoV infection cannot be presented because many causes of NCD present similar signs. The etiologic diagnosis is complicated and requires necropsy and laboratory assistance.

Differential Diagnosis

Differential diagnosis of BRoV-induced NCD includes dietary gastroenteritis, bacterial diarrhea, and numerous other entities. It is often difficult to sort out the role of diet, environment, colostrum deprivation, bacteria, and viruses in NCD. The principal bacterial agents requiring consideration in the differential diagnosis include many serotypes of the genus *Salmonella* and enteropathogenic strains of *Escherichia coli*. Some of these are human pathogens, but many other enteric bacteria can be involved. In addition, cryptosporidia, *Chlamydia,* and other organisms are frequently involved.

The viral infections considered in the differential diagnosis include parvovirus, coronavirus, bovine viral diarrhea, and enteroviruses. Not infrequently, more than one of these agents are present and the specific etiology remains undetermined. ELISA kits are available for screening feces for BRoV antigen and serum for antibody.

Laboratory Diagnosis

It is advisable to contact laboratories in advance to determine the availability of BRoV diagnostic service and the nature of specimens desired.

Electron microscopic examination of feces sometimes permits recognition of particles with typical rotavirus morphology. A variety of immunologic procedures for detecting BRoV and its antigens are applied to fecal specimens to provide specific identification of particles present (Mebus 1990). Numerous commercial test kits are available.

Virus isolation in cell cultures requires specific cell lines, is more time consuming, and is less apt to be successful than immunological microscopic procedures, because BRoV does not readily produce a characteristic CPE on primary inoculation.

The specimens of choice are feces or rectal swabs from early cases of diarrhea. The specimen should be taken soon after the onset of diarrhea and collected directly from the calf and promptly frozen, preferably at dry ice temperature. Lacking this capability, home-type freezer temperatures are adequate.

Sections of intestine from early cases are also suitable specimens but are more difficult to obtain and harder to ship.

Antibody against BRoV can be detected by ELISA tests or by serum neutralization procedures that employ serum virus mixtures inoculated into cell cultures.

Serologic tests have limited diagnostic value for individual cases of BRoV because the antibody prevalence is high, particularly in infected herds where many calves have humoral antibody after suckling immune dams. Calves with humoral antibody can develop clinical infection. Local immunity and antibody in the gut are more involved in protection than is humoral antibody.

When negative, serologic tests on paired samples collected 3 weeks apart from calves and dams can be an effective means of eliminating BRoV from diagnostic consideration.

Clinical pathologic changes accompanying NCD are not specific for BRoV infection. They consist of acidosis with low bicarbonate levels and hemoconcentration resulting in the elevated hematocrit, lymphocyte counts, hemoglobin, and plasma proteins. Glucose levels frequently drop, particularly as death approaches. Affected calves are frequently hypogammaglobulinemic as a result of insufficient colostrum intake or absorption.

EPIDEMIOLOGY

The high antibody prevalence among adult cattle and the early age at onset of disease suggest widespread distribution of virus, a carrier state, and a unique age susceptibility.

All indications suggest an incubation period measurable in hours, with variations relating to dosage and differences between calves. Some calves may take 2 to 3 days to develop clinical signs.

Adult cattle populations in many areas have an antibody prevalence approaching 100%. Although the details are unclear, it appears as if carrier cattle may be the reservoir and the source of infection for their own calves via fecal contamination or possibly even transplacentally. Undoubtedly, infected calves can be the source of infection for other calves. Fecal-oral transmission probably occurs.

Most clinical cases occur between 1 and 10 days of age, probably because of age at exposure and neonatal susceptibility. Endogenous steroid production by the fetus just prior to birth may cause temporary depression in cell-mediated immunity, permitting early infections to be more damaging than those occurring later in life (Tennant et al. 1978). In addition, declining levels of colostrally acquired antibody in the gut lumen at 4 to 6 days of age may contribute to the age distribution. Occasionally older calves are affected (Clark et al. 1996). Undiagnosed clinical infection of adult cattle may occur.

There are no indications that sex or breed is an important determinant of the incidence of infection or disease.

IMMUNITY

The nature of the bovine immune response to BRoV infection and the role of immunity in preventing infection and disease are not completely understood.

Colostrally acquired maternal antibody in the gut exerts a protective effect, which dissipates rapidly because cows' milk antibody declines to negligible levels within a week, and antibody soon dissipates from the calf's gut. In dairy calves removed from the dam when 24 hours old, gut antibody levels soon become negligible. The humoral antibody status of calves is probably unrelated to the outcome of exposure and infection.

There are several antigenic components present in BRoV including two external type-specific antigens that stimulate a neutralizing antibody and determine serotypes and a group-specific internal antigen detectable by other techniques.

VIRUS PERSISTENCE

The high antibody prevalence in most cattle populations suggests that persistent infections occur. Likewise, the resistance of BRoV to disinfectants and environmental influences suggests that contaminated premises may achieve the epidemiologic effects of carrier cattle.

The annual appearance of BRoV-induced NCD on beef ranches practicing seasonal calving also suggests that carrier cattle are common. The potential of persistent infections and a carrier state require more study.

PREVENTION AND CONTROL

Prevention of all NCD will probably never be achieved. While the role of management and sanitation cannot be overemphasized, even the best-managed calving operations can have serious outbreaks. Calves have the best chance of survival if parturition occurs in clean areas, the cows' vulvas and udders are scrubbed and disinfected, and a first-day colostrum meal is provided to newborn calves.

If it is determined that BRoV is present in herds, oral vaccination of newborn calves may be implemented using the combined rotavirus and coronavirus MLV vaccine. Vaccine should be administered immediately after birth to ensure maximum likelihood of vaccine efficacy. This regimen is a logistical challenge, but it can be accomplished. The presence of a trained attendant at birth can increase survival rates considerably by instituting hygienic measures for the cow, the calf, and the premises and by clearing the calf's airways, disinfecting the navel, and ensuring colostral intake.

A modified live virus (MLV) vaccine, released for sale in the United States in 1973 is administered orally to calves at birth. It can reduce morbidity and mortality in herds infected with BRoV if combined with management changes. The vaccine has been available in combination with coronavirus vaccine since 1976 and is believed to reduce economic losses from NCD.

Opinions vary on the efficacy of the vaccine in calves (Theil and McCloskey 1995). This uncertainty results from the difficulties in field evaluation of vaccines and the need for reapplication of orally administered MLV vaccine, which may be suppressed by colostrally acquired antibody in the calf's gut. Some uncertainty may result from serotype variations in BRoV involved in outbreaks (Clark et al. 1996) or overattenuation of vaccine.

The combined rotavirus-coronavirus vaccine was approved for use on pregnant cattle in 1979. This procedure is intended to stimulate high BRoV titers in colostrum so nursing calves are protected by the presence of antibody in the gut.

The multifactorial etiology of NCD ensures no single product or procedure will be a cure-all. Nevertheless, isolation of BRoV and development of the vaccine contribute to profitable calf production.

THERAPY AND MANAGEMENT OF OUTBREAKS

If a specific etiologic diagnosis of BRoV infection is obtained in a herd, it is imperative to immediately initiate programs for hygienic parturition, colostrum acquisition, extreme sanitary measures for rearing calves, and vaccination of newborn calves and pregnant cattle. Vaccination however, is no panacea and will not replace good management practices.

Therapeutic procedures for treating NCD are similar regardless of the etiology and must be instituted before laboratory diagnosis is available.

Antibiotics have traditionally been administered orally and systemically to calves with neonatal diarrhea. The wisdom of indiscriminate antibiotic therapy is questionable because of cost and the need for bacterial cultures and sensitivity testing to determine which antibiotics are effective against the specific bacterial strains present. It is also ill advised because antibiotic residues remain in the veal, the animal may develop antibiotic resistance, antibiotics alter normal intestinal flora and may cause negative disease outcomes. The quest for alternatives has stimulated the screening of numerous natural compounds for anti-BRoV activity (Clark et al. 1998).

Restoration of fluid volume and normalization of electrolyte balance should be major objectives of therapy. It is best accomplished by massive intravenous transfusion of balanced electrolyte solutions or oral electrolyte therapy.

Successful treatment requires early recognition of diarrhea and prompt initiation of therapy and electrolyte transfusions.

Control of outbreaks is largely dependent on correcting management deficiencies that permit BRoV transmission to stressed or colostrum-deprived calves and by initiating therapeutic and preventive measures including vaccines.

LIKELIHOOD OF ERADICATION

The widespread distribution of antibody, indicating BRoV is ubiquitous in cattle populations (Acres and Babiuk 1978), suggests a low probability of eradication.

IMPACT ON INTERNATIONAL TRADE

BRoV is not categorized as a List A or List B disease by the Office International Des Epizooties. Thus BRoV is unlikely to be the object of international trade measures.

PUBLIC RESPONSIBILITY

Veterinarians attempting to solve NCD situations should endeavor to obtain laboratory assistance in determining the etiology of problems. Workers must be counseled on the roles of stress control, sanitation, good management practices, and colostrum in minimizing calf losses. Vaccination should be employed where indicated, but there is an obligation to point out that vaccine alone will not eliminate NCD.

AREAS IN NEED OF RESEARCH

Research is needed to determine the mechanism of immunity and resistance to BRoV infections. The possibility of a persistent latent infection or other mechanism for maintenance of the carrier state must be studied, and alternatives to antibiotic therapy should be sought.

REFERENCES

Acres, SD, Babiuk LA, 1978. Studies on rotaviral antibody in bovine serum and lacteal secretions using radioimmunoassay. *J. Am. Vet. Med. Assoc.* 173:555–559.

Chinsangarum J, Akita GY, Osburn BI, 1994. Detection of group B rotaviruses in feces by polymerase chain reaction. *J. Vet. Diagn. Invest.* 6:302–307.

Clark KJ, Tamberollo TJ, Xu Z, Mann FE, Bonnot CE, Woode GN, 1996. An unusual group A rotavirus associated with an epidemic of diarrhea among three-month-old calves. *J. Am. Vet. Med. Assoc.* 208:552–554.

Clark KJ, Grant PG, Sarr AB, Belakere JR, Swaggety CL, Phillips TD, Woode GN, 1998. An in vitro study of theaflavins extracted from black tea to neutralize bovine rotavirus and bovine coronavirus infections. *Vet. Microbiol.* 63:147–157.

Gerdes GH, 1994. Rotavirus infections. In *Infectious Diseases of Livestock With Special Reference to Southern Africa,* edited by JAW Coetzer, GR Thomson and RC Tustin. Capetown: Oxford University Press, pp. 484–489.

Mebus CA, 1969. Further studies on neonatal calf diarrhea virus. *Proc. U.S. Anim. Health Assoc.* 73:97–99.

Mebus CA, 1975. Reovirus and rotavirus infections. *Proc. U.S. Anim. Health Assoc.* 79:345–349.

Mebus CA. 1990. Bovine and ovine rotavirus. In *Infectious Diseases of Ruminants,* edited by Z Dinter, B Morein. Amsterdam: Elsevier Scientific Publishers. pp. 239–244.

Mebus CA, Stair EL, Underdahl NR, Twiehaus MJ, 1971. Pathology of neonatal calf diarrhea induced by a reo-like virus. *Vet. Pathol.* 8:490–505.

Parwani AV, Munoz M, Tsunemitsu H, Lucchelli A, Saif, LJ, 1995. Molecular and serologic characterization of a group A bovine rotavirus with a short genome pattern. *J. Vet. Diagn. Invest.* 7:255–261.

Tennant B, Ward DE, Braun RK, Hunt EL, Baldwin BH, 1978. Clinical management and control of neonatal enteric infections of calves. *J. Am. Vet. Med. Assoc.* 173:654–661.

Theil KW, McCloskey CM, 1995. Rotavirus shedding in feces of calves orally inoculated with a commercial rotavirus-coronavirus vaccine. *J. Vet. Diagn. Invest.* 7:427–432.

29

VESICULAR STOMATITIS

INTRODUCTION

Vesicular stomatitis (VS), a zoonotic disease of swine, equines, and cattle is caused by the VS virus (VSV). While exotic elsewhere, VS is endemic in parts of Central America, South America, and southern portions of North America. It frequently appears in western United States where, in the 1990s, it has occurred mainly in horses.

VSV also causes an influenza-like illness in humans. It has been studied extensively, but questions remain about natural reservoirs, modes of transmission, and methods of perpetuation in nature.

In cattle, VS sometimes causes economic losses and sometimes is self-limiting and relatively benign. Its importance lies in trade restrictions imposed on infected countries, disruption of domestic animal movements (Mumford et al. 1998), and its ability to obscure the true identity of foot-and-mouth disease (FMD), from which it is clinically indistinguishable. FMD could make major expansions if incorrectly diagnosed as VS.

VS has been reviewed by Hanson and McMillan (1990), Wilks (1994), Mebus (1998), and Murphy et al. (1999).

ETIOLOGY

VSV was identified in 1925, has been the subject of extensive laboratory investigation, and has been a model for studies of viral morphology, replication, and genetics. Its physical, chemical, and biologic properties are well known, but its natural history and epidemiology remain unclear.

VSV is the type species and major member of the genus *Vesiculovirus* of the family Rhabdoviridae, a group of rod (Gr. *rhabdos,* a rod) or bullet-shaped RNA viruses that contains agents infective for fish, plants, and arthropods. Although VSV is referred to as a single virus, there are two immunologically distinct serotypes (New Jersey and Indiana) with slightly different geographic distributions but overlapping ranges.

There are three subtypes of Indiana VSV. Indiana-1 was the first VSV isolate. Indiana-2 was named Cocal virus by Jonkers et al. (1964); they isolated it from mites infesting rice rats in Trinidad. Indiana-3 (Alagoas) was isolated during an outbreak among horses, mules, and cattle in the Brazilian state of Alagoas.

Indiana VSV and New Jersey VSV have slightly different epidemiologic characteristics (but may occur on the same property) and vary slightly in their pathogenicity for cattle. New Jersey VSV infections are most common in cattle and are generally more severe with higher attack rates. They are more likely to be associated with lesions on the feet.

VSV can be propagated in many cultures and quantitated in plaque assays. It grows in chick embryos, guinea pigs, and suckling mice but frequently loses virulence after serial propagation in laboratory hosts. It is readily inactivated by heat, sunlight, and most disinfectants.

Virus fingerprinting reveals niche-adapted genetic-strain specificity traceable to 3 major regional ecosystems, namely South America, Central America, and Mexico–United States.

CLINICAL SIGNS AND LESIONS

In addition to causing clinical disease in horses, swine, cattle, and llamas (Thomas 1996), VSV infects sheep, goats, and a variety of arboreal animals.

In cattle, VS can occur as sporadic individual cases in endemic areas. Bovine VS gains notoriety when multiple case outbreaks occur during summer months in temperate zones and rainy seasons in the tropics.

The classic febrile vesicular disease is not always observed in the field because the fever is transient, vesicles are fragile and rupture easily, and there are few epithelial remnants to suggest prior vesiculation. Thus, the lesions are considered erosions or ulcers rather than vesicles.

The anatomic location of lesions varies, perhaps as a result of routes of inoculation. In pastured nonlactating cattle, the lesions are seen in the oral cavity. In milch cattle, teat lesions receive most attention, although oral lesions also occur. Vesicles on the coronary band or interdigital spaces are observed less commonly than mouth or teat lesions. Vesicles on the tongue, gums, or lips are associated with excess salivation, lip smacking, and anorexia.

The lesions begin as raised blanched areas of fluid buildup. They are rarely observed as blisters, because fluid is lost rapidly resulting in areas of necrotic mucosa that often slough prior to examination, exposing the underlying vascular submucosal tissues. For this reason, major outbreaks involving thousands of pastured cattle may occur over vast areas before the vesicular nature of the disease is appreciated. Examination of recently infected, normal-appearing herdmates may reveal vesicles. Sometimes, necrotic epithelium sloughs during examination of the oral cavity and large portions of the tongue or gums are denuded.

In milch cattle, teat lesions are common, and mastitis is a costly sequel, particularly when lesions encompass teat orifices. The teat lesions can be spread by milking machines. In some outbreaks, up to 80% of cattle may develop teat lesions. Human cases can occur in milkers of infected cattle.

Human VSV infection may accompany outbreaks among livestock and is frequently mild, inapparent, and unreported (Mumford et al. 1998).

After a 2-to-6-day incubation period, some human VSV infections produce an "influenza-like" disease characterized by fever, chills, headache, muscular pain, stiffness, backache, sometimes reddening of the eyes and a running nose, and occasionally blisters on the lips and in the mouth. It usually lasts 2 to 3 days and is followed by complete recovery. It is thought that inapparent human infections followed by seroconversion are common.

Laboratory workers can acquire infection (which may be undiagnosed) by aerosol means, from cultures, from handling tissues of experimental animals, or from accidental injection. Face shields and masks should be used when working with VSV-infected material. People with immunologic deficits should not work with VSV or handle infected animals.

Bovine VS is a key point in control and recognition of FMD. VS is benign except when it occurs in serious outbreaks. Cattle owners and veterinarians who have grown accustomed to its periodic appearance in an area sometimes tend to ignore or not report it to avoid disruptions in movement of cattle and horses. The lesions, however, are indistinguishable from those of FMD. Thus, FMD can become established when regulatory officials are not contacted.

EFFECTS ON THE DEVELOPING FETUS

VSV does not appear to be a cause of abortions or fetal anomalies.

NECROPSY FINDINGS

Death among cattle is rare or absent in most outbreaks. The lesions produced by experimental inoculation evolve rapidly from macule to papule to vesicles and soon rupture, leaving ulcerations that heal rapidly.

Histopathologically, there is intracellular and extracellular edema, ballooning and degeneration of epithelial cells, and vesicle formation accompanied by neutrophilic infiltration. There are no inclusion bodies. The characteristic bullet-shaped morphology of VSV can sometimes be seen upon electron-microscopic examination of fresh lesions or vesicular fluid.

DIAGNOSIS

The diagnosis of VS should not be attempted without laboratory support because of the danger that it could be confused with FMD. Clinically, the two are indistinguishable, affecting both swine and cattle. Only VS, however, affects horses. The presence of clinical disease in horses is not sufficient to rule out FMD, because both diseases can occur simultaneously.

VS should be suspected if vesicular or ulcerative lesions are found in the mouth or on the feet of horses, swine, or cattle or on the teats of cattle. Outbreaks appear to start among pastured cattle during periods of insect activity and spread without obvious animal-to-animal contact. Frequently there have been similar episodes in the pastures or the same area.

The mild nature of bovine VS sometimes permits it to become well established before professional assistance is sought. The clinical diagnosis is frequently missed, and VS spreads unsuspected because vesicles per se may be absent or unobserved.

Differential Diagnosis

The most crucial diagnostic element is differentiation from FMD, which should be attempted by laboratory procedures conducted in concert with regulatory officials.

When the teats are not involved and the condition is largely confined to the muzzle and oral mucosa, the diseases affecting the bovine mucosa (DABM) (see Chapters 6 and 13) and photosensitization figure heavily in the differential diagnosis.

When teat lesions are present, bovine herpes mammillitis, pseudo lumpy skin disease, cowpox, and pseudocowpox must be considered. When swine are involved, it must be distinguished from vesicular exanthema of swine (VES), which has presumably been eradicated from swine, and swine vesicular disease (SVD).

Laboratory Diagnosis

Laboratory diagnosis is aimed at identifying the virus and distinguishing it from FMD virus (FMDV). Historically, differentiation involved inoculation of susceptible cattle, horses, and swine. The differentiation was based largely upon susceptibility of horses to VSV but not to FMDV, susceptibility of cattle to FMDV and VSV, and susceptibility of swine to FMDV, VSV, VES, and SVD viruses.

Animal inoculations were complicated by variable susceptibilities to differing routes of inoculation and strain differences in pathogenicity among the viruses causing vesicular diseases. Less expensive, faster, and more reliable procedures have largely replaced animal inoculations.

If adequate virus is present in vesicular epithelium or vesicular fluid, electron-microscopic examination can distinguish the VSV by its bullet shape.

Usually infectivity patterns and characteristics of cytopathology in various cell cultures are used as preliminary procedures to distinguish among viruses causing vesicles in cattle. Tissue-culture isolates from vesicular epithelium or vesicular fluid must then be identified by virus neutralization, enzyme-linked immunosorbent assay (ELISA), complement fixation (CF), or fluorescent antibody (FA) tests utilizing specific reference serums.

Serologic diagnosis requires paired serums and a demonstration of seroconversion by agar gel diffusion, competitive ELISA (CELISA), virus neutralization, or indirect FA tests.

Procedures for diagnosing VS are detailed by the Office International Des Epizooties (OIE) in the *OIE Manual of Diagnostic Tests and Vaccines* (OIE 2000).

Vesicular fluids (if obtainable), unruptured or sloughing epithelium of vesicular lesions, or scrapings are needed for virus isolation. Clotted blood is sometimes used for virus isolation and the serum is used for serology.

Esophageal–pharangeal fluids collected from convalescing patients with a probang are useful for diagnosing FMD.

EPIDEMIOLOGY

The infection and the disease are apparently confined to North, South, and Central America. In tropical and subtropical habitats, VSV infects a variety of wild animals and is perpetuated by unknown mechanisms. Excursions from endemic foci occur irregularly in summer and are characterized by extensions northward through the United States, rarely into Canada, and southward into temperate zones of South America. These episodes frequently result in epidemics (Jenney 1967; Goodger et al. 1985; and Bridges et al. 1997) in somewhat predictable riverine locales.

DNA fingerprints indicate similarities of US isolates to VSV strains endemic in Mexico, giving rise to the possibility that it is introduced by imported feeder cattle. Equally logical is the assumption that Northern Mexico and Southwestern United States share an ecological niche supportive of VSV endemicity and when environmental conditions and insect population dictate, there is northward expansion of the endemic area.

The infection skips over large areas with unsuitable ecosystems, infecting animals miles apart and sparing some in relatively close proximity. VSV behaves like an arthropod-borne virus, with greatest endemic and epidemic activity in the rainy season in the tropics and during the summer in temperate regions. Usually the first cattle affected have recently been pastured. Recognizable activity seems to cease with the onset of drought or just before frost, but overwintering may result in disease in subsequent years.

All reports indicate that the incubation period ranges from 12 to 72 hours before development of fever and the beginning of vesicle formation.

The natural reservoirs are still uncertain, but virus probably persists in one or more natural hosts. Antibodies have been found in a wide variety of wild mammals (mostly arboreal or semiarboreal) in Panama (Tesh et al. 1969), and in feral swine in a unique ecosystem on Ossabaw Island, Georgia (Stallknecht et al. 1999). Early studies indicated evidence of VSV in white-tailed deer in Georgia and Louisiana (Jenney et al. 1970), and in wild turkeys in Texas. It is known that the feral swine population of Ossabaw Island, Georgia, remains an endemic focus of VSV–New Jersey (Stallknecht et al. 1999).

It was postulated that Indiana VSV may be a plant virus rendered infective for mammals after a suitable extrinsic incubation period in sandflies of the genus *Phlebotomus*. It has been suggested that the virus may be present in pastures and associated with forage (Hanson 1968).

The immediate source of infection also remains obscure. Certain pastures may be contaminated, but probably only provide settings needed for activity of suitable arthropod vectors. VSV has been isolated from phlebotomine sandflies that can serve as biological vectors (Stallknecht et al. 1999), mosquitoes, and eye gnats of the genus *Hippelates*.

The mode of transmission seems to vary with the situation. Both vector-borne and contact transmission seem likely. VSV appears to be transmitted mechanically by milking machines, but abrasions may be required for contact transmission.

Epidemiologic evidence suggests insect vectors, but the high levels of viremia, usually regarded as essential for vector transmission are usually absent. Other modes of transmission may occur.

In humans, transmission may occur by vectors, aerosol means, contact with infected tissues or laboratory cultures, or accidental injection.

There appears to be no unique distribution of infection or disease with respect to age, sex, or breed aside from immunity conferred by previous exposure or colostrum acquisition. In some outbreaks, however, disease is observed only in adult cattle.

IMMUNITY

Antibody detectable by virus neutralization tests appears within a few weeks of infection, and complement-fixing (CF) antibody can be detected earlier. The CF antibody wanes rapidly, but neutralizing antibody may persist for as long as 8 years.

Cattle with antibody have partial protection but can be reinfected with high doses of virus. Nursing calves acquire colostrally transferred neutralizing antibodies, which disappear around 4 months of age.

VIRUS PERSISTENCE

Persistence of viral RNA has been demonstrated for intervals inadequate to explain the virus's overwintering. A true carrier state may not occur (Letchworth et al. 1996). Prolonged maintenance of antibody titers suggests that either frequent reinfection or some mechanism of persistence may exist.

PREVENTION AND CONTROL

Because there appears to be multiple modes of transmission, no single procedure is available to limit introduction into new areas.

In affected areas reductions in the number of new cases may be achieved by removing cattle from pasture (pasturing is an identified risk factor for disease acquisition), confining them to buildings, and applying approved insecticides to individual animals (but not to premises) (Hurd et al. 1997).

Vaccination of cattle with inactivated or modified live virus vaccines is practiced to a limited extent in Central America. In 1995, USDA approved the use of inactivated autogenous vaccines prepared from isolates from outbreaks, but these vaccines were not widely used.

THERAPY AND MANAGEMENT OF OUTBREAKS

Upon suspicion of VS in the United States, state and federal regulatory agencies must be contacted, and herds quarantined until 30 days after the last clinical lesions are healed (Mumford et al. 1998).

If laboratory tests indicate VS, cattle should be removed from affected pastures. Sick cattle should be provided protection from the sun and given adequate water and feed. If secondary bacterial infections occur, antibiotics may be administered. Cows with teat lesions should be the last ones milked in order to minimize spread by milking equipment. Mortality is low and most animals recover within 1 to 5 weeks.

LIKELIHOOD OF ERADICATION

VS seems to be inexorably rooted in endemic areas of tropical and subtropical America. The presence of antibodies in a wide variety of wild animals suggests the presence of reservoirs. Natural disease cycles must be fully understood before the potential of eradication can be evaluated.

IMPACT ON INTERNATIONAL TRADE

VS is categorized as a List A disease by the OIE, but few countries impose major VS-based trade restrictions on commodities other than live animals. Because it is compulsorily reportable in United States (Mumford et al. 1998), only minor trade interruptions occur during outbreaks, but they are disconcerting to affected livestock, meat, and poultry exporters and to those moving horses internationally.

The OIE International Animal Health Code indicates that countries may be considered free when VS is notifiable and no clinical, epidemiological, or other evidence of VS has been found during the past 2 years. The code also lays out requirements for importing live animals from VS-infected or VS-free countries. The code does not suggest restrictions on importing meats and other animal products from VS-infected countries.

With respect to pork, swine are inefficient amplifiers of VSV. They can, however, be infected orally by meat scraps (Stahlnecht et al. 1999).

Contact transmission of the Ossabaw Island strain of VS New Jersey by sub-clinically infected pigs with tonsillar infections (probably via oral or fecal shedding) has been reported (Howerth et al. 1997).

PUBLIC RESPONSIBILITY

In FMD-free areas, all vesicular diseases require regulatory investigation and laboratory diagnosis. When it occurs in FMD-vaccinated cattle, clinical VS elicits concern about the effectiveness of FMD vaccines and possible introduction of new FMD strains.

Individuals suspecting VS or any vesicular disease are obligated to contact regulatory authorities so that laboratory diagnosis can be undertaken to rule out FMD.

The disease is transmissible to humans, and people working with infected cattle should be warned. Use of gloves and protective clothing may not be adequate to prevent human infection. If close contact with infected tissues is likely to occur, masks may be needed.

Immunologically compromised people should not work with the virus or infected animals or their tissues.

AREAS IN NEED OF RESEARCH

Although the biochemical and biophysical properties, cultural characteristics, and method of replication of VSV are well documented, extensive epidemiologic and pathogenesis studies are needed to identify natural reservoirs of the disease and modes of transmission.

REFERENCES

Bridges VE, McCluskey BJ, Salmon MD, Hurd HS, Dick J, 1997. Review of the 1995 vesicular stomatitis outbreak in the western United States. *J. Am. Vet. Med. Assoc.* 211: 556–560.

Goodger WJ, Thurmond M, Hehay J, Mitchell J, Smith P, 1985. Economic impact of an epizootic of bovine vesicular stomatitis in California. *J. Am. Vet. Med. Assoc.* 196:370–373.

Hanson RP, 1968. Discussion of the natural history of vesicular stomatitis. *Am. J. Epidemiol.* 87:264–266.

Hanson RP, McMillan B, 1990. Vesicular stomatitis virus. In *Infectious Diseases of Ruminants,* edited by Z Dinter, B Morein. Amsterdam: Elsevier Scientific Publishers, pp. 381–389.

Howerth EW, Stallknecht DE, Dorming M, Pisell T, Clarke GR, 1997. Experimental vesicular stomatitis in swine: effects of route of inoculation and steroid treatment. *J. Vet. Diagn. Invest.* 9:136–142.

Hurd HS, Norden DK, Hayek AM, 1997. Management factors associated with the spread of vesicular stomatitis–New Jersey. *Proc. U.S. Anim. Health Assoc.* 101:127–133.

Jenney EW, 1967. Vesicular stomatitis in the United States during the last five years (1963–1967). *Proc. U.S. Livestock Sanit. Assoc.* 71: 371–385.

Jenney EW, Hayes FA, Brown CL, 1970. Survey for vesicular stomatitis virus neutralizing antibodies in serum of white-tailed deer (*Odocoileus virginianus*) in southeastern United States. *.J Wildl. Dis.* 6:488–493.

Jonkers AH, Shope RE, Aitken TH, Spence L, 1964. Cocal virus, a new agent in Trinidad related to vesicular stomatitis virus. *Am. J. Vet. Res.* 25:236–242.

Letchworth GJ, Barrera JDC, Fishel JR, Rodriguez L, 1996. Vesicular stomatitis New Jersey RNA persists in cattle following convalescence. *Virology* 239:480–484.

Mebus CA, 1998. Vesicular stomatitis. *In Foreign Animal Diseases,* edited by WW Buisch, JL Hyde, CL Mebus. Richmond: US Animal Health Assoc. pp. 419–423.

Mumford EL, McClusky EW, Traub-Dargatz JL, Schmidt BJ, Salmon MD, 1998. Serologic evaluation of vesicular stomatitis virus exposure in horses and cattle in 1996. *J. Am. Vet. Med. Assoc.* 213:1265–1269.

Murphy FA, Gibbs EPJ, Horzinek MC, Studdert MJ, 1999. Vesicular stomatitis. *In Veterinary Virology,* 3rd ed. San Diego: Academic Press, pp. 439–441.

Office International Des Epizooties (OIE) 2000. Vesicular stomatitis. In *Manual of Diagnostic Tests and Vaccines,* 7th ed. with annual updates. Paris: OIE. Chapter 2.1.2 pp. 57–63.

Stallknecht DE, Howerth EG, Reeves CL, Seal, BS, 1999. Potential for contact and mechanical vector transmission of vesicular stomatitis New Jersey in pigs. *Am. J. Vet. Res.* 60:43–48.

Tesh RB, Peralta PH, Johnson KM, 1969. Ecological studies of vesicular stomatitis virus. I. Prevalence of infection among animals and humans living in an endemic area of VSV activity. *Am. J. Epidemiol.* 19:255–261.

Thomas LA, 1996. An interesting case of VSV and other diagnostic activities at FADDL. Report of the Committee on Foreign Animal Diseases. *Proc. U.S. Anim. Health Assoc.* 100:219–220.

Wilks CR, 1994. Vesicular stomatitis and other vesiculovirus infections. In *Infectious Diseases of Livestock With Special Reference to Southern Africa,* edited by JAW Coetzer, GR Thomson, RC Tustin. Capetown: Oxford University Press. pp. 363–366.

30

AKABANE AND BUNYAVIRUSES CAUSING BOVINE FETAL WASTAGE

INTRODUCTION

Akabane virus causes fetal wastage in cattle, sheep, and goats following inapparent insect-borne infections of pregnant animals in parts of Africa, Southeast Asia, Australia, and the Middle East.

The role of Akabane virus as a bovine pathogen came to light following epidemics of congenital arthrogryposis (joint immobility) and hydranencephaly (absence of cerebral hemispheres) in animals in Australia, Japan, and Israel (Nobel et al. 1971). Although other agents can cause similar defects, Akabane virus infection should be suspected when epizootics of congenital hydranencephaly and arthrogryposis occur.

Diagnosis is obtained by virus isolation or detection of neutralizing antibody in fetuses or neonates that have not acquired colostrum.

Akabane has been reviewed by Inaba and Matumoto (1990), Charles (1994), St. George and Standfast (1994), and St. George (1998).

ETIOLOGY

Akabane virus is named for a village in Japan where it was first isolated from mosquitoes (Oya et al. 1961). It is a member of the Simbu serologic subgroup of the genus *Bunyavirus* in the family Bunyaviridae, a group of over 200 heat- and pH-labile enveloped RNA viruses that agglutinate avian red blood cells and are transmitted by insects. The Simbu subgroup also includes Aino, Peaton, Douglas, and Timaroo viruses. While less prevalent, these viruses cause similar defects, have similar epidemiological characteristics, and should be regarded as "also ran" viruses in any discussion of Akabane.

Primary isolation is usually achieved by intracerebral inoculation of suckling mice. Some isolates have been adapted to grow in chick embryos, laboratory mice, and cell cultures in which cytopathic changes result.

Antibody surveys suggest that in addition to cattle, sheep, and goats in which it produces congenital defects, Akabane virus probably also has infectivity, without disease, for camels, dogs, horses, monkeys and pigs. Hamsters have proved to be an excellent experimental model for studying Akabane infections of pregnant animals and their fetuses.

CLINICAL SIGNS AND LESIONS

Akabane virus infections of cattle are generally inapparent and go unnoticed until abortions occur and calves with congenital anomalies are born.

EFFECTS ON THE DEVELOPING FETUS

Infection of susceptible pregnant cattle results in subsequent abortions, still-births, and birth of calves with a variety of congenital anomalies. These include a congenital arthrogryposis and hydranencephaly (AG/HE) syndrome (St. George and Standfast 1994) and a hydranencephaly–microencephaly (HE/ME) syndrome. These birth defects occur sporadically in endemic areas with high levels of population immunity and in massive epizootics when the virus first enters highly susceptible populations or when immunologically naive cattle are introduced into endemic areas. Arthrogryposis (fixation of joints), which occurs alone or in combination with hydranencephaly, can cause dystocia requiring fetotomy or cesarean section, which affected calves rarely survive.

The nature of anomalies is partially determined by the stage of gestation in which primary infection of the dam occurs. Observations of field cases and experimental data, however, have indicated large, sometimes overlapping, ranges of gestational ages of exposure associated with various anomalies. Thus, the nature of pregnancy outcomes and fetal lesions is not an accurate indicator of the stage of gestation when maternal infection occurred. If infection occurs simultaneously with insemination, Akabane virus can cause necrosis of the corpus luteum with failure to conceive (Foley 1996).

Most affected calves are dead at birth, but some survive for a short time if the condition is mild and the birth is uncomplicated.

Arthrogryposis causes joints to be fixed firmly in flexion and occasionally in extension. The joints are unmovable unless the tendons are severed, so affected calves, if born alive, are unable to stand or walk. The condition is usually bilateral, and the front legs are most commonly involved. Occasionally, scoliosis (lateral deviation of the spine), spina bifida (incomplete closure of the spinal canal), and muscle atrophy are present.

Neonates with the HE/ME syndrome have normal joints and only central nervous system involvement.

Although mildly affected calves may survive, most calves with serious HE/ME syndrome are aborted or they are stillborn or die shortly after birth. If carefully nursed, calves with serious brain lesions could conceivably survive, but many are severely disabled, frequently uncoordinated, blind or deaf, and lack avoiding and nursing reflexes.

NECROPSY FINDINGS

Necropsy examination of affected neonates reveals a variety of lesions including fixation of the forelimbs and sometimes of the hind limbs. Marked neurogenic muscle atrophy may be present. The muscles may be normal in size, with paleness, and have yellow interstitial edema.

Some calves have convex molding of the cranial and facial bones, lordosis, scoliosis, kyphosis, spina bifida, or cleft palate. Along with hydranencephaly, mild to severe cavitations in the cerebral hemispheres, pons, medulla, brainstem, and cervical spinal cord are sometimes present.

Histologic lesions correlate with gross findings. Atrophy and interstitial edema are present in muscles. Joints with persistent flexure or extension appear normal histologically.

In the brain, encephalitis, mild perivascular cuffing, and Wallerian degeneration may be observed in addition to massive cavitations. In the spinal cord there can be reduction in ventral horn neurones and demyelination of nerve fibers that supply areas of joint flexion or extension.

DIAGNOSIS

When AG/HE epizootics occur, Akabane is a primary diagnostic choice. However, sporadic and atypical cases and suspected incursions into previously free regions require laboratory confirmation to differentiate them from many other maternal conditions causing congenital anomalies. In the United States, Cache Valley virus causes similar lesions (Edwards et al. 1989).

Akabane virus infection of pregnant cattle should be suspected when congenital AG/HE or HE/ME syndromes appear sporadically or endemically along with stillbirths or abortions among cattle, sheep, and goats that have had no clinical signs and were pregnant during conditions suitable for insect transmission.

Clinical diagnosis is based on the appearance of classic signs and the typical epidemiologic pattern.

Differential Diagnosis

Abortions and stillbirths attributable to Akabane must be differentiated from the wide variety of other causes of these problems. Both AG/HE and HE/ME syndromes are characteristic but must be distinguished from other virus infections and sporadic idiopathic causes of congenital anomalies. These include genetic defects causing heritable joint deformities, vitamin and mineral deficiencies, maternal consumption of toxic plants, and environmental causes of congenital disorders that may emerge. They must also be distinguished from congenital defects caused by Aino, Douglas, Preston, and Timaroo (other Simbu subgroup viruses), Cache Valley virus (a *Bunyavirus* of the Bunyamwera subgroup that is present in the United States), occasional hydranencephaly that may be attributed to bluetongue virus, and cerebellum disorders produced by the virus of bovine viral diarrhea (Charles 1994).

Laboratory Diagnosis

In countries where Akabane virus exists, some laboratories are equipped for serologic tests to detect Akabane antibodies. In the United States, the US Department of Agriculture utilizes the Foreign Animal Disease Diagnostic Laboratory, which accepts specimens through state and federal regulatory channels.

Serum from aborted fetuses, stillborn calves, or calves definitely deprived of colostrum can be tested for neutralizing antibody. If it is present, presuckle antibody indicates intrauterine infection. This is convincing etiologic evidence of Akabane virus as a cause of AG/HE or HE/ME syndrome only if the serums are negative for antibody to other viruses producing similar syndromes. If antibodies are absent, Akabane cannot be positively ruled out because fetuses can be infected before they achieve immunocompetence, which occurs at about five months of gestational age.

In retrospective investigations where only maternal serums are available, comparison of antibody prevalence in dams of normal calves with that of dams producing anomalous calves can be deceiving unless differences are obvious. Some laboratories also use hemagglutination inhibition and agar gel diffusion tests for Akabane antibodies.

The Akabane virus can be isolated from placentas of aborting cows, fetuses, and stillborn calves, using cell culture or suckling mouse inoculation. The bovine fetus becomes immunocompetent at around five months of gestation, so virus isolation is difficult in calves born near term if their immune response has been adequate to clear the virus.

The virus can sometimes be isolated from blood of cattle in early stages of infection. Because the infection is inapparent in adults, frequent bleeding of sentinel cattle or fortuitous selection of cattle for testing is required to make this procedure useful. Isolation of Akabane virus from insects ensures its presence in an area and provides further evidence of its involvement in outbreaks.

Aseptically collected serums from aborted fetuses, stillborn calves, or calves with AH/ME or HE/ME syndrome are the specimens of choice. Because the serologic diagnosis is based on finding antibody produced before birth, there must be certainty that the calf has not acquired colostrum. If the calf is clearly incapable of nursing, this question won't arise. If there is doubt, examination of stomach contents for traces of milk is required, and if possible the dam's teats should be inspected for evidence of nursing. Any serum from a neonate should be accompanied by serum from its dam.

To isolate the virus, fetal spleen, blood, brain, spinal cord, cerebrospinal fluid, or muscle may be inoculated into suckling mice or Akabane-sensitive cell cultures, which can then be examined by fluorescent antibody techniques. Any collection of specimens should be preceded by consultation with the laboratory conducting the test.

EPIDEMIOLOGY

The AG/HE syndrome was reported prior to its association with Akabane virus. The virus was first isolated in 1959 from *Aedes* and *Culex* mosquitoes (Oya et al. 1961), and the epidemiologic details of the disease, recognized largely when massive epizootics occur in highly susceptible populations, have been explored since then.

Infected cattle are usually afebrile and asymptomatic. Within 1 to 6 days following exposure by insect bites, they develop a viremia that lasts up to 9 days before being cleared by host immune mechanisms (St. George 1998). The interval between exposure of the pregnant dam and expulsion of aborted fetuses or stillborn calves or the birth of anomalous calves varies. The gestational age of the fetus at the time of infection is a major determinant of the nature of the fetal disease and the anomalies induced.

The usual sources of infection are *Culex* and *Aedes* mosquitoes or gnats of the genus *Culicoides*. Biologic transmission in which the virus undergoes essential stages of multiplication in the insect is suspected but has not been established. Endemic areas may expand or contract as climatic pressures on vector populations vary from year to year and from decade to decade. If global warming causes expansion of tropical and semitropical zones, future centuries may experience major expansions of ecosystems supportive of Akabane and other vector-borne diseases.

Antibodies have been detected in cattle, horses, sheep, goats, pigs, dogs, and monkeys. This finding indicates only that these species are susceptible. They may be dead-end alien hosts that play no role in transmission or perpetuation of virus-insect-mammalian cycles of transmission or they may be essential components of viral survival.

All evidence indicates that transmission is by the bite of infected arthropods, which leads to brief viremia in pregnant cattle. Blood-borne distribution of the virus to the placenta results, where it replicates. It then goes to the fetus, where a brief fetal viremia permits distribution of virus to brain, muscle, and joints. This transmission process may occur when susceptible cattle are moved to endemic areas or when the virus enters hitherto uninfected areas because of climate-driven ecological changes permitting expansion of the range of competent vectors.

The clinical disease appears to be confined to neonates infected prenatally; these can be offspring of susceptible dams of all ages. In endemic areas, high percentages of mature cattle and even heifers become immune prior to pregnancy and produce normal calves, while nonimmune individuals infected during pregnancy abort or produce stillborn fetuses or calves with AG/HE or HE/ME syndromes.

Affected calves have been born to cattle of most dairy and beef breeds, including crossbred animals.

Although sporadic cases undoubtedly occur in endemic areas, major outbreaks are recognized when many deformed calves appear 4 to 6 months after periods of intense insect activity.

IMMUNITY

Actively induced serum antibody that persists for several years probably protects individuals from subsequent infections and helps to modulate epizootics.

Calves nursing immune cows acquire colostral antibody that usually wanes at about 4 months of age. Ingestion of colostrum undoubtedly provides calves with partial protection of variable duration. Colostrally acquired immunity can confuse efforts to diagnose the causes of congenital anomalies.

VIRUS PERSISTENCE

Akabane virus persists in endemic state in bovine populations through insect-cow-insect cycles. In pregnant cattle a brief persistent infection occurs in cotyledons of pregnant cattle and lingers there even after the cow develops circulating antibody and virus is cleared from other tissues (Charles 1994). Aside from that, classic persistent or latent infections of individual cattle have not been reported.

PREVENTION AND CONTROL

Control is based on insect control, vaccination, and controlling movement of livestock in and out of endemic areas. Control via insecticide application and elimination of breeding sites is usually unsuccessful. A formalin-inactivated vaccine requiring two initial doses 4 weeks apart and subsequent annual vaccination has been developed. An effective hamster-cell-propagated modified live virus vaccine is available that can be used safely on pregnant cows. The cost effectiveness of vaccination must be evaluated in differing ecological situations.

THERAPY AND MANAGEMENT OF OUTBREAKS

There is no treatment for abortions, stillbirths, or congenital anomalies. Mildly affected calves may go unnoticed or be maintained by careful nursing, but the latter is generally not practical. Handling of outbreaks requires obtaining a diagnosis. In areas currently free of Akabane, regulatory agencies should be involved at first suspicion of the disease. To be effective, vaccines must be administered prior to exposure.

LIKELIHOOD OF ERADICATION

Eradication measures cannot be realistically considered because of multiple competent vectors, the vast ecosystems that support vectors, and the lack of information on endemic cycles.

IMPACT ON INTERNATIONAL TRADE

Akabane is not categorized as a List B or List A disease by the Office International Des Epizooties. Because potential vectors are widely distributed, however, importing countries may require brief quarantines and tests to detect potentially viremic live cattle originating in endemic areas. Care must be taken to avoid moving immunologically naive susceptible cattle into endemic areas (Jagoe et al. 1993). As an insect-borne disease, transmission of Akabane by semen, meats, and other animal products is unlikely.

PUBLIC RESPONSIBILITY

If Akabane is suspected or diagnosed in a herd, the owner must be provided with a candid prognosis regarding the outcome of remaining pregnancies. In Akabane-free regions, regulatory officials should be notified on first suspicion of the disease.

AREAS IN NEED OF RESEARCH

Continued research is needed on the mechanisms of mechanical or biological transmission of Akabane by various vectors and on the potential emerging roles of closely related Bunya subgroup viruses.

REFERENCES

Charles JA, 1994. Akabane virus. Diagnosis of abortion. *Vet. Clin. North Am.: Food Animal Practice* 10:525–546.

Edwards JF, Livingston CW, Chung SI, Collinson EC, 1989. Ovine arthrogryposis and central nervous system malformations associated with in utero Cache Valley virus infection: Spontaneous disease. *Vet. Pathol.* 26:33–39.

Foley GL, 1996. Pathology of the corpus luteum of cows. *Theriogenology* 45:1413–1428.

Inaba Y, Matumoto M, 1990. Akabane virus. In *Infectious Diseases of Ruminants,* edited by Z Dinter and B Morein. Amsterdam: Elsevier Scientific Publishers, pp. 467–480.

Jagoe S, Kirkland PD, Harper PAW, 1993. An outbreak of Akabane-virus-induced abnormalities in calves after agistment in an epidemic region. *Aust. Vet. J.* 70:56–58.

Nobel TA, Klopfer U, Neumann F, 1971. Pathology of an arthrogryposis and hydranencephaly syndrome in calves in Israel 1969–1970. *Refu. Vet.* 28:144–151.

Oya A, Okuno T, Ogata T, Kobayashi T, Matsuyama T, 1961. Akabane virus: A new arbovirus isolated in Japan. *Jpn. J. Med. Sci. Biol.* 14:101–108.

St. George TD, 1998. Akabane. In *Foreign Animal Diseases,* edited by WW Buisch, JL Hyde, CL Mebus. Richmond: U.S. Animal Health Assoc. pp. 62–70.

St. George TD, Standfast HA, 1994. Diseases caused by Akabane and related Simbu-group viruses. In *Infectious Diseases of Livestock With Special Reference to Southern Africa,* edited by JAW Coetzer, GR Thomson, RC Tustin. Capetown: Oxford University Press. pp. 681–687.

31

EPHEMERAL FEVER

INTRODUCTION

Bovine ephemeral fever (BEF) is an acute, insect-transmitted disease characterized by periodic summer epizootics of fever, respiratory signs, depression, stiffness, lameness, and sometimes paralysis. It infects cattle and water buffalo in a variety of ecosystems in Australia and many parts of Africa, Asia and the Middle East, but is exotic to North and South America and Europe. Modified live virus and subunit vaccines are used for control. Despite extensive study, BEF remains an epidemiological enigma.

Ephemeral means *transient* or *short-lived*. The name fits the sudden onset and short course of the disease, and the animal's usual abrupt recovery. BEF has also been called three-day sickness, stiff-sickness, bovine epizootic fever, tongue fever of cattle, lazy man's disease, and drie-dae-stywesiekte (St. George 1994).

BEF has been reviewed by Combs (1978) and St. George (1990, 1994, and 1998). BEF virus (BEFV) and related Rhabdoviridae are discussed in detail in the proceedings of a 1992 symposium in Beijing, China (St. George et al. 1993).

ETIOLOGY

BEFV is a cone- or bullet-shaped single-stranded RNA virus of the genus *Ephemerovirus* in the family Rhabdoviridae. It is sensitive to most disinfectants and to changes in pH. It does not survive outside living hosts, in meat, or in the environment. It depends on insects for its transmission and is an infectious but noncontagious disease because of its lack of transmission by direct or indirect contact.

Experimentally, it is transmissible only by intravenous injection of BEFV into susceptible cattle. BEFV strains seem to vary in virulence.

The disease is propagated by intracerebral inoculation of mice and grows poorly in cell cultures. Similar clinical signs are sometimes attributed to two less-studied rhabdoviruses, namely Kotonkan virus found in parts of Africa and

Puchong virus in Malaysia. Other antigenically related, but less common and apparently nonpathogenic Rhabdoviridae include Kimberly, Berrimah, and Adelaide River viruses.

BEFV replicates in vascular epithelium and induces maximum interferon production.

CLINICAL SIGNS

BEF is sometimes described as an influenza-like disease because of its sudden onset and short duration and symptoms such as high fever and extreme debility. The analogy to flu weakens, however, because of the toxic, hypocalcemic, and paralytic components of BEF.

The fever associated with BEF is usually biphasic or triphasic with each phase peaking at 104° to 107° F and lasting 12 to 18 hours. With the exception of dropping milk production, which accompanies the first temperature rise, the onset of most clinical signs is associated with the second temperature rise (St. George 1998). The pathogenesis of the clinical disease has been categorized into five stages, namely toxic signs, inflammatory signs, hypocalcemic signs, emphysema, and prolonged paralytic signs (St. George 1993). The nature and severity of clinical signs vary among affected animals.

Some infected cattle experience a transient fever with few other overt clinical signs; antibody surveys indicate that subclinical infections occur. More seriously affected animals will have a rapid pulse, anorexia, excess salivation, lacrimation and nasal discharge, depression, decreased rumen activity, muscle tremors, and severe lameness in one or more legs. They may assume a sitting position or a short period of recumbency from which recovery may be spontaneous, unexpected, and sudden.

Some affected cattle have only slight lameness in one or more legs and recover promptly. Others experience total paralysis and have loss of reflexes, inability to swallow, and total rumen atony. These signs sometimes respond to intravenous calcium gluconate therapy or other therapies (Fenwick and Daniel 1996 and St. George 1997). Most uncomplicated cases recover spontaneously within 3 to 4 days of the first observed clinical signs. Signs persist longer and fatalities are most common in fattened steers, high-producing dairy cattle, and mature bulls in bull studs.

Death occurs in less than 1% of cases and is sometimes attributed to inhalation of medicines administered orally to cattle with impaired swallowing reflexes. Higher case-fatality rates may occur in remote areas where affected cattle cannot reach water.

Usually live animals have no observable gross lesions aside from occasional subcutaneous emphysema over the back or subcutaneous edema of the head.

EFFECTS ON THE DEVELOPING FETUS

Some cattle infected in the last two months of gestation may abort (St. George 1998). Early observations suggested that mummified fetuses and congenital abnormalities may have resulted from BEFV infections of pregnant cattle, but experiments indicated that this cause was unlikely (Parsonson and Snowdon 1974a) and such anomalies probably resulted from Akabane or Aino virus infections.

Although infected bulls may experience temporary drops in fertility, semen contamination with BEF virus is rare and appears to have minimal effect on fertility and pregnancy (Parsonson and Snowdon 1974b).

NECROPSY FINDINGS

Severe inhalation pneumonia is the cause of some deaths. Occasional animals have pulmonary edema and emphysema and subcutaneous emphysema over the back. Fibrinous fluids may be present in body cavities and joints.

Most lesions are associated with joints and muscles. There may be focal necrotic areas in muscle. There may be excess joint fluid, fibrin in synovial fluid, and inflammation and swelling of fascia or tendons. Lymph nodes may be swollen and edematous and may contain petechial hemorrhages. Slight pleural or pericardial effusion may be observed. Nonspecific agonal lesions such as hemorrhages in the trachea and heart may be observed.

Histopathologically, endothelial hypoplasia and perivascular infiltration with neutrophils is seen in synovial membranes and tendon sheaths.

DIAGNOSIS

Diagnosis is usually based on clinical signs. It can be challenging with individual cases because the clinical presentation varies in nature and severity among animals. Classic patterns emerge, however, when collections of cases appear in herd outbreaks. In areas considered free of BEF, laboratory confirmation is essential.

Differential Diagnosis

Where the typical classic outbreak pattern is absent, BEF can be confused with numerous causes of lameness and recumbency (St. George 1994). These could include plant poisonings, botulism, mycotoxin poisoning, and traumatic injuries.

Similar clinical signs are occasionally attributed to two less studied rhabdoviruses, namely Kotonkan virus found in parts of Africa and Puchong virus in Malaysia.

Laboratory Diagnosis

Confirmatory diagnosis can be obtained by inoculating susceptible calves with blood from acute cases and reproducing the classic clinical and hematological picture. Virus isolation attempts using cell culture inoculations are not always successful and sometimes must be preceded by intracerebral inoculation of suckling mice or intravenous inoculation of embryonating hens' eggs with subsequent inoculation into susceptible cell cultures.

Serologic tests include virus neutralization tests in suckling mice, the complement fixation, agar gel precipitin, plaque neutralization, and enzyme linked immunosorbent assays.

Early drops of blood lymphocytes and eosinophils and rising numbers of circulating leukocytes and a marked increase in the relative percentage of neutrophils in the blood are observed along with a marked drop in blood calcium.

EPIDEMIOLOGY

The epidemiology is characterized by periodic but unpredictable massive outbreaks that occur during periods of intense insect activity and cease at frost in temperate zones. Sporadic individual cases are not always recognized.

Although the details need elaboration, it appears that BEF maintains a state of endemicity with sporadic individual cases where suitable ecosystems exist. Periodically, after development of susceptible populations, the infection overflows during weather conditions supporting arthropod activity. It may be carried by wind-borne insect vectors (Murray 1970; Shirakawa et al. 1994) and spreads rapidly in areas where it has been absent for years. If arthropod activity is ideal, widespread infection produces a partially immune population, which, in the absence of wildlife reservoirs or appropriate vectors, eventually reverts to a total susceptibility to await the next epidemic.

In the naturally occurring disease the onset is sudden and the incubation period appears short. This phenomenon cannot be verified, however, because the bites of vectors are rarely observed. Experimental infection by intravenous inoculation of infective blood has produced signs between 2 and 4 days and rarely up to 9 days post inoculation.

BEFV infects cattle of all ages and breeds and both sexes.

Cattle are probably not the natural reservoir of BEFV because most bovine infections are followed by prompt immune responses that leave recovered animals free of persistent infection. Mosquitoes feed by direct penetration of vessels and appear to be the most efficient vectors (St. George 1993). They are probably the usual source of infection and the natural reservoir. Wind-borne insect vector migrations may explain some outbreaks (Shirakawa et al. 1994). BEFV has also been isolated from numerous midges of the genus *Culicoides*. The role (if any) of wildlife as perpetuating or amplifying hosts needs further exploration because when serosurveys are done, numerous wild ruminants and cervids have antibody.

IMMUNITY

Following natural infection, neutralizing antibody and protective immunity persists for several years and probably for the lifetime of most cattle. Immune cattle transfer immunity to calves that suckle colostrum on the day of birth, and the passive immunity so conferred appears to protect from clinical exposure but does not confer a lifelong immunity.

VIRUS PERSISTENCE

There is little clinical, epidemiological, or virological evidence of persistent or latent BEF virus infections in cattle.

PREVENTION AND CONTROL

Control by vector management will probably not be feasible unless future information reveals a specific vector involvement in given areas.

Attenuated live virus and subunit vaccines have been used in Japan, South Africa, and Australia (Inaba et al. 1974; St. George 1998). Vaccine studies are being continued.

THERAPY AND MANAGEMENT OF OUTBREAKS

Recovery is usually spontaneous. For serious cases, good nursing care and provision of shade and water are indicated. Oral feeding and medication administered by mouth is contraindicated because of the danger of inhalation pneumonia. In lame and recumbent animals, prompt recovery frequently follows intravenous administration of calcium gluconate.

Unlike many viral diseases, BEF cases seem to respond to early administration of antiinflammatory agents such as phenylbutazone and ketoprofen (Fenwick and Daniel 1996; St. George 1997).

LIKELIHOOD OF ERADICATION

Eradication efforts will probably not be undertaken until all wildlife reservoirs and competent vectors are identified and cost-benefit analyses indicate such efforts could be economically productive.

IMPACT ON INTERNATIONAL TRADE

BEF is not categorized as a List A or List B disease by the Office International Des Epizooties (OIE), but major outbreaks are usually reported. Importing countries often impose test or quarantine measures on live cattle from affected regions.

PUBLIC RESPONSIBILITY

When BEF is suspected in free regions, regulatory authorities should be contacted.

AREAS IN NEED OF RESEARCH

Further study is needed on the possible role of wildlife reservoirs and the mechanisms of survival in insect populations.

REFERENCES

Combs GP, 1978. Bovine ephemeral fever. *Proc. U.S. Anim. Health Assoc.* 82:29–35.

Fenwick DC, Daniel RCW, 1996. Evaluation of the effect of ketoprofen on experimentally induced ephemeral fever in dairy heifers. *Aust. Vet. J.* 74:37–41.

Inaba Y, Kurogi H, Takahashi A, Sato K, Omori T, Goto Y, Hanaki T, Yamamoto M, Kiski S, Kodama K, Harada K, Matumoto M, 1974. Vaccination of cattle against bovine ephemeral fever with live attenuated virus followed by killed virus. *Arch. Gesamte. Virusforsch* 44:121–132.

Murray MD, 1970. The spread of ephemeral fever of cattle during the 1967–1968 epizootic in Australia. *Aust. Vet. J.* 46:77–82.

Parsonson IM, Snowdon WA, 1974a. Ephemeral fever virus: Excretion in the semen of infected bulls and attempts to infect female cattle by the intrauterine inoculation of virus. *Aust. Vet. J.* 50:329–334.

Parsonson IM, Snowdon WA, 1974b. Experimental infection of pregnant cattle with ephemeral fever virus. *Aust. Vet. J.* 50:335–337.

Shirakawa H, Ishibashi K, Ogawa T, 1994. A comparison of the epidemiology of ephemeral fever in Japan and Korea. *Aust. Vet. J.* 71:50–52.

St. George TD, 1993. The natural history of bovine ephemeral fever. In *Bovine Ephemeral Fever Virus and Related Rhabdoviuses,* edited by TD St. George, MF Uren, PL Young, D Hoffman. Proceedings of the 1st International Symposium Held in Beijing, PRC, 25–27 August 1992. Canberra: Australian Centre for International Agricultural Research, pp. 13–19.

St. George TD, 1994. Bovine ephemeral fever. In *Infectious Diseases of Livestock With Special Reference to Southern Africa,* edited by JAW Coetzer, GR Thomson, RC Tustin. Capetown: Oxford University Press, pp. 404–415.

St. George TD, 1997. Effective treatment of bovine ephemeral fever. *Aust. Vet. J.* 75:221–223.

St. George TD, 1998. Bovine ephemeral fever. In *Foreign Animal Diseases,* edited by WW Buisch, JL Hyde, CL Mebus. Richmond: U.S. Animal Health Assoc. pp. 118–128.

St. George TD, 1990. Bovine ephemeral fever virus. In *Infectious Diseases of Ruminants,* edited by Z Dinter, B Morein. Amsterdam: Elsevier Scientific Publishers, pp. 405–415.

St. George TD, Uren MF, Young PL, Hoffman D (eds.), 1993. Bovine ephemeral fever virus and related Rhabdoviruses. *Proceedings of the 1st International Symposium Held in Beijing,* PRC, 25–27 August 1992. Canberra: Australian Centre for Intentional Agricultural Research.

32

FOOT-AND-MOUTH DISEASE

INTRODUCTION

Foot-and-mouth disease (FMD) (aftosa or aphthous fever), which affects all cloven-hoofed animals, is the most dreaded of cattle diseases. It is endemic in parts of South America, Africa, Asia, and Europe where it causes periodic losses through debility associated with formation of vesicles on the mouth, feet, and teats. Even greater losses can result from refusal of FMD-free countries to import livestock and livestock products from infected regions.

The clinical signs and lesions are similar to those of vesicular stomatitis (VS) and to a much lesser extent the other diseases affecting the bovine mucosa (DABM). Laboratory tests are required to identify the FMD virus (FMDV) and to distinguish among seven serotypes (each with multiple subtypes).

Spread occurs rapidly among susceptible cattle, and FMD is difficult to eliminate or control once established in an area, particularly if wild ruminants or feral swine become infected.

In endemic areas, FMD is partially controlled by vaccination. In FMD-free areas it is eradicated by slaughtering infected and exposed animals.

FMD has been reviewed by Mann and Sellers (1990), Thomson (1994), House and Mebus (1998) and Murphy et al. (1999).

ETIOLOGY

FMDV is a member of the genus *Apthovirus* in the family Picornaviridae. There are seven immunologically distinct types identifiable by a variety of procedures and requiring separate vaccines. The serotypes are designated A; 0; C; South African Territories (SAT) 1, 2, and 3; and Asia-1. Within these types are over 60 subtypes with differing nucleic acid and oligonucleotide sequences in their genomes.

FMDV subtypes overlap antigenically but can be distinguished by complement fixation (CF), immunodiffusion, neutralization and enzyme-linked immunosorbent assay (ELISA) tests. Some subtypes, such as that causing the 1997 swine specific outbreak on Taiwan, exhibit strict species preferences and will infect some species but not others. New subtypes occasionally arise spontaneously.

FMDV replicates and induces cytopathic changes in a variety of cell cultures, which yield large quantities of virus for use in research or vaccine production.

FMDV is exceedingly resistant to environmental influences. It will survive drying, can be carried on inanimate objects, and survives for prolonged periods in chilled and frozen meat (particularly lymph nodes and bone marrow) and in other animal products.

Many common disinfectants are ineffective against FMDV. While stable around neutrality (pH 7–9) it is inactivated by alkalis and acids including the lactic acid produced in muscles during rigor mortis and in meat after slaughter.

CLINICAL SIGNS AND LESIONS

Most cloven-hoofed animals can be infected, but sheep and goats experience less severe clinical signs than cattle and swine. These species may be infected for long periods before FMD is suspected.

FMD is clinically indistinguishable from VS. The signs, attributable to viral replication at sites of predilection and resultant vesicle formation, are preceded by a viremic stage characterized by fever, depression, anorexia, listlessness, and occasional shivering. As vesicle formation starts, excess salivation and nasal discharge are evident, and cattle may exhibit lip smacking, a classic early sign. Lameness, nasal discharge, drooling, and anorexia become more obvious as the vesicles mature and rupture.

The clinically visible lesions are rapidly rupturing vesicles filled with clear, straw-colored fluid. They vary in size from 0.5 to 10 cm in diameter and appear in areas where there is pressure, irritation, or friction on skin or mucosal surfaces—the interdigital spaces, heels, coronary band, teats, oral mucosa, nostrils and rumen pillars.

When first observed, the vesicles may have already ruptured, leaving erosions or ulcerations. When several animals are examined, however, it becomes apparent that the lesions begin as small blanched areas of epithelium that rapidly fill with fluid and promptly rupture. The epithelium soon separates and sloughs, leaving raw ulcers or erosions and tags of epithelial tissue. These heal rapidly, leaving a discolored area that fades until healing is complete. Eventually all traces are gone.

Death is uncommon except in neonatal calves. Many cattle are slaughtered, however, to prevent spread of the disease.

The debility that occurs during prolonged convalescence causes marked weight loss and decreased meat and milk production. Anorexia may be prolonged if the mouth lesions are extensive and painful. Lameness is common, and standing animals frequently kick their feet or shift their weight from foot to foot. Secondary bacterial infection of the hoof frequently occurs, and arthritis or abnormal hoof growth occasionally results.

Painful teat lesions in lactating cows may cause cows to refuse to be milked or to prevent calves from nursing. Mastitis of primary viral or secondary bacterial origin is a common sequel.

EFFECTS ON THE DEVELOPING FETUS

Abortion may occur during the acute stages of FMD or during convalescence. Calves nursing viremic dams can be infected and experience high fatality rates.

NECROPSY FINDINGS

Vesicular lesions appear in areas where there is pressure from walking (coronary band and interdigital spaces), chewing (oral mucosa), or digestive movements (rumen pillars).

In young cattle there may be a striped myocardial lesion called "tiger heart" resulting from degeneration and necrosis of cardiac muscle fibers. Similar lesions may be found in skeletal muscle.

Histologically, the vesicles of FMD are characterized by ballooning, cellular degeneration, intracellular and extracellular edema, and separation of superficial layers from basal epithelium (stratum germinativum), the sparing of which permits rapid healing. There is frequently hemorrhage or cellular infiltration of subcutaneous or submucosal tissues. No inclusion bodies are associated with FMD. The histopathologic picture is not sufficiently different from that of VS to be of diagnostic value.

Muscle lesions are characterized by necrosis or Zenker's degeneration of muscle fibers.

DIAGNOSIS

FMD should be considered whenever salivation and lameness occur simultaneously in cattle and vesicular lesions are seen or suspected. Laboratory tests are needed to differentiate FMD from VS. Precaution is advised about using the presence of vesicular lesions in horses (which are resistant to FMDV but not to VSV) as a differential feature, because FMD and VS can occur simultaneously.

In areas free of FMD, all suspected vesicular diseases must be promptly reported to subnational and national officials and investigated in depth. Efforts must be made to determine the source of infection and conduct appropriate laboratory tests.

In North America, specially trained foreign animal disease diagnosticians are available on short notice. They can collect proper diagnostic samples and send them to national laboratories for testing.

It is anticipated that rapid spread and high clinical attack rates will occur upon introduction of FMD into free areas. Relatively avirulent strains could appear, however, and the magnitude of clinical signs can vary.

Diagnosis of the vesicular diseases based on the differential susceptibilities of horses, cattle, and swine was formerly a standard procedure. Swine and cattle (but not horses) will develop lesions when inoculated with vesicular materials from animals with FMD. All three species should respond to inoculation with materials from VS cases. Animal inoculation is sometimes still done but more rapid laboratory tests are commonly used.

FMD should be suspected when typical signs and lesions occur. However, a specific etiologic diagnosis cannot be accomplished solely on clinical or epidemiologic observations.

Differential Diagnosis

Vesicular stomatitis has clinical signs and lesions identical to those of FMD. FMD must be considered, however, in the differential diagnosis of all cases of lameness, mucosal erosions, salivation, nasal discharge, and teat lesions.

Bovine viral diarrhea, rinderpest, malignant catarrhal fever, bluetongue, and papular stomatitis can be initially confused with FMD. FMD could be misdiagnosed as a respiratory disease if examination of oral mucosa is neglected. It could be mistaken for foot rot if the feet of lame cattle are not carefully examined. The teat lesions could be confused with poxvirus infections or bovine herpes mammillitis.

Laboratory Diagnosis

Laboratories undertaking differential diagnosis of vesicular diseases must have high-level biosecurity ratings and batteries of specific antiserums or monoclonal antibodies for identifying virus isolates. Laboratory procedures for FMD are detailed in the Office International Des Epizooties (OIE) *Manual of Standards for Diagnostic Tests and Vaccines* (OIE 2000).

If adequate virus is present and reagents are available, complement fixation (CF) or other tests can determine which (if any) FMDV serotype is present in vesicular tissues or fluids from suspect cattle. Once the presence of FMDV is determined, further CF or ELISA testing sequencing can determine the subtype.

Specimens are usually inoculated into cell cultures or experimental animals (or both) to ensure production of adequate virus stocks for subsequent testing.

Computerized sequence analysis of viral proteins after amplification by polymerase chain reactions (PCR) can determine the serotype but subtyping by this procedure requires further development (Stram et al. 1995)

Neutralization, gel diffusion, CF, or fluorescent antibody tests on cattle serums are of diagnostic value in FMD-free areas. In endemic areas, however, serologic reactions may result from vaccination or previous infection. Serologic tests are used to screen cattle intended for import into free areas.

A rapid non-type-specific virus infection associated antigen (VIAA) test is used for epidemiologic screening by some countries to detect serum antibodies resulting from infection or vaccination (OIE 2000).

Countries requiring laboratory support may consult the OIE for referral to designated reference laboratories and reference experts.

When possible, vesicular fluid is harvested from animals suspected of having FMD because it contains high quantities of virus. In addition, epithelium from early vesicles and epithelial tags from ruptured vesicles are useful specimens. There is a short-lived viremia, but unclotted blood from early cases can sometimes be a source of virus. Specimens from suspected FMD cases should be collected, packaged, and shipped in a manner to avoid spreading the disease and according to instructions from laboratories and regulatory authorities.

Esophageal–pharyngeal fluid is a useful specimen for virus isolation from acute, convalescent, or recovered animals. The esophageal–pharyngeal fluid is a mixture of saliva, postnasal drippings, and desquamated esophageal epithelium that is harvested with a probang, a metal cup attached to a flexible rod. This device, once used for collection of sputum samples for tuberculosis diagnosis, is passed down the esophagus, and the specimen is collected by gentle massage. Testing esophageal–pharyngeal fluid for FMDV or viral nucleic acid is used to detect carrier animals proposed for export.

FMDV can be isolated from lymph nodes, kidney, adrenal glands, heart, thyroid, or other tissues collected at necropsy. Specimens for virus isolation may be frozen for shipment to the laboratory. If dry ice is used, the specimen must be tightly sealed to prevent FMDV inactivation by lowered pH.

Live animals from which specimens are collected should be bled for serologic tests; when possible, another blood sample should be collected 3 weeks later for comparison.

EPIDEMIOLOGY

Epidemiologic discussions of FMD focus on its geographic distribution, high transmissibility, multiplicity of susceptible species and virus types and subtypes, and its refractoriness to control once established in an area.

While there is progress toward global eradication and control of FMD, there are areas of the world in which one or more FMDV types are still endemic. They include parts of South America (A, O, and C), Asia (Asia-1), Africa (SAT 1, 2, and 3), and portions of Europe.

Australia, New Zealand, Japan, many Pacific islands, the British Isles and most of Western Europe, and all of North and Central America are currently free of FMD.

Countries contiguous to infected areas or which regularly import animals or animal products from infected regions are at high risk and experience occasional costly FMD introductions.

Incubation periods can vary from 12 hours to 14 days but are usually 2 to 8 days.

The reservoir is cloven-hoofed animals. In Africa, Cape buffalo can be inapparently infected carriers presenting a reservoir that renders eradication unlikely (Thomson 1994).

The usual source of infection is actively infected cattle or swine. Contaminated bedding, feed, water, milk, equipment, or motor vehicles can carry FMDV. Meat or meat scraps from infected animals are common sources of infection for swine, which can subsequently transmit FMD to cattle by direct or indirect contact. Under certain circumstances, any product of animal origin including milk, meat, cheese, serum, hormones, or vaccines can serve as a vehicle for transmission to cattle.

Virus usually enters through the respiratory tract. Transmission can occur by direct or indirect contact with infected animals or their secretions, excretions, or tissues. Spread is rapid because infected animals shed large quantities of virus before clinical disease is evident.

Aerosol transmission occurs and wind-borne spread probably contributed to several European outbreaks (Mann and Sellers 1990). Aerosols exhausted by milk tankers moving from farm to farm have spread FMD.

FMDV infects semen, and transmission via artificial insemination is a potential hazard.

In susceptible populations, all ages and breeds and both sexes of cattle can become infected and develop clinical signs. Fatality rates are higher in calves than in adults.

IMMUNITY

Immunity to FMDV is type and subtype specific and of limited duration. Natural infection or vaccination affords partial rather than absolute protection from infection; subsequent clinical disease, although often mild, can occur. Calves being nursed by immune cattle acquire antibody that affords partial protection for up to 5 months.

Cattle recovered from infection with one serotype are usually susceptible to infection with others and can develop full-blown disease.

VIRUS PERSISTENCE

Following infection, surviving cattle generally clear virus from most tissues and organs within 2 weeks. However, a chronic infection of uncertain epidemiological significance may persist in the posterior pharyngeal area, with low levels of virus detectable for more than 2 years. These persistently infected cattle have not been shown to transmit FMD but their potential infectivity worries disease control officials.

When cattle are slaughtered during the active infection, virus may persist for several years in frozen tissues, particularly lymph nodes and bone marrow. Processed hides and tissues can also carry virus. All products from FMDV-affected areas must be regarded as potential sources of infection. Trade must be restricted to heat-processed products, carefully boned and lymphoid-tissue-depleted cured meats, or carefully tested and quarantined animals or germ plasm.

PREVENTION AND CONTROL

The prevention and control of FMD are based on excluding the virus from FMD-free areas. Virus exclusion requires strict import measures including processing, testing, and quarantine requirements; contingency plans involving diagnostic capacity, vaccine banks, test and slaughter and carcass disposal procedures; and preauthorized regionalization and quarantine authorities.

In endemic areas, vaccination is the basis of most control efforts. Vaccination reduces local disease losses but does not compensate for lost market access, which usually represents the greatest economic losses to the cattle industries of FMD-infected countries.

The easy transmission of FMDV requires total exclusion of animals and untreated animal products to protect FMD-free areas and causes a variety of barriers to trade.

Vaccines must be type and subtype specific. Many countries utilize trivalent inactivated vaccines against endemic serotypes. Vaccine-induced immunity is short-lived, and vaccination must be repeated 2–3 times annually. However, annual vaccination appears to be effective when highly potent vaccines are administered to 75% to 80% of cattle in an area. FMDV for vaccine production is propagated in bovine tongue epithelial tissues collected at slaughterhouses (Frenkle method) or in cell cultures.

FMD-free countries avoid vaccination and prefer the stamping out technique, because vaccination involves an endless outlay of resources. Vaccination also provides herd immunity that can mask clinical signs, permitting widespread dissemination before infection is recognized. Additionally vaccination limits the efficiency of serologic surveillance. Also, vaccination is discouraged because outbreaks have been traced to escape of FMDV from vaccine-production facilities and occasional failure of older inactivators like formalin have initiated vaccine-induced outbreaks.

Research projects are under way to develop improved products including subunit vaccines. These involve studies on new adjuvants, preservatives and viral inactivators. Efforts to develop safe modified live-virus vaccines have largely been unsuccessful.

THERAPY AND MANAGEMENT OF OUTBREAKS

In areas where FMD is endemic, local control or eradication efforts involve virus typing and vaccination or revaccination of local cattle against appropriate subtypes. When the presence of the disease is accepted, individual cases are treated symptomatically, and antibiotics may be given to limit secondary infections. Adequate food, water, and shade along with good nursing care are required.

In FMD-free areas, the slightest suspicion of FMD must be reported to regulatory officials. Immediately upon diagnosis, the so-called "stamping out method" is invoked. This method consists of immediate quarantine of all infected, exposed, and high-risk premises (usually involving area quarantines that restrict movement of animals, people, or vehicles). It also calls for depopulation of infected and exposed cloven-hoofed animals, disinfection of infected premises, and a period of 30 days or more, during which time no animals are permitted on the premises. This procedure is followed by a trial repopulation and eventual restocking. Thorough epidemiologic investigation is instituted to determine the immediate source of infection. Educational programs are undertaken along with strict controls on the movement of people, livestock, vehicles, and commercial or private undertakings that could expedite spread from the quarantined area.

If widespread infection occurs and the stamping out method becomes impossible to implement or if economic realities or public pressures force officials to cease eradication efforts, the affected area faces the possibility of permanent endemic status with all the economic and social disadvantages that status implies. The timing of any decision to abandon eradication and initiate vaccination is based on many factors. Ring vaccination around depopulated and infected areas can be used to limit spread until later efforts can narrow infected areas to a dimension permitting logistically feasible eradication approaches.

LIKELIHOOD OF ERADICATION

FMD has been successfully eradicated from Great Britain and parts of Western Europe, the United States, Canada, and Mexico by the stamping out method, which is feasible in newly infected areas only if prompt action is taken (Kitching 1990).

Once FMD is ensconced in an area, eradication requires monumental efforts and slaughter of entire populations including wildlife reservoirs. Eradication programs in endemic areas must be preceded by careful study of the logistic, environmental, and economic feasibility of the project. If resources and infrastructure are available and domestic industry and neighboring countries are cooperative, the long-range economic benefits of FMD eradication are considerable.

Experience in South America and elsewhere indicates that progress from programs based on governmental partnerships with producers and industry groups is greater than when regulatory authorities adopt govern-and-command tactics.

Eradication by developing countries seems unlikely especially in Africa where wildlife reservoirs exist. South Africa has used extensive testing, surveillance, and control of wildlife movements by fencing to eradicate FMD from the entire country, except in the Kruger National Wildlife Preserve.

IMPACT ON INTERNATIONAL TRADE

FMD is categorized as an OIE List A disease. Cattle and related products from infected regions are excluded from major world markets or subjected to stringent risk-reduction measures such as special processing, quarantines, and testing.

Many FMD-free countries have protected themselves from a variety of diseases by restricting commerce in most bovine and porcine commodities from FMD-infected regions. As eradication efforts succeed, more specific disease-by-disease measures must be designed to replace these blanket measures.

PUBLIC RESPONSIBILITY

The greatest public responsibility regarding FMD involves the obligation to report suspected cases and comply with regulatory decisions.

In rare cases, humans become infected in laboratories or slaughterhouses, on farms, or by drinking infected milk. Human FMD is usually characterized by inapparent infection accompanied by brief periods during which the infected person may serve as the immediate source of infection for livestock. Rarely, humans develop sore throats, headaches, and vesicles on the hands, feet, and oral mucosa. So-called epidemic hand-foot-and-mouth disease of humans is a Coxsackievirus infection and is not caused by FMDV.

AREAS IN NEED OF RESEARCH

FMD is of such international importance that ongoing research is required on almost all aspects of the disease until technologies evolve to make world eradication a feasible goal.

There is continued need for improved diagnostic procedures, epidemiologic surveillance strategies, improved vaccines, and environmentally sound carcass-disposal methods.

REFERENCES

House J, Mebus CM, 1998. Foot and mouth disease. In *Foreign Animal Diseases,* edited by WW Buisch, JL Hyde, CL Mebus. Richmond: U.S. Animal Health Assoc., pp. 213–224.

Kitching RP, 1990. A recent history of foot and mouth disease. *J Comp Pathol* 118: 89–108.

Mann JA, Sellers RF, 1990. Foot and mouth disease. In *Infectious Diseases of Ruminants,* edited by Z Dinter, B Morein. Amsterdam: Elsevier Scientific Publishers. pp. 503–512.

Murphy FA, Gibbs EPJ, Horzinek MC, Studdert MJ, 1999. Foot and mouth disease. In *Veterinary Virology*. 3rd ed. San Diego: Academic Press, pp. 521–528.

OIE, 2000. Foot-and-mouth disease. In *OIE Manual of Standards for Diagnosic Tests and Vaccines*. Paris: Office International Des Epizooties.

Stram Y, Molad T, Chai D, Gelman B, Yadin H, 1995. Detection and sub typing of foot-and-mouth disease virus in infected cattle by polymerase chain reaction and amplified VP1 sequencing. *J. Vet. Diag. Invest.* 7:52–55.

Thomson GR, 1994. Foot and mouth disease. In *Infectious Diseases of Livestock With Special Reference to Southern Africa*, edited by JAW Coetzer, GR Thomson, RC Tustin. Capetown: Oxford University Press, pp. 825–852.

33

LUMPY SKIN DISEASE

INTRODUCTION

Lumpy skin disease (LSD) a poxvirus infection also called pseudo-urticaria, exanthema nodularis bovis, knopvelsickte, and Neethling virus disease, occurs in much of Africa, Kuwait, and Egypt and is unreported or believed to be exotic elsewhere.

It is characterized by nodular cutaneous eruptions accompanied by lymphadenitis, edema of the legs or brisket, and sometimes respiratory involvement and abortion.

There is confusion in some early accounts of LSD because for years it was confused with pseudo lumpy skin disease (PLSD), which is caused by bovine herpesvirus-2 (BHV-2) also the cause of bovine herpes mammillitis (BHM). LSD and PLSD can be distinguished histopathologically and virologically.

LSD is not highly fatal but is economically important because of its prolonged debilitating effects, its association with infertility and abortion, and the damage it causes to hides. In LSD-free areas it is regarded as a serious exotic disease.

LSD has been reviewed by Woods (1990), Davies (1991), Barnard et al. (1994), and House (1989 and 1998).

ETIOLOGY

The lumpy skin disease virus (LSDV), also called the Neethling virus, is a large DNA virus classified in the genus *Capripoxvirus* in the family Poxviridae. It is closely related to the sheep pox and goat pox viruses, from which it may have arisen by transspecies adaptation. The three viruses have immunological similarities and sometimes cross-protect against one another and cross-neutralize in serologic tests. They are, however, distinct in finer genetic and antigenic detail.

LSDV grows in a variety of cell cultures, producing cytopathic changes and intracytoplasmic inclusion bodies. It is relatively resistant to physical and chemical agents and can survive in dried scabs for prolonged periods.

Impala, onyx, and giraffes are susceptible to experimental infection but don't appear significant as reservoirs for cattle.

CLINICAL SIGNS AND LESIONS

LSD can be an acute disease, but more commonly it is subacute and evolves into a chronic debilitating condition. While mainly a dermatitis characterized by nodules that develop into cutaneous ulcers, it can have systemic manifestations including fever, nasal discharge, pneumonia, reduced milk production, abortion, and mastitis secondary to teat lesions. It is usually accompanied by swollen lymph nodes and edema of dependent areas, particularly the legs, dewlap, and brisket.

The onset may be acute, characterized by fever (104–107° F), anorexia, excess lacrimation, and nasal discharge that is initially serous or mucoid and later becomes mucopurulent. Enlargement of superficial lymph nodes is common.

The nodular skin lesions are sometimes visible from a distance as erect tufts of hair and may cover the entire body. More often, they are confined to the skin of the head, legs, and lower body. They involve all layers of the skin and frequently penetrate to the subcutaneous tissues.

In naturally occurring cases, the lesions vary in diameter from 0.5 to 5 cm, but in cattle experimentally infected by intradermal inoculation, the lesions may be 2 to 3 times that size. The cutaneous nodules may ooze serum and ulcerate, leaving necrotic open sores. Frequently there is minimal ulceration, merely a dry scab that persists for several weeks before falling off. Some nodular lesions become hard and persist for years as knots in the skin.

Yellowish white nodular lesions may be present in the visible portions of the nasal and oral mucosa. They slough, leaving mucosal erosions and ulcers that may cause difficulty in eating or breathing. Clinical cases are frequently complicated by diarrhea.

Except in unusual situations, the case fatality rarely exceeds 2% to 3%.

EFFECTS ON THE DEVELOPING FETUS AND REPRODUCTION

Pregnant cows affected with LSD may abort and infected cows may experience temporary infertility. Bulls may become temporarily or permanently infertile.

NECROPSY FINDINGS

In addition to skin and mucosal lesions visible in the intact animal, nodular lesions are occasionally distributed throughout internal organs and tissues, particularly pharynx, larynx, trachea, rumen, abomasum, uterine wall, and sometimes skeletal muscle or lungs. These are firm, dense masses containing exudate, which may be serous or serohemorrhagic.

Histopathologically, there is inflammatory infiltration of skin or mucosa with neutrophils, lymphocytes, mast cells, and macrophages; perivascular cuffing; and a proliferative fibroblastic reaction. This event is followed by coagulative and liquefactive necrosis and sloughing.

Eosinophilic intracytoplasmic inclusion bodies are present in some cells within lesions and on their periphery.

DIAGNOSIS

In endemic areas, the classic clinical signs (nodular dermatitis, lymphadenitis, and edema) and random spread to cattle without direct contact are usually adequate to permit diagnosis.

In LSD-free areas, a specific etiologic diagnosis is required and regulatory intervention with laboratory support is essential.

A classic LSD outbreak would include multiple cases of nodular dermatitis with lymphadenitis and edema of the legs and brisket. These lesions may be preceded by an acute, febrile episode characterized by excess nasal discharge, salivation, and lacrimation. Cases frequently occur in noncontiguous herds or areas with no known cow-to-cow contact.

Differential Diagnosis

If characteristic signs, lesions, and epidemiologic patterns appear and multiple cases are present, experienced diagnosticians can usually render a clinical diagnosis that would withstand histopathologic and virologic scrutiny. In individual or sporadic cases it may be difficult to differentiate LSD from PLSD and numerous other conditions.

PLSD, the cutaneous disease caused by bovine herpesvirus-2 (see Chapter 17) has occurred simultaneously with LSD but is relatively uncommon outside Africa. However, BHM is also caused by BHV-2, and is present in Europe and North America.

PLSD is usually milder than LSD. The lesions are more superficial, shallower, and less likely to ulcerate than those of LSD and are distinguishable from LSD lesions by their flat surface and depressed centers. They can be distinguished histopathologically by the inclusion bodies, which are intranuclear in PLSD and intracytoplasmic in LSD.

Sometimes differentiation between LSD and PLSD can be accomplished only in the laboratory. The generalization that LSD lesions penetrate deeper and are more nodular than those of PLSD, which tend to be flat with depressed centers, may be dangerous because of extreme individual variations. PLSD can have a generalized distribution and occasionally occurs on the oral mucosa, particularly in suckling calves.

PLSD lesions generally involve only the superficial skin layers. Unlike LSD lesions, which tend to indurate and persist, PLSD lesions appear to undergo necrosis and regress, leaving dried necrotic skin that cracks and sloughs and then forms hair-free areas that heal without scarring.

Cutaneous streptothrichosis, *Dermatophilus congolensis* infection, occurs worldwide but mostly in the tropics. It is a superficial cutaneous encrustation that is generally more benign than LSD but can sometimes be widely distributed over the skin areas and be debilitating. It is usually less nodular and accompanied by less necrosis than seen in LSD. The mycelia may be demonstrable in stained skin scrapings, and the causative actinomycete can be cultured from macerated lesions or encrustations.

Photosensitization usually causes nonnodular, less discrete, cutaneous necrosis and pityriasis confined to nonpigmented areas. Cattle grubs, the larvae of flies of the genus *Hypoderma,* cause nodules over the backs of cattle. These nodules can be identified by the central orifice through which the larva emerges. Insect bites usually involve less reaction and necrosis and persist for a shorter time. Demodectic mange can be diagnosed by skin scrapings.

Laboratory Diagnosis

Visualization of virions by transmission electron microscopy and histologic examinations for characteristic lesions and intracytoplasmic inclusions (see Necropsy Findings) are key to diagnosis.

The LSD virus can be isolated by inoculation of primary lamb or calf cell cultures with fluid from swollen lymph nodes or properly prepared lesions. LSDV produces cytopathic changes and intracytoplasmic inclusion bodies. Specific identification of LSDV in cultures requires immunofluorescent or immunoperoxidase staining.

Paired serums can be tested for seroconversion using serum neutralization or indirect fluorescent antibody tests in which LSDV may cross react with other poxviruses.

Frozen lesions for virus isolation and fixed lesions for standard histopathology or electron microscopy are useful for laboratory diagnosis.

EPIDEMIOLOGY

The epidemiology and details of postulated vector transmission are not completely understood.

Incubation periods vary, but usually an initial temperature rise occurs within 4 to 14 days after experimental inoculation. A local reaction follows shortly, and generalized infection occurs within another 2 days. The incubation period following natural infection probably ranges from 1 to 5 weeks.

Cattle are believed to be the natural host, reservoir, and usual source of infection for other cattle. LSDV infection can be established experimentally in goats, sheep, giraffes, and impala.

The exact mode of transmission is uncertain. Insect vectors are suspected because the disease seems to spread to herds without direct contact with affected cattle, it seems to be prevalent in insect-infested lowland areas, new cases cease shortly after killing frosts, and quarantine measures are frequently ineffective in limiting spread.

LSD virus has been isolated from flies. New infections seem to accompany cattle movements and vector migrations unaccompanied by cattle. Experimentally, LSD can be transmitted readily by intradermal inoculation.

While traditionally considered a disease of southern and eastern Africa, LSD is now established in western Africa and Egypt. Potential for spread to other regions exists.

If immune status is comparable, LSD infects all ages equally, but calves usually have more serious clinical signs. All breeds and sexes appear to be equally susceptible but thin-skinned European breeds appear to be more seriously affected than thick-skinned African breeds.

IMMUNITY

Following nursing of immune dams, calves with colostrally acquired maternal antibody are usually able to resist serious clinical signs for several months.

It is believed natural infection confers lifelong resistance in most cattle. Artificial infection with some strains of sheep poxvirus also confers resistance and has been used as a vaccination.

VIRUS PERSISTENCE

Virus persists in skin lesions for 33 days and in semen for 22 days after appearance of clinical signs. LSDV may survive in scabs on the ground for prolonged periods.

PREVENTION AND CONTROL

In general, segregation and isolation have not been regarded as successful control measures, and hygienic measures are largely ineffective because noncontact transmission occurs. Vaccination with attenuated modified live-virus vaccine and sheep and goat pox vaccines have been successfully employed in South Africa. An apparently successful recombinant capripox vaccine using rinderpest fusion protein protects against both diseases (Romero et al. 1994).

Strict testing and quarantine procedures should be undertaken before LSD-free countries import cattle or germ plasm from infected regions.

THERAPY AND MANAGEMENT OF OUTBREAKS

In endemic areas, therapy involves good nursing care, protection from sun and provision of adequate food and water, which enables cattle to recover and convalesce with minimal debility. If possible, infected cattle should be segregated. Where practical, insect control programs should be instituted.

In LSD-free areas, regulatory officials should investigate suspected cases. Laboratory methods should be employed to determine the etiology and eradication procedures should be considered. Prompt slaughter resulted in eradication after a one-time incursion into Israel (Shimshony 1989), despite rapid spread in dairy herds (Yeruham et al. 1995).

LIKELIHOOD OF ERADICATION

Although eradication was achieved after a single introduction into Israel by stamping out all affected and contact animals (Shimshoni 1989), eradication has not been accomplished in Africa.

IMPACT ON INTERNATIONAL TRADE

LSD is categorized as a List A disease by the Office International Des Epizooties (OIE). Caution is advised against unrestricted importation of live cattle from infected regions.

PUBLIC RESPONSIBILITY

In LSD-free areas, people who suspect the disease are obligated to contact regulatory authorities.

AREAS IN NEED OF RESEARCH

Research is needed to clarify the mode of transmission.

REFERENCES

Barnard BJH, Muntz E, Dumbell K, Prozesky L, 1994. Lumpy skin disease. In *Infectious Diseases of Livestock With Special Reference to Southern Africa,* edited by JAW Coetzer, GR Thomson, RC Tustin. Capetown: Oxford University Press, pp. 605–612.

Davies FG, 1991. Lumpy skin disease, an African capripox virus disease of cattle. *Br. Vet. J.* 147:489–503.

House JA, 1989. Lumpy skin disease. *Proc. U.S. Anim Health Assoc* 93:305–314.

House JA, 1998. Lumpy skin disease In *Foreign Animal Diseases,* edited by WW Buisch, JL Hyde, CL Mebus. Richmond: U.S. Animal Health Assoc. pp. 303–310.

Romero CH., Barret T, Kitching RT, Carn VM, Black DN, 1994. Protection of cattle against rinderpest and lumpy skin disease with a recombinant capripox vaccine expressing the fusion protein of rinderpest virus. *Vet. Rec.* 137:152–154.

Shimshony A, 1989. Lumpy skin disease: Israel. Report of the Committee on Foreign Animal Diseases. *Proc. U.S. Anim. Health Assoc.* 93:334–335.

Woods JA, 1990. Lumpy skin disease virus. In *Infectious Diseases of Ruminants,* edited by Z Dinter, B Morein. Amsterdam: Elsevier Scientific Publishers. pp. 53–67.

Yeruham I, Nir O, Braverman Y, Davidson M, Grinstein H, Haymovich M, Zamir O, 1995. Spread of lumpy skin disease in Israeli dairy herds. *Vet. Rec.* 137:91–93.

34

RIFT VALLEY FEVER

INTRODUCTION

Rift Valley fever (RVF) is a zoonotic mosquito-borne disease that causes devastating epidemics among sheep, goats, cattle, and humans. It is confined to Africa but has the potential for spread from that continent if viremic animals or humans are introduced into suitable ecosystems with competent vectors (House et al. 1992). Described by Daubney et al. (1931) in the Rift Valley in Kenya, RVF has expanded its range to include much of Southern, Eastern, Western, and Central Africa (Walsh 1987; Olaleye et al. 1996a).

RVF, sometimes called infectious enzootic hepatitis of sheep and cattle, is more serious in sheep than in cattle. In bovine outbreaks, losses result from abortions and an acute, highly fatal, necrotic hepatitis in calves.

Control is via mosquito abatement measures, vaccination, and avoiding human contact with infected tissues.

RVF has been reviewed by House et al. (1992), Wood et al. (1990), Swanepoel and Coetzer (1994), and Mebus (1998).

ETIOLOGY

RVF virus (RVFV) is a member of the *Phlebovirus* genus of the family Bunyaviridae, which contains many arthropod-borne viruses infecting mammals and insects. The virus has a broad host range and causes clinical or subclinical infections in ruminants, dogs, and cats (Walker et al. 1970a, b), rodents, and bats and has been isolated from numerous insects.

The RVFV is readily propagated in mice, hamsters, rabbits, and lambs, in which it produces a fatal hepatitis. It also grows in chick embryos and a variety of cell cultures (Johnson and Orlando 1968), producing variable cytopathic effects. It is relatively stable at a pH range between 7 and 8.

Strains with slightly differing amino acid or nucleotide sequences vary in pathogenicity but are immunologically similar (Swanepoel and Coetzer 1994). RVFV shows minimal potential for mutation. Wesselsbron virus is an immunologically distinct flavivirus that causes a similar disease in sheep and cattle.

CLINICAL SIGNS AND LESIONS

Although widespread epidemics involving sheep, cattle, and humans are common, individual sporadic cases undoubtedly occur in endemic areas. Abortion is usually the dominant feature of RVF in adult cattle. In addition, there is frequently an elevated temperature and a catarrhal stomatitis, with buccal erosions accompanied by excess salivation and bloody or fetid diarrhea. Lameness resulting from laminitis or coronitis may be present.

In adult cattle the case fatality rate rarely exceeds 10%. In calves RVF is a highly fatal fulminating condition characterized by sudden onset, extreme depression, collapse, and death within 24 to 48 hours.

In humans, who contact infected animals or sleep outside in mosquito-infested areas, there is sudden onset of fever, muscle aches, headache, retroorbital pain, transient loss of visual acuity, prostration, and sometimes fatal encephalitis and hemorrhagic fever (Swanepoel and Coetzer 1994).

EFFECTS ON THE DEVELOPING FETUS

Primary infection of pregnant cattle usually results in abortion.

NECROPSY FINDINGS

At necropsy, cattle dying of RVF have focal hepatic necrosis and varying degrees of hepatic congestion. Jaundice is usually absent. There may be edema, congestion, or hemorrhage of the gallbladder, as well as scattered hemorrhages throughout the body, including subcutaneous tissues and gastrointestinal mucosa. There may be excess pericardial fluid, subendocardial hemorrhage, and enlargement and hemorrhage or necrosis of the spleen. The mesenteric lymph nodes may be enlarged and moist and there may be ascites. The white focal areas in the liver contain necrotic hepatic cells and inflammatory cells.

DIAGNOSIS

RVF epidemics are generally recognized by their sudden appearance and rapid spread. Introduction into free areas involves large numbers of sick and dying animals of many species. There is sickness and abortion among sheep and goats, with mortality rates approaching 90% among lambs. Adult sheep and cattle are less seriously affected, but calves may experience high death rates.

Such outbreaks are usually accompanied by influenza, dengue, or yellow-fever-like disease in people and sometimes by involvement of dogs and cats, with high fatality among puppies. Outbreaks usually occur during the rainy season or periods of high insect activity. Clinical diagnosis is based on the epidemiologic picture, clinical signs, and extensive focal hepatic necrosis found at necropsy.

RVF is similar to Wesselsbron disease, which also affects sheep, goats, and cattle (Mushi et al. 1998). However, RVF is more common, has higher abortion and mortality rates and rarely produces icterus in neonates, a finding common in Wesselsbron disease. Confirmation of a diagnosis requires laboratory tests.

RVF is characteristically marked by simultaneous appearance of an acute febrile disease in sheep, goats, cattle (with high fatality rate in calves), and people following periods of rainfall.

Differential Diagnosis

Despite a characteristic diagnostic profile, the diagnosis of RVF in sheep is sometimes delayed because of its similarities to bluetongue, Wesselsbron disease, and enterotoxemia. In bovine epidemics, concurrent disease among sheep, goats, and humans is a diagnostic clue.

Sporadic cases, however, can easily be confused with cases of ephemeral fever and the diseases affecting bovine mucosa (DABM), especially rinderpest and foot-and-mouth disease. Because abortion is a principal manifestation, brucellosis and other causes of abortion storms must be considered. Despite the nearly pathognomonic lesions and epidemiologic pattern, laboratory tests are essential for a definitive diagnosis.

Laboratory Diagnosis

RVFV can be isolated by inoculation of chick embryos, mice, or cell cultures. Isolates can be identified serologically or by immunofluorescent techniques on sections or impressions of liver, spleen, or brain. Paired serums can be tested by neutralization, complement fixation, or hemagglutination inhibition tests.

In Africa, all classic serologic tests have been adopted to detect rising RVFV antibody titers. Except for neutralization tests, all can be done using inactivated antigens to increase laboratory safety. Detection of early antibody by ELISA technique permits diagnosis using a single serum sample.

Frequently, susceptible lambs are inoculated with materials from suspected cases; development of characteristic lesions aids in diagnosis. Unless laboratories have experienced personnel and appropriate reagents, the diagnosis may be delayed. In the United States, the National Veterinary Services Laboratories high security Foreign Animal Disease Diagnostic Laboratory at Plum Island, New York has diagnostic capability.

Early leukopenia followed by leukocytosis and altered liver enzymes occur, but these are rarely used for diagnostic purposes because the clinical, epidemiologic, and pathologic features are distinctive.

Blood for serology and liver, spleen, kidney, or lymph nodes for virus isolation are the specimens of choice. If possible, entire animals can be submitted for necropsy to permit diagnosticians to harvest specimens most suited to available laboratory procedures.

EPIDEMIOLOGY

The salient epizootiologic features of RVF are widespread geographic distribution in sub-Saharan Africa (with absence elsewhere) and serological evidence of extensive undiagnosed infections in humans and high levels of interepidemic immunity in livestock (Olalaye et al. 1996a, b). Also important are interepidemic maintenance in specific forest and grassland ecosystems, and appearance in devastating mosquito-borne epizootics associated with vector population surges during times of excess rainfall at 4-to-15-year intervals. Subsequent contact transmission to humans working with infected animals and their tissues and abrupt cessation of new cases with the onset of killing frost are other significant factors.

Ecosystems suitable for virus amplification may exist outside Africa.

The incubation period ranges from several hours to several days.

Many species are susceptible to RVFV. At times it has been suggested that dogs, monkeys, rodents, or various forest mammals (or birds) may support sylvatic mammal-insect-mammal cycles in Africa.

The immediate source of infection is usually mosquitoes or other insects. Most varieties of mosquitoes can transmit RVFV. Mosquito larvae feeding on infected tissues, aborted fetuses, or in virus-contaminated water can mature into infective adults (Turell et al. 1990) and may serve as maintenance vectors. A small percentage of transovarian transmission occurring in mosquitoes and virus acquisition by mosquito larvae (which survive for long periods between rainfalls) may explain interepidemic virus survival.

From all indications, RVF is largely mosquito transmitted and RVFV has been isolated from numerous mosquitoes in Africa. Members of the *Culex* species appear to be the principal vectors (House et al. 1992). Biological transmission by mosquitoes and possibly some mechanical transmission by biting flies and midges appear to be major modes of transmission. RVFV has been recovered from ticks, but they are probably unimportant as vectors.

Evidence indicates that spread to humans by contact with meat or tissues of infected animals also occurs. Experimentally it can be transmitted by aerosol means, and non-arthropod contact transmission in nature may be significant. Compared to ruminants, humans are probably not a significant source of infection for mammals or for mosquitoes.

Although cattle of all ages, sexes, and breeds become readily infected during outbreaks, the disease is more severe and the fatality greater in calves than in adult cattle. In the field, fatality rates among calves may range from 10% to 100%. A 70% death rate among experimentally infected calves has been reported.

IMMUNITY

All evidence suggests that a relatively solid and potentially lifelong immunity follows recovery from natural infection (Wilson 1994) or successful vaccination. The duration of immunity resulting from natural infection is probably at least 2 to 3 years. Colostral transfer of maternal antibody affords passive immunity to calves that nurse immune dams during the first day of life.

VIRUS PERSISTENCE

The possibility of persistent RVFV infection needs exploration.

PREVENTION AND CONTROL

The usual control procedures applicable to mosquito-borne viral infections, such as spraying, use of screened buildings, movement of susceptible cattle to higher ground where mosquito activity is less likely, and other mosquito control procedures, must be invoked early in epizootics. These measures are frequently ineffective because of the sudden onset and rapid spread.

Preexposure vaccination is the preferred control measure (Morrill et al. 1997a, b). It is, however, difficult to persuade owners to vaccinate during prolonged interepidemic periods (Swanepoel and Coetzer 1994). Vaccination with both inactivated and modified live (abortigenic) vaccines is practiced in Africa. An inactivated vaccine produced in monkey kidney cell cultures is sometimes used in humans. A mutagen-attenuated vaccine developed for human use, tested successfully in cattle appears non-abortigenic and would likely be used if RVF became established in the United States (Morrill et al. 1997a, b).

LIKELIHOOD OF ERADICATION

Until the natural host reservoir and the details of interepidemic survival are understood, there is little likelihood of successful eradication from any sizable area in which RVF becomes established.

IMPACT ON INTERNATIONAL TRADE

RVF is categorized as a List A disease by the Office International Des Epizooties (OIE). The OIE International Animal Health Code considers countries RVF-free if RVF is compulsorily reportable and they have had neither clinical signs nor have imported animals from RVF-infected countries for 3 years. Because of the risk of introduction and establishment of RVF (House et al. 1992), non-African countries impose a variety of RVF-based import measures on live ruminants and animal products from infected areas.

PUBLIC RESPONSIBILITY

People diagnosing RVF in Africa are obligated to alert livestock owners to initiate vaccination and mosquito control measures, and issue alerts that contact with sick and dying animals (particularly their tissues) invariably causes human infection. People suspecting RVF in free areas should contact regulatory officials.

AREAS IN NEED OF RESEARCH

Major research efforts are needed to determine the natural host reservoir and the method by which the disease is perpetuated in nature.

REFERENCES

Daubney R, Hudson JR, Carnham PC, 1931. Enzootic hepatitis or Rift Valley fever: An undescribed virus disease of sheep, cattle and man in East Africa. *J. Pathol. Bacteriol.* 34:545–579.

Johnson RW, Orlando MD, 1968. Growth of Rift Valley fever virus in tissue culture. *Am. J. Vet. Res.* 29:463–471,

House JA, Turell MJ, Mebus CA, 1992. Rift Valley fever: present status and risk to the western hemisphere. *Ann. N.Y. Acad. Sci.* 653: 233–242.

Mebus CA 1998. Rift Valley fever. In *Foreign Animal Diseases,* edited by WW Buisch, JL Hyde, and CL Mebus. Richmond: U.S. Animal Health Assoc. pp. 353–361.

Morrill JC, Mebus CA, Peters CJ,1997a. Safety and efficacy of a mutagen-attenuated Rift Valley fever vaccine in cattle. *Am. J. Vet. Res.* 58:1104–1109.

Morrill JC, Mebus CA, Peters CJ, 1997b. Safety of a mutagen-attenuated Rift Valley fever vaccine in fetal and neonatal bovids *Am. J. Vet. Res.* 58:1110–1114.

Mushi, EZ, Binta MG, Raborokgwe M, 1998. Wesselsbron disease virus associated with abortions in goats in Botswana. *J. Vet. Diagn. Invest.* 10:191.

Olaleye OD, Tomori O, Ladipo MA, Schmitz H, 1996a. Rift Valley fever in Nigeria: infections in humans. *Rev. Sci. Tech. Off. Int. Epiz.* 15:923–935

Olaleye OD, Tomori O, Schmitz H, 1996b. Rift Valley fever in Nigeria: infections in domestic animals. *Rev. Sci. Tech. Off. Int. Epiz.* 15:937–946.

Swanepoel R, and Coetzer JAW, 1994. Rift Valley fever. In *Infectious Diseases of Livestock With Special Reference to Southern Africa,* edited by JAW Coetzer et al. Capetown: Oxford University Press, pp. 688–717.

Turell MJ, Linthicum KJ, Beaman JR, 1990. Transmission of Rift Valley fever virus by adult mosquitoes after ingestion of virus as larvae. *Am. J. Trop. Med. Hyg.* 43:677–680.

Walker JS, Renitnele NS, Carter RC, Mtten JQ, Schu LG, Stephen EL, Klein F, 1970a. The clinical aspects of Rift Valley fever virus in household pets. I. Susceptibility of the dog. *J. Infect. Dis.* 21:9–18.

Walker JS, Renitnele NS, Carter RC, Mtten JQ, Schu LG, Stephen EL, Klein F, 1970b. The clinical aspects of Rift Valley fever virus in household pets. II. Susceptibility of the cat. *J. Infect. Dis.* 21:19–24.

Walsh J, 1987. Rift Valley fever rears its head. *Scienc*e 24:1397–1399.

Wilson ML, 1994. Rift Valley fever virus ecology and epidemiology of disease emergence. *Ann. N.Y. Acad. Sci.* 740:169–180.

Wood OL, Meegan JC, Morrill JHC, Stephenson EH, 1990. Rift Valley fever. In *Infectious Diseases of Ruminants,* edited by Z Dinter, B Morein. Amsterdam: Elsevier Scientific Publishers, pp. 481–494.

35

RINDERPEST

INTRODUCTION

Rinderpest (RP), or cattle plague, a usually fatal condition caused by the RP virus (RPV) is often considered the most devastating bovine disease. RPV also infects sheep, goats, buffaloes, yaks, and most wild ungulates.

Fear of RP stimulated establishment of the Office International Des Epizooties (OIE) and the first European veterinary colleges. RP is endemic to India, the Middle East, and parts of northern, eastern, and western Africa but exotic in Europe, Australia, North America, and South America.

RP is rapidly transmitted within herds and areas and easily introduced into free areas by military campaigns or cattle movements. It is currently excluded from RP-free areas by embargoes on livestock and livestock products from enzootic regions in which it is partially controlled by vaccination.

Rinderpest has been reviewed by Scott (1990), Rossiter (1994), Mebus (1998) and Murphy et al. (1999).

ETIOLOGY

RPV is a single-stranded, enveloped RNA virus that is the prototype virus of the genus *Morbillivirus* of the family Paramyxoviridae. It is related to the viruses of canine distemper, human measles, and peste des petits ruminants (PPR) and is probably their historic progenitor.

Most RPV strains are immunologically similar, but may vary in pathogenic potential. Genetic analyses indicate subtle differences between lineages prevailing in Africa and Asia (Scott 1998).

RPV grows in embryonated eggs and in cell cultures producing cytopathic changes characterized by syncytium formation and intranuclear and intracytoplasmic inclusions. It is antigenically stable and readily neutralized by specific immune serums.

RPV is similar but distinct from the virus of PPR, also called pseudorinderpest, which causes a rinderpest-like disease in sheep and goats (Rossiter and Taylor 1994).

RPV is relatively sensitive to environmental influences, being inactivated readily in processed meat or putrefying flesh. In tropical settings it is usually rendered noninfective in 12 hours (Scott 1998). Thus RP modified live-virus (MLV) vaccines are temperature labile and require constant refrigeration. RPV is susceptible to common disinfectants.

CLINICAL SIGNS AND LESIONS

Clinical RP is characterized by sudden onset, fever, leukopenia, anorexia, severe depression, erosion and hemorrhage of alimentary tract mucosa, nasal and ocular discharges, diarrhea, dehydration, and death.

The disease pattern differs in susceptible and endemic populations and strains vary in virulence. Therefore, a gamut of signs and lesions can be seen depending on the circumstances.

Peracute cases may die within 2 to 3 days without diarrhea or mucosal erosions (Mebus 1998).

RP is often described as a drastic version of bovine viral diarrhea (BVD). The first clinical sign is fever, which is followed by excess serous ocular and nasal discharges that soon become mucopurulent. Many affected cattle assume a languid attitude, standing with head and neck slightly extended, with salivation and excess nasal discharge evident.

The pulse rate is accelerated, and the respirations are rapid and labored as death approaches. After 5 to 6 days diarrhea begins and the temperature drops. The diarrhea may be bloody and it contributes to severe dehydration that precedes death. Both the feces and breath can be extremely fetid.

Careful examination usually reveals ulcers or erosions in the oral mucosa. They begin as elevated gray or white necrotic foci that slough, exposing underlying tissues and giving a red color to sharply delineated erosions. They may coalesce, leaving large areas devoid of epithelium in the entire oral cavity including the sides and under surface of the tongue.

The anterior one third of the dorsal surface of the tongue is generally spared. Frequently there is diffuse congestion on the gums, and reddening at the point of emergence of incisor teeth.

Interruptions of mucosal integrity, leukopenia, and lymph node damage set the stage for opportunistic bacteria and coinfecting viruses (Murphy et al. 1999).

Some less virulent RPV strains cause inapparent infection or very mild signs and lesions. Some breeds are less severely affected than others are (Scott 1998).

EFFECTS ON THE DEVELOPING FETUS

Occasionally, acutely infected cattle abort after appearance of clinical signs. Little is known of the effects mild infection may have on fetal development.

NECROPSY FINDINGS

Necropsy findings indicate a severe systemic infection with affinity for lymphoid tissues and alimentary tract epithelium.

Fatal cases present a feces-soiled, dehydrated carcass, a roughened hair coat, and evidence of rapid weight loss. The nasal passages may be plugged with mucopurulent material. Frequently a trail of wet or matted hair extends anteroventrally from the medial canthus delineating flow of excess conjunctival fluid.

In peracute cases, mucosal lesions may be absent. However, most animals live long enough to develop erosions and hemorrhages throughout the alimentary tract.

There are discrete and coalesced, red-bottomed erosions on the ventral surface of the tongue (rarely the anterior portion), the gums, and both the hard and soft palate, extending back into the pharynx and upper third of the esophagus, where they are aligned in linear fashion.

Erosions are less common in the rumen and reticulum and are uncommon in the omasum. There may be hemorrhages and erosions in the abomasum. The pyloric region frequently has hemorrhages, edema, and massive epithelial necrosis.

The small and large intestines have hemorrhage, congestion, and erosions. The Peyer's patches frequently have hemorrhage, erosions, necrosis, or severe lymphoid depletion. There is generally diffuse congestion and hemorrhage throughout the large intestine. Hemorrhages along the longitudinal folds of the terminal ileum and the rectum result in lesions called tiger or zebra stripes.

The lesions mostly involve the digestive tract. Lesions of other organs are generally nonspecific or secondary in nature and include congestion, hemorrhage, and edema (frequently agonal in nature). Occasionally, eczematous skin lesions are seen, particularly in buffaloes, but these are unusual and nonspecific lesions in cattle.

Histopathologically, there is massive destruction of lymphoid tissues and disappearance of mature lymphocytes in Peyer's patches, lymph nodes, and spleen. Most alimentary tract lesions are histologically denoted erosions rather than ulcers, because the basement membranes are usually intact. Throughout the intestines, congestion and hemorrhage predominate.

Giant cells containing intranuclear and intracytoplasmic inclusion bodies develop in epithelial and lymphoid tissues (Scott 1990).

DIAGNOSIS

The diagnosis of RP requires experience. Descriptions of the drastic disease could lead to complacency, because variable clinical forms occur. Any suggestion of RP in free areas requires regulatory intervention and laboratory tests.

The similarity to BVD offers a perfect avenue for misdiagnosis, particularly if mild strains are introduced initially. In RP-free areas, any diseases affecting bovine mucosa (DABM) mandate inquiries about possible connections with RP-infected areas.

Rinderpest should be suspected whenever acute febrile diarrhea is accompanied by erosions of the oral mucosa, particularly if rapid spread is present and animals of all ages sicken and die.

In endemic areas, clinical diagnosis can be based on presence of diarrhea and fever seen concomitantly with oral erosions. In RP-free areas, clinical diagnosis requires immediate laboratory confirmation.

Differential Diagnosis

RP must be differentiated from BVD. In individual cases differentiation is impossible on a clinical basis. If several cases are present, the history of the disease in the area, the epidemiologic pattern, and the generally more drastic nature of rinderpest help to distinguish it from BVD. On necropsy, BVD rarely has diffuse hemorrhages in the pyloric portion of the abomasum.

In addition to BVD, RP must be distinguished from all other DABM, the collection of infections that cause crusting of the muzzle and ulceration, erosion, vesiculation, necrosis, or hemorrhage in the bovine alimentary tract. DABM include malignant catarrhal fever, bluetongue, RP, foot-and-mouth disease, papular stomatitis, vesicular stomatitis, and sometimes infectious bovine rhinotracheitis. Acute salmonellosis, arsenic toxicosis, and other poisonings can be confused with rinderpest.

Differentiation from peste des petits ruminants (PPR) is crucial in some circumstances. PPR is an RP-like disease of sheep and goats but does not produce clinical signs in cattle (Rossiter and Taylor (1994). Because RP causes illness in sheep and goats, the two immunologically related Morbilliviruses must be distinguished in areas where eradication is undertaken or in situations where sheep and goats are infected with a newly appearing rinderpest-like disease. The specific etiology can be determined by virus isolation and identification procedures such as capture enzyme linked immunosorbent analysis or reverse transcriptase polymerase chain reaction methods.

Laboratory Diagnosis

Laboratory diagnosis requires identification of RPV, RPV antigens, or virus-specific nucleic acids in lymphoid tissues or nasal or ocular secretions.

Virus can be isolated in tissue cultures and identified by neutralization or competitive ELISA with known immune serums. Suspension of spleen, lymph nodes, and blood may have adequate viral concentration for detection in agar gel immunodiffusion and complement fixation tests using known RP hyperimmune serum. Also fluorescent antibody (FA) reagents can detect high quantities of virus in infected tissues.

Inoculation of susceptible cattle can be used as a diagnostic procedure. Sometimes however, incubation is extended and more rapid procedures are indicated.

Serological diagnosis can be accomplished by neutralization tests on paired serums, but this is usually impractical due to diagnostic urgency and because many cattle succumb before a second serum is collected. Therefore, virus isolation and identification are essential.

A marked leukopenia occurs shortly after infection and accompanies the initial fever. Within 2 to 3 days there is a lymphocytic response, with an outpouring of immature lymphocytes. In cattle that survive, the total white blood cell count returns to normal coincident with complete recovery. This event usually takes several weeks.

Laboratory diagnostic procedures for RPV are detailed in the Manual of Diagnostic Tests and Vaccines published by the OIE (OIE 2000).

In rinderpest-free areas, blood, spleen, lymph nodes, bone marrow, and sections of alimentary mucosa should be collected by regulatory officials from acutely ill cattle, shipped rapidly, and processed promptly.

EPIDEMIOLOGY

RP typifies a virulent, highly fatal virus infection bestowing relatively solid immunity upon survivors and possessing a capacity for readily evolving into an endemic state after introduction into free areas.

The incubation period varies with virus strain, dosage, and route of exposure. Sudden onset of fever usually occurs 3 to 15 days after exposure.

Most domestic and wild ruminants are susceptible, but cattle and buffaloes probably constitute major reservoirs in Africa. Sheep and goats can be infected and develop clinical signs, which must be distinguished from PPR. Serious clinical RP among sheep and goats is uncommon, however, and many breeds show few clinical signs. The source of infection is nasal discharge and other secretions and excretions. These contain large quantities of virus during the early stages of the infection. Swine can be infected but rarely develop serious disease.

In nature RP is usually transmitted by direct or indirect contact with excretions (particularly nasal discharge) of live infected animals. Infectivity can be maintained for short periods on contaminated equipment, clothing, fences, buildings, or vehicles. The portal of entry is probably the respiratory tract, with nasal epithelium being the site of the first infection.

Virus multiplication occurs in lymph nodes draining the upper respiratory tract. Viremia occurs and widespread viral distribution throughout the body follows.

Swine can be infected by eating meat of infected cattle and then transmit RPV to cattle. The virus can be isolated from a variety of insects, which are probably insignificant in transmission.

Susceptible cattle of all ages and breeds and both sexes can be infected and develop clinical disease. Zebu breeds maintained for generations in enzootic areas have more resistance than newly introduced breeds. European breeds have been seriously affected in outbreaks that were relatively mild among native African cattle. Some African breeds retain susceptibility and suffer losses from clinical disease and modified live virus (MLV) vaccines, which are relatively avirulent for Zebu cattle (Scott 1998).

Generally, rinderpest appears to spread rapidly by contact. Because incubation periods can be as long as 12 to 15 days, the interval between index cases and secondary cases may approximate 2 weeks, and rapidity of intraherd spread following introduction is an inconsistent diagnostic feature. Nevertheless, most cattle in involved herds become infected within 3 to 4 weeks.

RP is transmitted between herds and regions principally (but not exclusively) by trade in cattle and movement of nomads seeking fresh pasture and water for their herds.

IMMUNITY

Natural infection or successful vaccination usually leaves cattle solidly immune and resistant to subsequent infection. Calves being nursed by immune cattle in the first 12 to 24 hours after birth acquire passive immunity that is protective for several months.

VIRUS PERSISTENCE

Most evidence suggests that cattle clear the virus following recovery and develop neutralizing antibody that persists for life without virus shedding.

PREVENTION AND CONTROL

In enzootic areas, RP is successfully controlled by mass vaccination programs using MLV vaccines of cell culture origin. These vaccines are effective if properly refrigerated to ensure vaccine virus infectivity. Recombinant and vectored vaccines are under development.

In RP-free areas, cattle and unprocessed animal products from enzootic regions must be excluded.

RP has characteristics that make it amenable to control. Past introductions into Australia, Europe, and North and South America have been eradicated by drastic slaughter. RP has been subsequently excluded by quarantines and import restrictions.

RP-free countries fear its introduction because totally susceptible populations can experience high mortality and rapid spread. Delay in diagnosis of incursions is likely because extreme variation in pathogenicity occurs between RPV strains, and susceptibility may vary among breeds of cattle, and because RP may resemble BVD and other DABM.

THERAPY AND MANAGEMENT OF OUTBREAKS

Generally, there is little use in attempting treatment. A high percentage of affected cattle die. In enzootic areas, immediate vaccination of herdmates and nearby herds is essential as soon as rinderpest is suspected. When the disease is suspected in rinderpest-free areas, regulatory officials must be notified immediately and quarantines imposed on animals, people, and equipment. If RP were diagnosed in the United States, an animal health emergency would be declared and eradication by the stamping-out method would be initiated.

LIKELIHOOD OF ERADICATION

Aside from a variety of susceptible wildlife ruminant reservoirs and a potential reservoir in swine, rinderpest possesses most characteristics required of an eradicable disease. Current disarray in infrastructure and social conditions in Africa limit the likelihood of eradication (Scott 1998).

The virulent RPV strains spread rapidly, leaving few survivors, and recovered animals are immune and apparently rarely shed virus. Infected or exposed cattle can be easily identified serologically. Therefore in free areas, rinderpest is amenable to eradication by drastic slaughter and subsequent intensive clinical and serologic surveillance.

The United Nations Food and Agriculture Organization (FAO) is attempting global eradication by the year 2010, but skepticism remains as to the feasibility of the project (Scott 1998).

Where already established, rinderpest can be reduced to tolerable levels by vaccination.

Control is probably more feasible than eradication in areas where wild ruminants abound on vast open ranges and there are uncontrolled nomadic wanderings, or where cattle are sacred.

In regions where it is believed RP no longer exists and vaccination has been discontinued, OIE recognition of RP-free status can be requested if clinical and serological surveillance and reporting systems are implemented (James 1998).

IMPACT ON INTERNATIONAL TRADE

RP is an OIE List A disease; most RP-free countries impose strict import measures to ensure its exclusion.

PUBLIC RESPONSIBILITY

In RP-free areas, anyone suspecting the disease is obligated to contact regulatory authorities immediately. The owners of animals with DABM should be queried about possible contacts with Asia or Africa. In enzootic areas, outbreaks should be reported so that vaccination procedures can be initiated.

AREAS IN NEED OF RESEARCH

Research is needed to continually upgrade diagnostic procedures and improve vaccines.

REFERENCES

James AD, 1998. Guide to epidemiological surveillance for rinderpest. *Rev. Sci. Tech. Off. Int. Epiz.* 17:796–809.

Mebus CA, 1998. Rinderpest. In *Foreign Animal Diseases* edited by WW Buisch, JL Hyde, CL Mebus. Richmond: U.S. Animal Health Assoc. pp. 362–371.

Murphy FA, Gibbs EPJ, Horzinek MC, Studdert MJ, 1999. Rinderpest. In *Veterinary Virology,* 3rd ed. San Diego: Academic Press, pp. 421–423.

Office International Des Epizooties (OIE) 2000. Rinderpest. In *Manual of Diagnostic Tests and Vaccines* (6th ed.) with annual updates. Paris: OIE, pp. 81–89.

Rossiter PB, 1994. Rinderpest. In *Infectious Diseases of Livestock With Special Reference to Southern Africa,* edited by JAW Coetzer, GR Thomson, RC Tustin. Capetown: Oxford University Press, pp. 735–757.

Rossiter PB, Taylor WP, 1994. Peste des petit ruminants. In *Infectious Diseases of Livestock With Special Reference to Southern Africa,* edited by JAW Coetzer, GR Thomson, RC Tustin. Capetown: Oxford University Press, pp. 758–765.

Scott GR, 1990. Rinderpest virus. In *Infectious Diseases of Ruminants,* edited by Z Dinter, B Morein. Amsterdam: Elsevier Scientific Publishers, pp. 341–354.

Scott GR, 1998. Global eradication of rinderpest yea or nay? *Ann. N.Y. Acad. Sci.* 849:293–298.

36

BOVINE SPONGIFORM ENCEPHALOPATHY

INTRODUCTION

Bovine spongiform encephalopathy (BSE) is not a classic viral disease but belongs to a group of unconventional subviral disorders known as transmissible spongiform encephalopathies (TSE) or prion diseases (Weissmann et al. 1998).

BSE, an insidious, chronically progressive, inevitably fatal neurodegenerative disease, is manifested by behavioral, postural, and locomotor disorders.

BSE has caused international concern and distrust, politically and economically motivated trade barriers, uncertainty within veterinary services worldwide, and dissension within the European Community (EC). It is also the reason for efforts by the Office International Des Epizooties (OIE) to develop standards for safe movement of animals and animal products and criteria in order for countries to be recognized as BSE-free.

BSE was first recognized in the UK in 1985–86 (Wells et al. 1987) where it was called "mad cow disease." Starting as a few cases, it soon became a major epizootic that by 2000 had killed over 200,000 cattle and caused slaughter of almost 4 million exposed animals. By 1996, veterinarians acknowledged that BSE was a European problem and not confined to the UK.

Although debated in some circles (Wilesmith et al. 1991; Lacy 1995), BSE probably originated from protein supplementation of cattle diets with meat and bone meal containing rendered offal from scrapie-affected sheep (Taylor, 1991). Later, meat and bone meal produced from BSE-infected cattle probably amplified the epidemic (Kimberlin and Willesmith 1994).

In the early 1980s, the UK instituted energy-saving measures that lowered rendering temperatures by eliminating fat extraction. This method used organic solvents and subsequent prolonged exposure to steam needed to drive solvent residues from rendered products. It may have permitted survival of the scrapie agent (or a mutation thereof) and its dissemination among cattle that acquired it in feed and developed clinical signs after 2-to-8-year incubation periods.

Like other TSE, BSE causes spongy degeneration of neurons in the brain and spinal cord. The result is gradual loss of body condition and progressive loss of neurologic function causing behavioral changes, incoordination, staggering, recumbency, and death.

Except for a 1993 single Canadian case in a cow imported as a 3-month-old calf from England in 1987, as of December 2000, BSE had not occurred in North or South America. The absence of BSE in the United States as compared with the UK was postulated to be due to the fact that the US has a smaller sheep population. For that reason it has fewer scrapie-infected sheep and less feeding of ovine offal to cattle. Also, there may be strain differences between UK and US scrapie agents. The US rendering industry has not used fat solvent extraction since the 1970s.

The transmissible spongiform encephalopathies (TSE), a perplexing group of slowly progressive fatal diseases characterized by gradual loss of neurologic function and body condition, have been described in several animal species and humans.

These conditions, originally called slow virus infections because of their long incubation periods and progressive clinical courses, are now called TSE because classical viruses have not been isolated and other etiologies have been proposed.

Some TSE occur sporadically and widely separated in time and space and appear unrelated. Others are geographically clustered and associated with unique exposure factors such as cannibalism, transspecies carnivorousness, and protein supplementation of animal diets with ruminant offal.

The TSE share common characteristics. They are all progressive, ultimately fatal neurologic disorders attributable to spongiform degeneration of neurons. They sometimes appear to have a familial or species-related susceptibility component that is difficult to distinguish from epidemiologic patterns produced by common exposures to common sources of infection, toxicosis, or deficiency.

The human TSE include kuru, fatal familial insomnia, Gerstmann–Straussler–Scheinker syndrome, and Creutzfeldt–Jakob disease (CJD). Until recently, human TSE have occurred sporadically and have generally been regarded as nontransmissible biochemical defects. An exception is kuru, which was virtually eliminated when the custom of eating brains of dead relatives ceased among affected populations in Papua–New Guinea.

Creutzfeldt–Jakob disease (CJD) is a chronic degenerative human neurologic disorder that occurs sporadically worldwide with attack rates of approximately one case per million people. It was regarded as a noninfectious genetic or metabolic defect until 1993 when a new variant form of CJD (VCJD) was recognized in England (Will et al. 1996). VCJD is a fatal psychiatric locomotor disorder that differs from classic CJD by having earlier age of onset, and slightly different clinical signs and microscopic lesions.

VCJD probably occurs when people eat BSE-contaminated meat. Experimental evidence indicates the agents of CJD and VCJD are probably biologically indistinguishable (OIE 1998).

Upon appearance of VCJD, human health concerns caused further bans on cattle and beef from the UK. There were also criticism of British handling of BSE, allegations that protection of agricultural interests caused neglect of consumer safety, and a shifting of some animal health responsibilities from agricultural to consumer-oriented agencies in European Union (EU). Milk, milk products, gelatin, and properly rendered tallow were considered safe, but cosmetics, pharmaceuticals, and products using animal-derived materials or glands became suspect.

The TSE of animals include scrapie, BSE, feline spongiform encephalopathy, chronic wasting disease (CWD) of deer and elk, and transmissible mink encephalopathy (TME).

Scrapie, the prototype spongiform encephalopathy, occurs in sheep and rarely in goats. It has been endemic in Great Britain for several centuries. It was first diagnosed in the United States in 1947, presumably introduced by Suffolk sheep imported from the UK. Following an incubation period of 1 to 2 years or more, affected sheep develop locomotor incoordination and behavioral changes including rubbing against objects and staggering. Other symptoms include tremors, walking in circles, and progressive weight loss. These end in death. Scrapie is seen mostly in black-faced sheep that are 2 to 8 years old and has received revived attention because of the relationship of BSE to VCJD.

Chronic wasting disease (CWD) of deer and elk is a fatal chronic progressive debilitating disease first identified in the United States in 1977. CWD is characterized by weight loss and emaciation. Clinical signs have appeared in elk, mule deer, and black-tailed deer in the western United States and Canada in animals ranging from 17 months to 15 years of age. Affected animals drink more frequently than usual and salivate and urinate excessively. They may have blank stares in both eyes, and develop life-threatening pneumonia, which is frequently the cause of death.

The differential diagnosis of CWD includes malnutrition, parasitism, chronic pneumonia, renal, or enteric disease; weather stress; or inhalation pneumonia, which frequently causes death. Although they have spongiform brain lesions, CWD patients only occasionally exhibit behavioral changes, nervousness, hyperexcitability, hyperesthesia, teeth grinding, or pelvic ataxia. Preliminary studies indicate the etiologic agent is probably distinct from both scrapie and BSE. Knowledge of CWD will probably expand with further surveillance and advancing diagnostic technology.

Transmissible mink encephalopathy (TME) is a rare, fatal neurodegenerative disease of mink with clinical signs and lesions similar to other TSE. It was speculated that TME may result from feeding mink with meat from downer (nonambulatory) cows (Marsh 1990). This conjecture has been used by the EU as evidence that BSE is present in the United States.

BSE has been reviewed by Detwiler and Rubenstein (1998), Murphy et al. (1999), and the OIE (OIE 1998).

ETIOLOGY

The causative agent of TSE has not been visualized microscopically nor definitively isolated and characterized. There are three hypothesized causes of TSE.

The virus theory suggests the etiologic agents are small unconventional viruses (slow viruses) that behave differently from classic viruses and whose mysteries will be unraveled by advancing technology.

The virino theory suggests TSE are caused by nucleic acids imbedded in host protein.

The most popular hypothesis says TSE are caused by replicating, nucleic-acid-deficient, proteinaceous infectious particles, prions, sometimes called prion proteins (PrP). Some prions are normal brain constituents that become abnormal on exposure to infectious prions. This theory says that BSE emerged in the UK via abnormal scrapie prions present in rendered ovine offal fed to cattle as a protein supplement.

Until the issue is resolved, the etiologic agents of the TSE will likely be referred to as prions. Like viruses, distinguishable prion strains infect different animal species. These strains may have evolved from common ancestors through interspecies transmission and genetic adaptation. The BSE PrP has infected captive wild felidae and ruminants and domestic cats in the United Kingdom.

Strain differences within and between TSE-producing prions are determined by western blot analysis on proteinase K treated brain material or by experimental mouse inoculations. Mice injected intracerebrally with distinct PrP strains differ in incubation period, duration, nature, and fatality rates of experimentally induced disease. They also differ as to the extent, distribution, and microscopic appearance of neuronal degeneration and the immunohistochemical specificity of resulting PrP plaques.

Prions are not inactivated by the temperatures attained in autoclaves or some rendering processes and are unaffected by radiation, ultraviolet light, disinfectants, antibiotics, and known medications. Because PrP do not stimulate classic inflammatory or immunologic responses, the TSE are difficult to diagnose in live animals and are unlikely to be amenable to prevention by classical vaccines.

CLINICAL SIGNS AND LESIONS

Affected cattle have normal temperatures and exhibit a variety of neurological dysfunctions. Experienced observers first notice subtle behavioral changes such as licking, wrinkling of the nose, head rubbing, grinding of teeth, abnormal head carriage, ear and tail twitching, and excessive salivation. Affected animals are likely to stand quietly with necks extended, heads lowered, and a blank stare in the eyes; they are easily startled.

Affected cattle may be unusually apprehensive, reluctant to approach familiar objects, and aggressive toward humans or other animals. Shortly, the neurologic deficits become more obvious and progress to incoordination (first noticed in the hind legs and later in front) and locomotive deficits with hypermetria, ataxia, staggering, stumbling, and eventual recumbency. These signs appear along with reduced milk production and loss of condition. Death usually occurs within 6 months of the onset of signs.

EFFECTS ON THE DEVELOPING FETUS

To date, no specific fetal disorders have been reported. If transplacental infection from dam to developing fetus or vertical transmission to suckling calves occurs at all, it is uncommon (Hoinville et al. 1995) and difficult to substantiate because of the long incubation period.

NECROPSY FINDINGS

Aside from emaciation, agonal findings, and occasional injuries there are no gross lesions.

Histologically, there are degenerative microscopic spongiform lesions characterized by intracytoplasmic vacuoles in the gray matter, but virtually no evidence of inflammatory or immunological responses.

Immunohistochemical staining of brain and spinal cord material reveals accumulations of PrP that appear as fibrils on electron microscopic examination. The presence of BSE specific PrP can be demonstrated by western blot technology.

DIAGNOSIS

Diagnoses based on clinical signs and epidemiological patterns are confirmed at postmortem by microscopic and histochemical brain and spinal cord examinations or by time-consuming and expensive inoculations of brain tissues into experimental animals. Biopsied lymph nodes or tonsils can be examined histochemically (Schreuder et al. 1996). Although third-eyelid biopsies and other live-animal procedures are under development, rapid tests to detect the presence of the agent(s) in tissues or blood of live presymptomatic but incubating animals are needed.

In BSE-endemic regions, the profile includes presence of the disease in the area or herd, a history of feed supplemented with ruminant-origin protein, and classic clinical signs supported by postmortem pathologic findings.

In regions considered BSE-free, initially animals will present suspicious neurological signs or recumbency. The disease will be detected only if specific surveillance programs and laboratory support are available.

Although there are no pathognomonic signs, herdsmen and veterinarians in endemic areas gain proficiency in clinically identifying cases that are ultimately confirmed.

Differential Diagnosis

The differential diagnosis includes listeriosis, rabies, pseudorabies, nervous acetonemia, grass tetany, brain/spinal cord tumors, abscesses or infestation with migrating hypoderma larvae, thromboembolic meningoencephalitis; milk fever, obturator paralysis, various toxicoses (Weaver 1992; Robinson and Gorham 1992), and other causes of down cows (Cox 1998).

Laboratory Diagnosis

Histopathologic exams reveal spongiform changes and occasional hypertrophy of astrocytes (star-shaped nerve cells) in gray matter and vacuolization in neurons. Immunohistochemical examination of brain and spinal cord can be used to detect abnormal accumulations of PrP.

Clinical pathological parameters, including examinations of cerebrospinal fluid, are usually within normal ranges.

Procedures for laboratory diagnosis are detailed in the OIE *Manual of Standards for Diagnostic Tests and Vaccines* (OIE 2000).

The desired specimens, brain, spinal cord, and lymph nodes should be collected promptly after death by people wearing protective clothing and face masks (Detwiler and Rubenstein 1998). The carcass must be held in a secure place until the diagnostic procedures are completed; it must be incinerated if BSE is diagnosed.

EPIDEMIOLOGY

Current hypotheses about the cause of BSE and its transmission within and between species, and the most appropriate methods of control are largely founded on epidemiological evidence but are nonetheless convincing. Without exact knowledge of the etiological agent and lacking live animal tests, control measures and regulatory actions must be based on precautionary principles; only time will tell if they are sufficient and effective.

The incubation period ranges from 2 to 8 years. In experimental animals inoculated intracerebrally, the incubation period ranges from 6 months to two years.

It is believed that tissues (brain, spinal cord, intestines, spleen, lymphoid and ocular tissues, and perhaps placenta) of infected animals are the source of infection.

Although ingestion of infected tissues appears to be the natural mode of entry into new susceptible hosts, this scenario does not explain all cases. Contact transmission does not appear to occur. Maternal and vertical transmission appear to play a minor (if any) role in transmission of BSE (OIE 1998), and there is minimal risk of transmission by embryo transfer. Semen is probably safe if handled under conditions outlined in the OIE International Animal Health Code.

Most animal TSE can be transmitted experimentally by intracerebral inoculation of brain tissue from affected individuals into experimental animals, which then develop characteristic signs and lesions. Inferences derived by such studies, however, must be hedged with the realization that this is a most unnatural mode of transmission in terms of both route and dosage of exposure.

The onset of clinical signs has been observed in animals from 22 months to 15 years of age. Although more common in dairy than in beef cattle, BSE seems to affect all breeds of cattle (Willesmith et al. 1991).

As of December 1999, BSE has been confirmed in indigenous cattle in Great Britain, Ireland, France, Belgium, Luxembourg, Portugal, the Netherlands, and Switzerland. Imported cases have been diagnosed in Canada, Denmark, Oman, and elsewhere. The lack of indigenous cases in other European countries may be due to faulty surveillance or reporting. The number of cases in these areas may ultimately expand because of the alleged dumping of contaminated feed after the 1988 UK ban on feeding of specified bovine offal (SBO) to ruminants (Butler 1996).

IMMUNITY

All observations indicate that BSE does not stimulate immune responses that are measurable by present techniques.

VIRUS PERSISTENCE

It appears that prions or other agents triggering clinical BSE persist permanently in brain, spinal cord, and lymphoid tissues of infected animals.

PREVENTION AND CONTROL

Lacking convenient antemortem diagnostic tools, the causes and modes of transmission of TSE are subject to speculation, controversy, and political manipulation, all of which handicap eradication or control programs.

Preventing establishment of BSE in regions can be attempted by monitoring and surveillance programs and by strict import controls on live animals, germ plasm, and animal products including meat and bone meal. Border security measures and a ban on feeding ruminant protein to animals will also be helpful.

THERAPY AND MANAGEMENT OF OUTBREAKS

As the 1986–2000 epizootic evolved, the United Kingdom invoked stepwise and increasingly stringent measures on BSE-affected herds. These measures ultimately progressed to extensive surveillance, trace-back to herds of origin, quarantine, slaughter, incineration of infected herds, and a ban on the feeding of ruminant brain and spinal cord and ultimately other SBOs (spleen, intestines, tonsils, thymus and other lymphoid tissues) in 1989. There was a decrease in the incidence in calves born after the effective implementation of the SBO ban, but subsequent increased exportations of meat and bone meal raised questions about the future health of livestock in recipient countries.

As the significance of the spreading European BSE epizootic became more apparent, the United States developed constantly updated BSE Emergency Disease Guidelines (USDA 1996) and gradually instituted measures to prevent BSE from entering the country. Many of these measures required time-consuming rule-making procedures that included review by multiple branches of government and publication for public comment. In 1989, the USDA Animal and Plant Health Inspection Service (APHIS) banned importation of live cattle from the United Kingdom and placed under surveillance the 499 UK-origin cattle imported after 1981. These animals were traced and in so far as possible; upon their death, their brains have been examined for microscopic evidence of BSE without detecting any cases.

Since 1989, the USDA has sought to identify any BSE cases in the United States through cooperative surveillance programs by which the brains of all rabies-negative mature non-ambulatory cattle are subjected for histopathological examination for BSE.

In 1996, the USDA restricted the importation of all live ruminants and ruminant products from countries where BSE was known to exist and later added all European countries to the list of affected countries. Countries can be removed from the list by fulfilling strict criteria. Products derived from ruminants, such as fetal bovine serum, meat and bone meal, blood meal, offal, fats, and glands, cannot be imported into the United States from these countries except under a special permit for scientific research purposes. Few slaughter plants in BSE-affected countries are currently approved to export ruminant products to the United States.

In addition to import restrictions, the United States has developed an educational program to alert the animal-health community to report suspicious animals. There is a rigorous BSE surveillance program involving accredited veterinarians, meat inspectors, and more than 250 APHIS and state veterinarians specially trained to diagnose foreign animal diseases. They regularly conduct field investigations of suspicious disease conditions, including cattle displaying signs of central nervous system disorders. In 1999, the US Food and Drug Administration placed a precautionary ban on blood donations from individuals who had lived in Britain for more than 6 months.

LIKELIHOOD OF ERADICATION

Until reliable live animal tests are developed, the most effective control strategies will probably fall short of global eradication. The establishment of low-incidence regions with strong animal health infrastructures may eradicate BSE and prevent its reintroduction. Only time will tell if drastic test and slaughter programs as undertaken in the United Kingdom will achieve elimination of BSE from all of Europe.

IMPACT ON INTERNATIONAL TRADE

BSE is an OIE List A disease. Officials engaged in international discussions regarding BSE and TSE must respect other countries' right to be concerned about possible introduction, establishment, and amplification of BSE or other TSE in their territories and about potential TSE-associated human health hazards. These concerns are particularly legitimate in countries with bona fide surveillance programs. Under such programs, countries document their contentions that they are not affected with BSE, scrapie, or other TSE. The EU and many countries have excluded live cattle, meat, and bone meal from BSE-affected countries. Some scrapie-affected countries restrict importation of sheep and other ovine products from scrapie-affected regions for fear of importing exotic scrapie strains that may cause BSE.

PUBLIC RESPONSIBILITY

The responsibilities for dealing with BSE fall upon all segments of the livestock economy including the veterinary profession and the rendering industry. Regulatory agencies are responsible for developing and implementing policies and procedures to make sure that BSE is not introduced and amplified in the United States, North America, or elsewhere. It is, however, laboratory diagnosticians, private practitioners, food inspectors, and livestock owners in each country who will be the heroes that recognize the first cases and implement eradication procedures.

In regions considered BSE-free, suspicious clinical signs require regulatory action, epidemiologic investigation, careful postmortem examinations, and efforts to find an animal's birthplace to determine if cases are indigenous or imported.

AREAS IN NEED OF RESEARCH

Research is needed to identify and further characterize the etiologic agent and to develop live animal tests to identify incubating animals.

REFERENCES

Butler D, 1996. Did UK dump contaminated feed after the ban? *Nature* 381: 544–545.

Cox VS, 1998. The many causes of down cows. *Proc. Ann. Conf. Bov. Pract.* 31:164–166.

Detwiler LW, Rubenstein, R, 1998. Bovine spongiform encephalopathy. In *Foreign Animal Diseases*, edited by WW Buisch, JL Hyde, CL Mebus. Richmond: US Animal Health Assoc. pp. 129–146.

Hoinville LJ, Wilesmith JW, Richards MS, 1995. An investigation of risk factors for cases of bovine spongiform encephalopathy born after the feed ban. *Vet. Rec.* 136: 312–318.

Kimberlin RH, Willesmith JW, 1994. Bovine spongiform encephalopathy (BSE): epidemiology, low dose exposure and risks. *Ann. N.Y. Acad. Sci.* 724:210–220.

Lacy RW, 1995. Bovine spongiform encephalopathy—the disputed claims. *J. Nutrit. Environ. Med.* 5:401–408.

Marsh RF, 1990. Bovine spongiform encephalopathy in the United States. *J. Am. Vet. Med. Assoc.* 196:1677.

Murphy FA, Gibbs EPJ, Horzinek MC, Studdert MJ, 1999. Bovine spongiform encephalopathy. In *Veterinary Virology,* 3rd ed. San Diego: Academic Press, pp. 576–578.

OIE, 1998. Bovine spongiform encephalopathy. In Report of the Meeting of the OIE Animal Health Code Commission. Paris: OIE.

OIE, 2000. Bovine spongiform encephalopathy. *In Manual of Diagnostic Tests and Vaccines* (6th ed) with annual updates. Office International Des Epizooties. Paris: pp. 1–389.

Schreuder BEC, van Keulen LJM, Vromans MEW, Langeveld JPM, Smits MA, 1996. Preclinical test for prion disease. *Nature* 381:563.

Taylor KC, 1991. The control of bovine spongiform encephalopathy in Great Britain. *Vet. Rec.* 129:522–526.

United States Department of Agriculture, 1996. Bovine Spongiform Encephalopathy Emergency Disease Guidelines, prepared by the Animal and Plant Health Inspection Service. Riverdale, Maryland.

Weaver DA, 1992. Bovine spongiform encephalopathy: Its clinical features and epidemiology in the United Kingdom and significance for the United States. *Compendium for Continuing Education* 14:1647–1656.

Weissmann C, Fischer M, Raeber A, Bueler H, Sailer A, Schmerling D, Rulicke T, Brandner S, Aguzzi A, 1998. The use of transgenic mice in the investigation of transmissible spongiform encephalopathies. *Rev. Sci. Tech. Off. Int. Epiz.* 17:278–293.

Wells GAH, Scott AC, Johnson CT, Gunning RF, Hancock RB, Jeffrey M, Dawson ME, Bradley R, 1987. A novel progressive spongiform encephalopathy in cattle. *Vet. Rec.* 121: 419–420.

Wilesmith JW, Ryan JBM, Atkinson MJ, 1991. Bovine spongiform encephalopathy: epidemiologic studies on the origin. *Vet. Rec.* 128:199–203.

Will RG, Ironside JW, Zeidler M, Cousens SN, Estibeiro K, Alperovitch A, Poser S, Pocchiari M0, Hofman A, Smith A, 1996. A new variant of Creutzfeldt–Jakob disease in the UK. *Lancet* 347:921–925.

INDEX

Printed and bound by CPI Group (UK) Ltd, Croydon, CR0 4YY

16/04/2025

14658458-0004